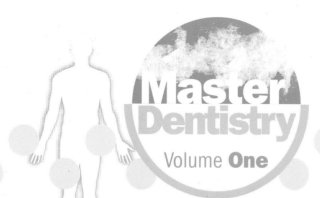

Master Dentistry

Volume One

Oral and Maxillofacial Surgery, Radiology, Pathology and Oral Medicine

Dedication

Our partners and Matthew, Francesca and Imogen

Commissioning Editor: Alison Taylor
Development Editor: Clive Hewat
Project Manager: Christine Johnston
Design Direction: Stewart Larking
Illustration Manager: Merlyn Harvey
Illustrator: Graeme Chambers

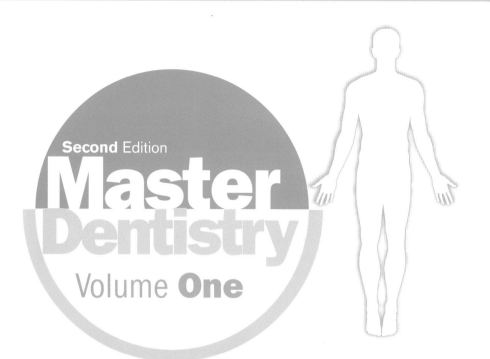

Second Edition

Master Dentistry

Volume One

Oral and Maxillofacial Surgery, Radiology, Pathology and Oral Medicine

Paul Coulthard
BDS MFGDP MDS FDSRCS PhD
Professor of Oral and Maxillofacial Surgery,
The University of Manchester;
Honorary Consultant, Central Manchester
and Manchester Children's University
Hospitals NHS Trust

Keith Horner
BChD MSc PhD FDSRCPS FRCR DDR
Professor of Oral and Maxillofacial Imaging,
The University of Manchester;
Honorary Consultant, Central Manchester
and Manchester Children's University
Hospitals NHS Trust

Philip Sloan
BDS PhD FRCPath FRSRCS
Consultant Histopathologist, Royal Victoria
Infirmary, Newcastle upon Tyne;
Honorary Professor, School of Dental
Sciences, Newcastle University

Elizabeth D. Theaker
BDS BSc MSc MPhil
Senior Clinical Teaching Fellow in
Oral Medicine and Senior Tutor for
Undergraduate Dental Studies,
The University of Manchester

CHURCHILL LIVINGSTONE

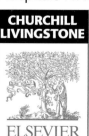

ELSEVIER

Edinburgh   London   New York   Oxford   Philadelphia   St Louis   Sydney   Toronto   2008

CHURCHILL
LIVINGSTONE
ELSEVIER

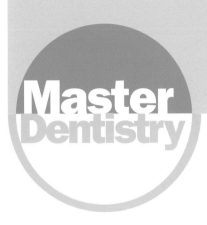

First edition 2003
Second edition 2008

ISBN: 978-0-443-06896-6

British Library Cataloguing in Publication Data
A catalogue record for this book is available from the British Library

Library of Congress Cataloging in Publication Data
A catalog record for this book is available from the Library of Congress

Note

Knowledge and best practice in this field are constantly changing. As new research and experience broaden our knowledge, changes in practice, treatment and drug therapy may become necessary or appropriate. Readers are advised to check the most current information provided (i) on procedures featured or (ii) by the manufacturer of each product to be administered, to verify the recommended dose or formula, the method and duration of administration, and contraindications. It is the responsibility of the practitioner, relying on their own experience and knowledge of the patient, to make diagnoses, to determine dosages and the best treatment for each individual patient, and to take all appropriate safety precautions. To the fullest extent of the law, neither the Publisher nor the Authors assumes any liability for any injury and/or damage to persons or property arising out of or related to any use of the material contained in this book.

The Publisher

ELSEVIER your source for books, journals and multimedia in the health sciences
www.elsevierhealth.com

Working together to grow libraries in developing countries
www.elsevier.com | www.bookaid.org | www.sabre.org

ELSEVIER BOOK AID International Sabre Foundation

The publisher's policy is to use **paper manufactured from sustainable forests**

Printed in China

Contents

Preface

This book is written for clinical students, undergraduate and postgraduate, as an aid to understanding clinical dentistry. Our purpose is to present our specialties in an integrated patient-focused way. The disciplines of oral and maxillofacial surgery, oral and maxillofacial radiology, oral and maxillofacial pathology and oral medicine have been brought together to provide an understanding of clinical problems. We have therefore worked together to compile chapters, although we have each taken a lead in coordinating particular chapters (Paul Coulthard chapters 1,3,4,6,8,9; Keith Horner chapters 2,5,7,15,16; Philip Sloan chapters 10,11,12,13; and Elizabeth Theaker chapter 14). This new edition has been thoroughly updated since the publication of the earlier popular text and has an introductory chapter about evidence-based practice that we believe is important for clinicians to understand. This book deals primarily with those clinical problems that would traditionally come under the 'surgical and medical umbrella'.

We did not presume to trespass into other areas of dentistry; these are dealt with in the accompanying volume of this series – *Master Dentistry 2: Restorative Dentistry, Paediatric Dentistry and Orthodontics*, edited by Peter Heasman. We hope that the format is fresh and stimulating with ample opportunity for readers to test their knowledge.

Whilst this book will act as a core text for undergraduates approaching final examinations, it will also be useful for dental students at any stage of the course who want to expand their knowledge. Postgraduates approaching professional examinations such as MJDF should find the book particularly appropriate.

Paul Coulthard
Keith Horner
Philip Sloan
Elizabeth Theaker
2008

Introduction

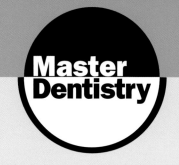

Using this book

Philosophy of the book

This book brings together core text from the traditional subject areas of oral surgery, oral medicine, oral pathology and radiology to help readers to organise their knowledge in a useful way to solve clinical problems. We believe that this core text of knowledge is essential reading for university undergraduate final examination success and will also be of help to graduates undertaking vocational training, their trainers and those preparing for postgraduate professional examinations such as the MJDF in the UK or international equivalent. This book will also be helpful as a reference for those undertaking university higher degrees such as MSc and specialist clinical training.

During your professional education, you will be gaining knowledge of oral surgery, oral medicine, oral pathology and radiology and also developing your clinical experience in these areas of dentistry. You may, however, be anxious to know how much you should know to answer examination questions successfully. The aim of this book is to help you to understand how much you should know. However, we also believe that learning is for the purpose of solving clinical problems rather than just to pass examinations and we, therefore, hope to help you to develop understanding. To ensure examination success, you will need to integrate knowledge and experience from different clinical areas so that you can solve real clinical problems. If you aim to do this, then you will be able to cope with the simulated ones in examinations.

You are required to be competent to practise dentistry on graduation and this requirement is directly related to how to be successful in the Finals examinations. Your examiners will wish you to demonstrate to them that you will make sensible and safe decisions concerning the management of your patients. So demonstrate that to them! Your clinical judgement may not be based on a lot of experience but it will be sound if you stick to basic principles. Ensure that you can take a logical, efficient history from a patient and that you are confident in your clinical examination. You will be required to use your findings together with your knowledge and the results of appropriate investigations to reach a diagnosis and suggested treatment plan. Various aspects of this process are examined in different ways but to be successful in final university and postgraduate examinations you must appreciate that there is a difference between learning and understanding. Being able to regurgitate facts is

not the same as applying knowledge and will not help your patients.

It is important that you understand what you would be expected to know and manage for your particular working situation. We have, therefore, been explicit about the knowledge and skills required of those graduates working in primary care and the areas that you need to know about but do not need to understand to the same degree. There is often confusion about the role-play in an examination, and candidates attempt to avoid further questioning by stating that they would refer the patient to a specialist rather than manage them themselves! In reality, there are clearly some things that you must know and others that you need only to be aware of; it is important to know when to refer. However, even if you are not working in a hospital environment you need to be able to explain to your patient what is likely to happen to them. For instance, if a patient experiences intermittent swelling associated with a salivary gland, then you will need to refer the patient to hospital for investigation but you also need to be able to give your patient an idea about the most likely pathosis and management. Also, when deciding that your patient requires general anaesthesia for their treatment, you need sufficient knowledge to make an appropriate sensible referral and to provide the relevant information for your patient even though you will not be providing the anaesthesia.

Layout and contents

We have presented the text in a logical and concise way and have used illustrations where appropriate to help understanding. Principles of diagnosis and management are explained rather than stated and where there is controversy, this is described. The contents cover the broad areas of subjects of relevance to oral surgery, oral medicine, oral pathology and radiology but are approached by subject area rather than by clinical discipline. We deliberately present an integrated approach, as this is more helpful when learning to solve clinical problems. The artificial boundaries of specialities do not assist the clinician learning to deal with a patient's problems.

Many of the answers to the questions in the self-assessment sections present new information not found in the text of the chapter so to get the most out of this book, it is important to include these assessment sections. While it may be tempting to go straight to the answers, it would be more beneficial to attempt to write down the answers before turning to them, or at least think about the answers first.

Approaching the examinations

The discipline of learning is closely linked to preparation for examinations. Give yourself sufficient time. Superficial memorising of facts may be adequate for some multiple choice examinations but will not be adequate when understanding is required. Spending time to acquire a deeper knowledge and understanding will not only get you through the examination but will have long-term use solving real problems in clinical practice. It is useful to discuss topics with colleagues and your teachers. Talking through an issue will let you know very quickly whether or not you understand it, just as it will in an oral examination!

This book alone will not get you through an examination. It is designed to complement your lecture notes, your recommended textbooks, past examination papers and your clinical experience. Large reference textbooks are of little use when preparing for examinations and should have been used to supplement your notes and answer particular questions during the course. Short revision guides may have lists of facts for cramming but will not provide sufficient information to facilitate any understanding and will not be enough for finals and postgraduate examinations. Medium-sized textbooks recommended by your teachers will, therefore, be the most useful. This book will help to direct your learning and enable you to organise your knowledge in a useful way.

The main types of examination

Make sure that you are familiar with the examination style and look at past examination papers if possible.

Multiple choice questions

Multiple choice questions (MCQs) are usually marked by computer and are seen to be a good method of examining because they are objective, but they do not often check understanding. They do require detailed knowledge about the subject. Be sure to read the stem statements carefully as it is possible to know the answer but not score a point because you misunderstand the question. Calculate in advance how much time you have for each question and check that you are on schedule at time intervals during the examination. Find out if a negative marking system is to be used, such that marks are lost for incorrect answers, as this will determine whether it is worth a guess or not when you do not know the answer.

Extended matching items

Extended matching items (EMIs) are thought to be valuable in assessing both the level and application of knowledge. They may be based around a theme, such as a diagnosis, a set of investigations or a symptom or sign. Identify the theme, then carefully read the introductory 'lead in' statement. Note that an option to be matched with each vignette or case may be used once, more than once or not at all. On occasions when more than one option could be correct, choose the best option available.

Short notes

Do not waste time writing irrelevant text. Short note questions are marked by awarding points for key facts. While layout is always important to allow the examiner to identify these facts easily, a logical approach is less important than for an essay. Give each section of the question the correct proportion of time rather than spending too long on one part in an attempt to get every point. It is more efficient to get the easiest points down for every question rather than all for one part and none for another.

Essays

Answer the number of essays requested. It is dangerous not to answer a question at all and many marking systems will mean that you cannot pass even if you answered another question rather well. Quickly plan your answer so that you can present a logical approach. The use of subheadings will guide your examiner through the essay, indicating that you have an understanding of the breadth of the question and score you points on the way. A brief introduction to set the scene will produce a good impression. Describe common factors first and rare things later. Try to devote a similar amount of text to each aspect of the answer. Maintain a concise approach even for an essay. Finish the essay with a conclusion or summary to draw together the threads of the text or describe the clinical importance.

Vivas

The viva is probably the most anxiety inducing of all types of examinations. It can be very difficult to know how well or not you are doing, depending on the attitude of the examiners. The examiners usually begin with general questions and then move on to requests for more detailed information and continue until you reach the limit of your knowledge. It is useful to have pre-prepared initial statements on key subjects, which might include a definition and a list of causes or types of pathology. This can help you to be articulate at the start of the viva until you settle into things.

There is frequently more than one answer to a question of patient management and it is not wrong to state this in an examination. To explain that a particular area is not well supported by scientific evidence and describe the alternative views will be respected and appreciated. Students are often advised to lead the direction of the viva, but in practice this may be difficult to do. In reality, the examiner may insist that you follow rather than lead. Remain calm and polite and do not hold back on showing off what you know.

Evidence-based practice

Overview

Evidence-based medicine and dentistry is not new but is not always well understood. It is a way of thinking that should permeate every aspect of clinical practice. This chapter describes this philosophy, provides an overview of its components, and provides an approach on how to make best use of the scientific literature and the benefits of evidence-based medicine.

1.1 Decision making

Learning objectives

You should:

- know what influences clinical decisions
- understand what evidence-based practice is
- understand the advantages and limits of using an evidence-based approach to practice.

Clinical decision making is influenced by many factors, including expert opinions, experience, expectations, financial constraints and political pressures, in addition to research evidence.

Evidence-based medicine is the explicit and judicious use of current best evidence to guide health-care decisions. It integrates this best research evidence with clinical expertise and patient values. The aim of evidence-based medicine is to optimise clinical outcomes and quality of life for patients.

This approach may be used for individual patients, or for planning and purchasing care for groups of patients. Patients will benefit if their clinician is abreast of the latest data but he or she also needs to be able to take a good history, carry out a good examination, and have an understanding of the patients' values and preferences.

Evidence-based medicine

Best research evidence

When working with patients there is a constant need to seek information before making a clinical decision and professionals need to develop the habit of learning by inquiry so when confronted with a clinical question they can look for the current best answer as efficiently as possible. It can be difficult to find the current answer in a large database such as MEDLINE with over ten million references and a specialised database such as the Cochrane Library or Best Evidence can be a better place to start. Best-evidence resources are growing in number and are accessible as never before.

Best research evidence is clinically relevant research from basic science and clinical research. It either validates previously accepted diagnostic tests, preventive regimens and treatments, or replaces them with new ones that are more powerful, more accurate, more effective and safer. The strength of evidence from various study designs is shown in Figure 1.

Do not look at promotional brochures, which often contain unpublished material and ignore anecdotal 'evidence' such as the fact that a dental celebrity is using the product. Do not accept the newness of a product as an argument for changing to it as the opposite might have good scientific argument.

Clinical expertise

Clinical expertise is the ability to use clinical skills and past experience to rapidly identify each patient's unique oral health state and diagnosis, their individual risks and benefits of potential interventions and their personal values and expectations.

Patient values

Patient values are the unique preferences, concerns and expectations each patient brings to a clinical encounter and which must be integrated into clinical decisions if they are to serve the patient. It is usual practice for the clinician to describe the diagnosed condition or disease to the patient and then describe the treatment available together with the harms that the treatment may potentially cause. To determine the patient values, the clinician could go on to ask the patient to make a value judgement about these two, that is, which is worse and by how much. The patient may need to think about this or discuss with family members. The clinician may also describe the outcomes of forgoing or accepting treatment. For example, when the consultation concerns the removal of a lower wisdom tooth, the clinician may ask the patient to compare the distress caused by the pericoronitis with the anticipated distress of temporary pain and swelling and possible altered sensation. The patient should also take into account the likelihood of future episodes of pericoronitis if they forgo surgery.

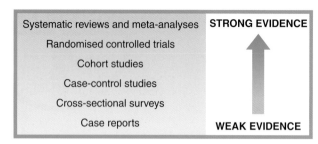

Systematic reviews and meta-analyses — **STRONG EVIDENCE**

Randomised controlled trials

Cohort studies

Case-control studies

Cross-sectional surveys

Case reports — **WEAK EVIDENCE**

Fig. 1 Strength of evidence from some research designs.

Benefits and limitations of evidence-based medicine

The aim of evidence-based medicine is to improve clinical outcomes for patients and there is plenty of evidence that this is the case. One example is that myocardial infarction survivors who are prescribed aspirin or beta-blockers have lower mortality rates that those who aren't prescribed these drugs. Another example would be the benefit of using streptomycin for pulmonary tuberculosis as demonstrated by the historic Medical Research Council trials. These are generally regarded as the first of the modern randomised controlled trials.

The randomised controlled trial provides the underlying basis for evidence-based medicine and the number of trials is growing exponentially with more than 150 000 listed by the Cochrane Library. However, there are limitations to evidence-based medicine. There is a shortage of consistent scientific evidence, difficulties in application of research evidence to individual patients, and barriers to the practice of high-quality care. Some clinicians misunderstand the philosophy of evidence-based medicine and incorrectly believe that it means a loss of clinical freedom, or that it ignores the importance of clinical experience and of individual values.

1.2 Randomised controlled trials

Learning objectives

You should:
- know what a randomised controlled trial is
- understand what the components of a trial are
- have knowledge of the different types of trial
- understand the importance of minimising bias in trials.

Randomised controlled trials may be used to compare health screening, diagnostic and preventative strategies in addition to different treatments. They are recognised to be one of simplest yet most powerful and revolutionary clinical research tools that we have. People are allocated at random to receive one of several clinical interventions, and comparisons are made (Fig. 2).

Components of the randomised controlled trial

- The patients who take part in the trial are referred to as 'participants' or the study population. Participants don't have to be ill as the study can be conducted in healthy volunteers or members of the general public.

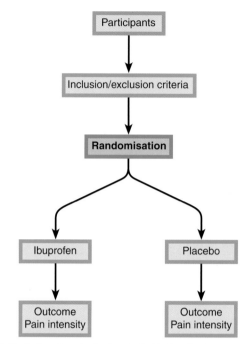

Fig. 2 Illustration of randomised controlled trial method.

- The investigators are those that design the study, administer the interventions, and analyse the results.
- One of the interventions is usually regarded as the standard of comparison or 'control', hence the name randomised *controlled* trial, and the group of participants who receive the control are known as the 'control group'. The control may be conventional treatment, placebo or no treatment.
- Outcomes are measures, so randomised controlled trials are regarded as quantitative studies. They compare two or more interventions and so are regarded as comparative studies. Case-series studies may also be quantitative but do not include comparisons among groups.

Randomisation and allocation concealment

Random allocation means that all participants have the same chance of being assigned to each of the study groups. This ensures that the groups are balanced for the disease severity or other predictors of prognosis and not biased. The randomisation should be concealed from the clinicians who entered patients into the trial so they don't know which treatment the patient will receive, otherwise they may consciously or unconsciously distort the balance of the groups being compared.

The best method for allocation to study group is to use random-number tables or computer-generated sequences. Some investigators report using 'odd or even' birth year or hospital number but there may be problems with these 'quasi-randomisation' methods. The investigator may subvert the allocation because he or she knows which group the patient will be in and the study results could be biased as the groups are not properly balanced. For example, if comparing different surgical techniques for the removal of wisdom teeth, it would be important to have an equal mix of simple and difficult cases in the different groups and not all the simple cases in one group and all the difficult cases in another. If the groups are kept as similar as possible at the start of the study then it will be easier to isolate and quantify the impact of the intervention.

Blinding

Ideally all patients and clinicians involved in the trial should be blind to the intervention so that all groups are treated equally apart from the experimental treatments that are being compared. If this isn't the case then the study may be biased by patients who report symptoms, and clinicians who interpret them, influenced by their hunches and opinions about the anticipated treatment effectiveness. It is, however, not always possible to blind all trials. In surgical trials, for example, the surgeon will be aware of which technique of the alternatives he or she is using, but it may be feasible to have clinicians other than the operating surgeon, who are blind to the study group, carrying out the postoperative assessments. This would be described as a single-blind trial.

A trial is described as 'double-blind' when both the participants and the investigator are blind to the intervention. Some trials require a double-dummy. This may be the case, for example, in an oral medicine trial when two or more mouthrinse interventions need to look and taste the same. The double-blind, double-dummy randomised controlled trial can also be useful when, for example, a drug in tablet form is to be compared with a drug in injection form. Participants in one of the study groups would receive a tablet containing the active drug together with an injection of placebo, and the other study group would receive a placebo tablet with an injection of the active group.

A study is described as 'triple-blind' when the statistician who is analysing the data is blind to the identification of the study group in addition to the investigator and participants.

Completeness of follow-up

All patients entered to the study should be accounted for at its conclusion. Ideally no patients should be lost to follow-up because these patients could have had outcomes that would affect the conclusions of the study. They may have dropped out because of an adverse outcome. One way of dealing with the data where there are patients who have been lost is to assign the worst-case outcome to all of those lost to follow-up. However, some consider that a loss of more than 20% is unacceptable.

Sample size calculation

A clinical trial should be large enough to have a high chance of detecting, as statistically significant, a benefit from the treatment. Many trials are too small to be sure that no benefit exists. The authors may conclude that the intervention had no benefit but if they had calculated in advance the appropriate sample size, and recruited more participants, then they may have observed an effect.

Inclusion and exclusion criteria

The criteria used to determine who can enter the trial and who should be excluded shouldn't be too restrictive. If they are restrictive then the conclusions can only be used to guide decisions for the narrow group of patients who also fit the criteria.

Estimate of effect

The estimate of effect or treatment effect is the relationship observed between the intervention and outcome. There are various methods available to describe the results in clinically useful ways, including the risk ratio and a number needed to treat to benefit. The risk ratio is the ratio of the risk in the intervention group to the risk in the control group. A risk ratio of one indicates no difference between comparison groups. The number needed to treat to benefit (NNT) is an estimate of how many people need to receive a treatment before one person would experience a beneficial outcome. The NNT for 1 g oral paracetamol compared to placebo to achieve at least 50% relief of severe or moderate pain after surgery is about 3.8. Ibuprofen at 400 mg compared to placebo has an NNT of 2.4 and is therefore a more effective oral analgesic.

The confidence interval (CI) provides a measure of the precision or uncertainty of study results for making inferences about the population of patients. As CIs indicate strength of evidence about quantities such as treatment benefit, they are of particular relevance to practitioners of evidence-based medicine.

Different types of randomised controlled trial

Efficacy and effectiveness

Efficacy refers to whether an intervention works in people who receive it. In an efficacy trial the investigators completely control the administration of the intervention given to the participants. Surgical trials comparing different surgical techniques are efficacy trials. Trials investigating analgesics for pain control after wisdom tooth surgery are often efficacy trials too, when patients are usually kept on the study premises so that investigators can ensure that the study medication is taken properly. Even if participants go home a high compliance is expected and will usually be aided by contacting the participants by telephone to prompt this.

Effectiveness refers to whether an intervention works in people to whom it has been offered. These effectiveness trials try to evaluate the effects of an intervention in a similar environment to that found in usual clinical practice. The inclusion criteria are likely to be less strict as the intention is to mimic the real world. Participants may accept or refuse the intervention, which is likely to already have a proven efficacy.

Phase I, II and III trials

Trials designed for evaluation of new drugs are described as Phase I, II and III trials. Following the investigation of safety and potential efficacy in animal studies, the first human trials are conducted. These are known as Phase I studies and are carried out with healthy volunteers as participants and focus on safety and establishing the appropriate dose level. These are followed by Phase II studies that investigate efficacy of the chosen dose or a dose range. Participants will be patients who have a condition requiring the drug, for example, pain after surgery, requiring an analgesic. Phase III studies are effectiveness studies comparing the new drug with an existing similar drug.

Once the new drug has been approved for marketing, there is likely to be a phase of monitoring. This phase is sometimes called a Phase IV trial, although it is not a randomised controlled trial but rather a survey.

Parallel, cross-over and split-mouth design

When participants are exposed to only one of the study interventions, for example a new analgesic or placebo, the study is described as a parallel trial or trial with parallel group design. An alternative design, used less frequently, is when the participant is given one intervention followed by another in random order, that is, each participant receives both interventions. This is called a 'cross-over' trial. This has been used for comparing patient satisfaction after provision of a conventional denture versus an implant-retained denture. Participants are randomised to receiving a conventional denture, or implant-retained denture. Then after an evaluation period, those with the conventional denture receive dental implants and a new or modified denture. Those participants with implants have the abutments only removed, so that the soft tissues heal over the implants (implants are allowed 'to sleep'), and then have a conventional denture made. In this way patients can experience both interventions and report their satisfaction in a better way.

In a split-mouth design each patient acts as his or her own control. The different treatment options are carried out on different sides of the mouth. The advantage of this type of design is that the influence of host-related factors, such as general health, age, or oral hygiene, on the interventions are reduced. The split-mouth design could not be used for the comparison of two mouthrinses as the effect of each could not be limited to one side or the other but is excellent for procedural treatments such as placement of dental implants. The intervention is randomised to the right or left side of the patient's mouth.

Bias and assessment of randomised controlled trials

Bias

Bias in health-care research refers to any process or factor that causes the results of a trial to deviate away from the truth. It usually occurs unconsciously rather than because the investigators are making a deliberate attempt to falsify the conclusions. Bias can be introduced at any stage, in the planning, conducting or analysis of a trial. A bias known as 'selection bias' is described when patients are entered into a trial such that the groups are not properly balanced. For example, an investigator may believe that a new implant system is better than an existing one but is anxious that it may not actually work so well for the more complex cases. If the clinician has prior knowledge as to which implant group a particular patient will be in, then he or she may present study information in such a way to the complex patients that they are discouraged from entering the trial altogether when they were due to enter the new implant system group. This should not occur if the randomisation and allocation procedure is good.

Bias can also occur in the publication and dissemination of trials. Authors are more likely to submit and editors are known to be more likely to accept papers for publication when the findings are positive. This is referred to as 'publication bias'. It would be helpful if high-quality trials were published irrespective of the direction of their findings.

Assessing the quality of RCTs

Not all published trials are perfect and so if you want to be confident about the conclusions drawn from a trial in guiding your clinical decision making, then the quality of the paper should be assessed. The degree to which the trial has been designed, conducted and analysed well is described as the 'internal validity' of the trial. The precision and extent to which it is possible to generalise the results of the published trial to other settings is known as the 'external validity'. There are various assessment tools available to determine the quality, although these are likely to be modified as needed. It may, for example, be important to know that a trial comparing different analgesics for pain after wisdom tooth surgery was blinded properly. However, blinding of participants would not be important in a trial comparing lingual nerve protection with no protection during wisdom tooth surgery when measuring postoperative tongue sensation as the patient is unlikely to introduce bias. It is necessary therefore to consider what parts of any assessment tool are important and relevant to the research question being asked.

The outcomes measured should be meaningful and provide direct information about benefit or harm. Outcome measures may be described as 'true' and 'surrogate' outcomes. A 'true' outcome provides unequivocal evidence of tangible benefit for the patient. An example in a dental implant trial would be the presence or absence of a functioning implant-supported prosthesis. A 'surrogate' outcome is a predictor of the true outcome. In the dental implant trial, the number of surgical visits required or the presence of plaque, bleeding of probing, or radiographic marginal bone changes, would be described as surrogate outcomes.

Outcomes should be reliable, reproducible, easily quantifiable and affordable.

1.3 Other research methods

A multicentre double-blind placebo controlled trial is not the only way to answer a therapeutic question. There are some questions that cannot be answered by randomised controlled trials usually because it would be inappropriate for the investigator to influence the aetiology or natural history of the disease. For example, we believe from observational studies that dental implant osseointegration is significantly impaired in patients who smoke, thus reducing implant success. It would not be ethical to randomise patients to smoking and non-smoking groups and so a randomised controlled trial cannot be undertaken. We must be content with observational studies. Similarly it may not be feasible to study an intervention that may not show effects for many years because of the difficulty in funding and high drop-out.

Also, some things are so obvious that there doesn't need to be a randomised controlled trial. There has never been a randomised controlled trial to show that defibrillation of the heart in ventricular fibrillation saves more lives that doing nothing, or to demonstrate that antibiotics are beneficial in treating pneumonia.

Cohort studies

In a cohort study, two or more groups of individuals are selected on the basis of difference in their exposure to a particular agent and followed up to determine how many in each group develop a particular disease or other outcome.

The evidence that there is a causal, rather than coincidental, link between smoking and ill health was produced by the world-famous cohort study that followed up 40 000 British doctors divided into four cohorts (non-smokers and light, moderate and heavy smokers). The authors published their 10-year interim results in 1964, which showed a substantial excess in both mortality from lung cancer and all-cause mortality in smokers with a 'dose–response' relation. They went on to publish 20-year and 40-year results, with an impressive 94% follow-up, that confirmed the dangers of smoking.

Case-control studies

Case-control studies like cohort studies are usually concerned with the aetiology of a disease rather than its treatment. Patients with a particular disease are 'matched' with controls in the general population. Data are collected (from medical records or by asking the individuals) about past exposure to a possible causal agent for the disease.

Cross-sectional surveys

In a cross-sectional survey, data are collected from a representative sample of subjects or patients by interview, examination or some other means. The collection is at a single time point, although this may be in the past when this is commonly extracted from the medical records. Most surveys do not have a comparison or control group but rather, internal comparisons are made.

Case reports

A case report describes in detail the history of a single patient to illustrate a rare condition, treatment or adverse reaction to treatment. Whilst considered to be relatively weak in the hierarchy of clinical evidence, they are useful to highlight to colleagues a new development or important observation that would otherwise be lost in a clinical trial.

A case report was used to highlight a doctor's observation of two newborn babies in his hospital that had absent limbs and that both mothers had taken a new drug in early pregnancy called thalidomide.

1.4 Systematic reviews

Learning objectives

You should:
- know what a systematic review is
- understand the importance and use of systematic review.

A systematic review uses a predefined methodology to bring together randomised controlled trials on a similar topic, which have been systematically identified, appraised and summarised to give a summary answer. The methods used include steps to minimise bias in all parts of the process: identifying relevant studies, selecting them for inclusion, and collecting and combining their data. Reviews aim to minimise standard error by amassing very large numbers of individuals. They may include statistical methods for combining the results of individual studies called 'meta-analysis'. Systematic review of the effects of health care is the most powerful and useful evidence available for decision making.

Cochrane Collaboration

The Cochrane Collaboration is an international organisation that aims to help people make informed decisions about health, by preparing, maintaining and ensuring the accessibility of rigorous, systematic and up-to-date reviews (and where possible, meta-analysis) of the benefits and risks of health-care interventions. The collaboration consists of an international network of researchers, physicians, dentists and other health-care professionals. Since its creation in 1993, the Cochrane Collaboration has undergone an unprecedented growth and has such potential to influence decision making that it has been described as a rival of the Human Genome Project in its implications for modern medicine. The main product is the electronic Cochrane Library, which contains four databases. Cochrane reviews represent the highest level of evidence on which to base clinical treatment decisions. The typical components of a review are shown in Box 1.

Box 1 Components of a Cochrane systematic review

- Background
- Objectives
- Criteria for considering studies for this review
- Types of studies
- Types of participants
- Types of interventions
- Types of outcome measures
- Identification of studies for inclusion
- Search strategy
- Databases searched
- Any language restrictions
- Any unpublished studies
- Study selection
- Quality assessment
- Data collection and analysis
- Main results
- Discussion
- Reviewers' conclusions for practice and research.

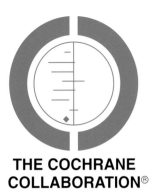

**THE COCHRANE
COLLABORATION**®

Fig. 3 Cochrane Collaboration logo.

In many meta-analyses, 'non-significant' trials contribute to a pooled result that is statistically significant. A famous example of this is a pooling of seven trials of the effect of giving steroids to mothers who were expected to give birth prematurely. Only two of the trials showed a statistically significant benefit (in terms of survival of the infant) but the improvement in precision (that is, the narrowing of the confidence intervals) in the pooled results, shown by the narrower width of the diamond compared to individual lines, demonstrates the strength of the evidence in favour of this intervention. This meta-analysis showed that infants of mothers treated with steroids were 30% to 50% less likely to die than infants of control mothers. The results are typically displayed in a graph called a forest plot that makes it easy for the reader to see the amount of variation between the results of the studies, as well as an estimate of the overall result of all the studies together. The forest plot from this review has been adopted as the logo for the Cochrane Collaboration (Fig. 3).

A more recent systematic review in 2005 based on 139 studies showed that there was 'no credible evidence' that the vaccine against measles, mumps and rubella was involved in the development of either autism or Crohn's disease.

1.5 How to read a paper

Learning objectives

You should:
- understand the importance of critical appraisal.

The medical and dental literature is vast and growing rapidly, so the reader should be clear about why he or she is reading to avoid getting lost. Reasons may include keeping up-to-date, to find an answer to a specific clinical question or to undertake research. There are many poor-quality studies published, so once the reader has identified papers of potential interest, it is important to assess their methodological quality or 'critically appraise', and note their clinical applicability.

Appraisal questions

When seeking to provide the best possible care for patients, clinicians need to know what works, what doesn't and how to distinguish between the two. When reading a paper it is useful to ask particular questions (see Box 2) but remember that it is easier to criticise the research of others than to undertake a perfect piece of research oneself.

CONSORT

The CONSORT (Consolidation of the Standards of Reporting Trials) statement was published in 1996 by a group of biostatisticians, clinical epidemiologists and journal editors to help authors with the reporting of randomised clinical trials for publication in journals. The statement consists of 22 items on a checklist (Table 1) and flow diagram (Fig. 4).

Many journals, including the *British Dental Journal, JAMA, British Medical Journal* and *The Lancet,* require that papers submitted reporting randomised controlled trials should adhere to the recommended presentation. The intention is that this initiative will improve the quality of RCTs and their reporting in publications.

1.6 Clinical practice guidelines

Learning objectives

You should:
- know what clinical guidelines are
- understand the advantages and limits of guidelines.

Guidelines are systematically developed statements to assist practitioner and patient decisions about appropriate health care for specific clinical circumstances. Their purpose is to make evidence-based clinical standards explicit and accessible so that a decision in the clinic or at the chairside will be easier and more objective. Guidelines have two components: an evidence summary, and detailed instructions on how to apply to the patient. They can also be used as a standard for assessing professional performance, to delineate the division of labour, for example, between primary care (general practice) and secondary care (hospital), to educate patients and professionals about current best practice, and to improve the cost-effectiveness of health services.

Valid guidelines create their evidence components from systematic reviews of all the relevant worldwide literature.

Table 1 CONSORT checklist of items to be included when a randomised trial is reported

Paper section	Item	Description
Title & Abstract	1	How participants were allocated to interventions (e.g., 'random allocation', 'randomised', or 'randomly assigned').
Introduction		
Background	2	Scientific background and explanation of rationale
Methods		
Participants	3	Eligibility criteria for participants and the settings and locations where data were collected
Interventions	4	Precise details of the interventions intended for each group and how and when they were actually administered
Objectives	5	Specific objectives and hypotheses
Outcomes	6	Clearly defined primary and secondary outcome measures
Sample size	7	How sample size was determined
Randomisation – Sequence generation	8	Method used to generate the random allocation sequence
Randomisation – Allocation concealment	9	Method used to implement the random allocation sequence clarifying whether the sequence was concealed until interventions were assigned
Randomisation – Implementation	10	Who generated the allocation sequence, who enrolled participants and who assigned the participants to their groups
Blinding	11	Whether or not participants, those administering the interventions, and those assessing the outcomes were blinded to the group assignment
Statistical methods	12	Statistical methods used to compare groups for primary outcomes
Results		
Participant flow	13	Flow of participants through each stage (a diagram is strongly recommended). Specifically, for each group report the numbers of participants randomly assigned, receiving intended treatment, completing the study protocol, and analysed for the primary outcome.
Recruitment	14	Dates defining the periods of recruitment and follow-up
Baseline data	15	Baseline demographic and clinical characteristics of each group
Numbers analysed	16	Number of participants in each group
Outcomes and estimation	17	For each primary and secondary outcome, a summary of results for each group and the estimated effect size and its precision (e.g., 95% confidence interval).
Ancillary analyses	18	Address multiplicity by reporting any other analyses performed including subgroup analyses and adjusted analyses, indicating those pre-specified and those exploratory.
Adverse events	19	All important adverse events or side-effects in each intervention group
Discussion		
Interpretation	20	Interpretation of the results taking into account study hypotheses, sources of potential bias or imprecision and the dangers associated with multiplicity of analyses and outcomes.
Generalisability	21	Generalisability (external validity) of the trial findings
Overall evidence	22	General interpretation of the results in the context of current evidence

However, guidelines may also use less robust evidence. Each recommendation should be tagged with the level of evidence on which it is based and the recommendation can then take this into account (Table 2).

Problems with guidelines

Health-care managers tend to welcome guidelines more than many clinicians who may distrust them. The concern is that in the absence of best evidence, guidelines may be produced anyway using poor evidence such as 'expert opinion' and the clinician may feel under pressure to adhere to these. Guideline development usually involves a small number of individuals with a consequent limited range of views and skills, so it is important that the recommendations are evaluated and modulated by external review and comment and tested in the field in which they are to be implemented.

Clinical guidelines have also been criticised for inhibiting innovation and preventing individual cases from being dealt with discretely and sensitively.

Also, nationally developed guidelines may not reflect local needs, or those developed in primary care may not reflect secondary care and vice versa. Some may consider that they may lead to an undesirable shift in balance of power between purchasers and providers, and may be perceived to be politically motivated.

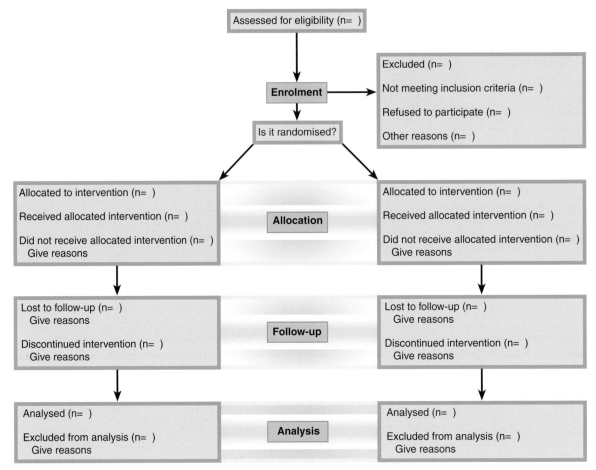

Fig. 4 The CONSORT flowchart.

Table 2 Levels of evidence and grades of recommendations for therapies

Grade of recommendation	Level of evidence	
A	1a	Systematic reviews of randomised controlled trials
A	1b	Individual randomised controlled trial with narrow confidence interval
A	1c	All or none
B	2a	Systematic reviews of cohort studies
B	2b	Individual cohort study and poor quality randomised controlled trial
B	2c	'Outcomes' research
B	3a	Systematic reviews of case-control studies
B	3c	Individual case-control study
C	4	Case series and poor quality cohort and case-control studies
D	5	Expert opinion without explicit critical appraisal

Assessing patients

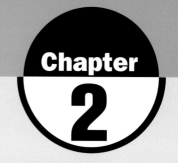

Overview

This chapter describes the basic principles of assessing a dental patient. A history should include significant medical and social facts as well as the dental problem. An initial extra-oral examination covers both the visual appearance of the patient and features such as swellings and nerve dysfunction. Once these aspects are completed, the intra-oral examination will attempt to identify any lumps or swellings and to differentiate these into dental and non-dental origins. Features such as ulcers and motor or sensory nerve dysfunction will also be noted before the detailed examination of the troublesome tooth or teeth. The physical examination of the teeth is described. Specific investigations must be chosen for their suitability both in terms of the usefulness of the results and the medicolegal aspects of their use. For example, both HIV testing and the use of X-rays have implications beyond the results that they provide. The relative merits of the various investigations are described.

2.1 History

Learning objectives

You should:
- understand what information should be elicited in history taking
- develop a questioning style that is consistent, thorough and obtains the most information.

A full and accurate history is of paramount importance in assessment of a patient. In some cases, the history may provide the diagnosis while in the remainder it will give essential clues to the nature of the problem. The approach to history taking needs to be tailored to the type of complaint being investigated.

It is important to have a systematic approach to taking a history. A consistent series of questions will avoid inadvertently missing an important clue. Use 'open' rather than 'closed' (those usually eliciting a yes/no response) questions wherever possible to avoid leading the patient. Record the patient's own responses rather than paraphrasing. The history will cover:

- the complaint
- the history of the complaint
- past dental history
- social and family history
- medical history.

The complaint

'What is the problem?' Record the patient's symptoms. If there are several symptoms make a list, but with the principal problem first.

History of the complaint

'When did the problem(s) start?' Identify the duration of the problem. Also remember to ask whether this is the first incidence of the problem or the latest of a series of recurrences.

Past dental history

'Do you see your dentist regularly?' Establish whether the patient is a regular or irregular attender. Obtain a general picture of their treatment experience (fillings, dentures, local and general anaesthetic experience).

Social and family history

'Just a few questions about yourself.' The importance of recording such basic details as the age of the patient is self-evident. Other factors such as marital status and job help to gain a picture of the patient as a person rather than a mere collection of symptoms. Occupation can have direct relevance to some clinical conditions but may also reveal aggravating factors such as physical or psychological stress. Record alcohol consumption (units per week) and smoking. Family history may be relevant in some instances, for example in some genetic disorders such as amelogenesis imperfecta.

Medical history

'Now some questions about your general health.' This is obviously important. Some medical conditions may have oral manifestations while others will affect the manner in which dental treatment is delivered. Even if the patient volunteers that they are 'fit and healthy' when you say you are going to ask them a few medical questions, you must persist and enquire specifically about key systems of the body:

- cardiovascular (heart or chest problems)
- respiratory (chest trouble)
- central nervous system (fits, faints or epilepsy)
- allergies

- current medical treatment: a negative response should be further confirmed by asking whether the patient has visited their general practitioner recently
- current and recent drug therapy
- past medical history: previous occurrences of hospitalisation or medical care
- bleeding disorders
- history of rheumatic fever
- history of jaundice or hepatitis
- any other current health problems: a negative response can be confirmed, with a final 'so you are fit and well?'.

See Chapter 3 for a more detailed discussion of the medical aspects of dental care.

2.2 Extra-oral examination

Learning objectives

You should:
- know how to palpate lymph nodes
- be able to identify and assess swellings, sensory disturbance and motor disturbances
- understand what to look for based on the history.

Like history taking, examination necessitates a systematic approach. As a general rule, use your eyes first, then your hands to examine a patient. Start with the extra-oral examination before proceeding to examine the oral cavity.

Take time to look at the patient. This may seem obvious but will identify swellings, skin lesions and facial palsies. Facial pallor may indicate anaemia, or that the patient may be about to faint. This process of observation will start while you are taking the history.

Visual areas would cover:

- general patient condition
- symmetry
- swellings
- lips/perioral tissues.

Palpation would cover:

- lymph nodes
- temporomandibular joint (TMJ)
- salivary glands
- problem-specific examination.

Lymph node examination

The major lymph nodes of the maxillofacial region and neck are shown in Figure 5. The submental, submandibular and the internal jugular nodes (jugulo-digastric and jugulo-omohyoid node being the largest) are of particular importance because these receive lymph drainage from the oral cavity. Examination of the nodes should be systematic, although the order of examination is not critically important. To palpate the nodes, the examiner should stand behind the patient while he/she is seated in an upright position. Use both hands (left hand for the left side of the patient etc.). A common sequence would be to start in the submental region, working back to the submandibular nodes then further back to the jugulo-digastric node (Fig. 5).

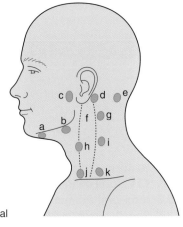

a Submental
b Submandibular
c Preauricular
d Postauricular
e Occipital
f Jugulo-digastric
g Jugulo-omohyoid
h Mid jugular
i Midposterior cervical
j Lower jugular
k Lower posterior cervical

Fig. 5 Principal lymph nodes in the head and neck. The dotted lines indicate the outline of the sternocleidomastoid muscle.

Then continue by palpation of the parotid region downwards to the retromandibular area and down the cervical chain of nodes. When a node is perceived as enlarged, record the texture: a hard node of a metastasising malignancy contrasts well with a tender, softer node in an inflammatory process.

Temporomandibular joint

A detailed examination of the TMJ is probably only needed when a specific problem is suspected from the history. Details of examination of this joint and the associated musculature is given in Chapter 15.

Salivary glands

As with the TMJ, examination of the salivary glands is only required when the history suggests this is relevant. Chapter 13 describes the examination of the major salivary glands.

Problem-specific examination

The examination will be made in the light of the symptoms reported by the patient but the examiner may detect swelling, sensory or motor disturbance that the patient has not noticed.

Swelling/lump

The procedure for examination of a swelling or a lump must encompass a range of observations:

- anatomical site
- shape and size
- colour
- single or multiple
- surface texture/warmth
- tenderness
- fluctuation
- sensation/pulsation.

Consistency can be informative, ranging from the soft swelling of a lipoma, through 'cartilage hard' pleomorphic adenomas and 'rubbery hard' nodes in Hodgkin's disease to the 'rock hard' nodes of metastatic malignancy. Tenderness and warmth on palpation usually indicates an inflammatory process, while neoplasms are commonly painless unless secondarily infected. Fluctuation indicates the presence of fluid. To assess fluctuation, place two fingers on the swelling and press down with one finger. If fluid is present the other finger will record an upward pressure. Pulsation in a swelling will indicate direct (i.e. it is a vascular lesion) or indirect involvement (i.e. in immediate contact) of an artery.

Paraesthesia/anaesthesia

The presence of sensory disturbance is usually identified initially by the patient in the history. It is important to identify the *extent* of the affected area and the *degree* of alteration in sensation. It is best to use a fairly fine, but blunt-ended, instrument for this at first, for example the handle of a dental mirror. First, run the instrument gently over what is assumed to be a normal area of skin so that the patient knows what to expect. Then repeat this over the symptomatic area, asking the patient to say whether they can feel anything. Record the area of altered sensation in the notes using a drawing.

The degree of alteration in sensation can be assessed by using different 'probes'. A teased-out piece of cotton wool can be used or, where anaesthesia appears to be profound, a sharp probe can be (carefully) tried.

The extent of the area of paraesthesia or anaesthesia will tell you the particular nerve, or branch of a nerve, involved (Fig. 6). This will, in turn, inform you about the possible location of the underlying lesion. For example, a patient with disturbed sensation of the upper lip has a lesion affecting the maxillary division of the trigeminal nerve. If this is the sole site of sensory deficit, it suggests a lesion closer to the terminal branches of this cranial nerve (e.g. in the maxillary sinus). In contrast, if sensory deficiencies are simultaneously present in other branches of the nerve, it suggests that the lesion is more centrally located.

Paralysis/motor disturbance

While paralysis or motor disturbance may be reported as a symptom by the patient, it may initially be identified during an examination. In the maxillofacial region, the motor nerves that are likely to be under consideration are the facial nerve, the hypoglossal nerve (see below) and the nerves controlling the muscles that move the eyes.

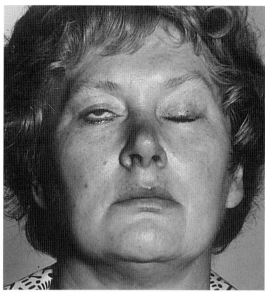

Fig. 7 Patient with Bell's palsy.

Disturbance in function of the facial nerve will result in effects on the muscles of facial expression. Paralysis of the lower face indicates an upper motor neurone lesion (stroke, cerebral tumour or trauma). Paralysis of all the facial muscles (on the affected side) indicates a lower motor neurone lesion. The latter is seen in a large number of conditions but, for the dentist, important causes include Bell's palsy (Fig. 7), parotid tumours, a misplaced inferior dental local anaesthetic and trauma.

2.3 Intra-oral examination

Learning objectives

You should:
- be able to differentiate dental and non-dental sources of symptoms
- understand the significance of features of ulcers such as form, site and pain
- be able to examine for motor and sensory nerve dysfunction
- know how to examine a tooth.

Again, a systematic approach is essential to avoid being distracted by the first unusual finding you encounter. The examination must include lips, cheeks, parotid gland orifices, buccal gingivae, lingual gingivae and alveolar ridges in edentulous areas, hard palate, soft palate, dorsal surface of the tongue, ventral surface of the tongue, floor of mouth, submandibular gland orifices and, finally, the teeth. Different clinicians will have their own sequence of examination, but it is the thoroughness of the examination that is important, not the order in which the regions of the mouth are examined.

Once the general intra-oral examination is complete, a problem-specific examination can proceed. This is tailored to the clinical problem.

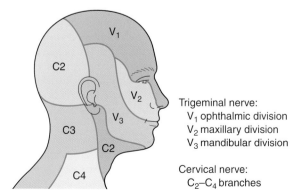

Trigeminal nerve:
V₁ ophthalmic division
V₂ maxillary division
V₃ mandibular division

Cervical nerve:
C₂–C₄ branches

Fig. 6 Cutaneous sensory innervation of the head and neck by the trigeminal and cervical nerves.

Swelling/lump

The examination of an intra-oral swelling or lump is essentially the same as that described above as part of the extra-oral examination. Most oral swellings are inflammatory, caused by periapical or periodontal infections. However, the minority of oral swellings and lumps that are non-dental encompasses a wide range of conditions, the details of which form a significant part of this book.

Ulcer

Examination of an ulcer should include assessment of eight important characteristics:

* site
* single/multiple
* size
* shape
* base of the ulcer
* edge
* pain
* time period.

Visual inspection is essential but palpation is also an important part of the examination of an ulcer. Gloves must be worn for palpation and the texture of the ulcer base, margin and surrounding tissues should be ascertained by gentle pressure. Malignant neoplasms tend to ulcerate, and these often feel firm, hard or even fixed to deeper tissues. A raised margin is a suspicious finding, as is the presence of necrotic, friable tissue in the ulcer base and bleeding on lightly pressing (Fig. 8). Healing traumatic ulcers tend to be painful on palpation and they feel soft and gelatinous.

The finding of an ulcer on examination may necessitate taking additional history; for example, if a traumatic ulcer is suspected, direct questioning may prompt the patient to recall the injury (Fig. 9). If multiple ulcers are detected, this may lead to further enquiries about any previous history of recurrent oral ulceration or specific gastrointestinal diseases. It is surprising how often ulceration is discovered that the patient is not aware of. When an ulcer is found, it is vital that a detailed record of the history and examination findings is made. Any oral mucosal ulcer that does

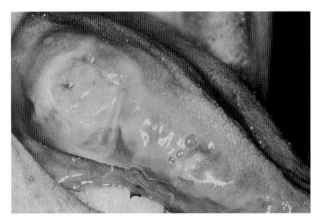

Fig. 9 Clinical photograph of a traumatic ulcer of the lingual mucosa. Note the superficial nature of the ulcer. Its base is covered by fibrous exudates and the surrounding area is inflamed.

not heal within 3 weeks should be considered as possibly malignant and urgent referral must be arranged.

Certain ulcers have a tendency to occur in particular oral sites; for example, squamous cell carcinomas are most common on the lower lip, in the floor of mouth and the lateral border of the tongue. On the other hand, traumatic ulcers are most common on the lateral border of the tongue and buccal mucosa in the occlusal plane. Ulceration on the lower lip is also a common site for traumatic ulceration, particularly following administration of an inferior dental block or after a sports injury. Site is also important in diagnosis; for example, minor aphthae are restricted to lining mucosa and can be ruled out if ulceration is occurring on the hard palate or gingivae.

Size and shape can also be helpful; for example, linear fissure-type ulcers may be seen in Crohn's disease, though aphthae are more usual. The shape of a traumatic ulcer may reveal the cause; for example, semicircular ulcers are sometimes caused by the patient's fingernail. Bizarre persistent ulceration is sometimes a result of deliberate self-harm, unusual habits or taking recreational drugs; in such cases, diagnosis can be difficult as the patient may deny knowledge of the causation. Minor aphthae have characteristic size and site features, which can distinguish them from major and herpetiform aphthae (see Ch. 11).

Pain, as mentioned above, is a feature of inflammatory and traumatic ulcers, while in the early stages a malignant ulcer is often painless. Advanced malignant ulcers eventually tend to become painful as a result of infection and involvement of adjacent nerves. Presentation with a painful traumatic ulcer is common in dentistry. The cause should be eliminated if possible (e.g. smoothing or replacement of an adjacent fractured restoration), symptomatic treatment such as analgesic mouthwash prescribed and most importantly, review arranged to ensure that healing has occurred.

Paraesthesia/anaesthesia

The principles of examination are those described above for extra-oral examination. Once again, you need good anatomical knowledge of the nerves supplying different parts of the oral cavity to interpret the possible site of the underlying pathological process (Fig. 10).

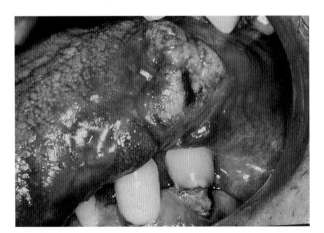

Fig. 8 Clinical photograph of a squamous cell carcinoma of the tongue. Note the raised edges and necrotic centre.

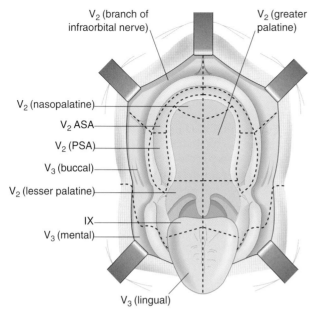

V₂ (branch of infraorbital nerve)
V₂ (greater palatine)
V₂ (nasopalatine)
V₂ ASA
V₂ (PSA)
V₃ (buccal)
V₂ (lesser palatine)
IX
V₃ (mental)
V₃ (lingual)

ASA = Anterior superior alveolar nerve
PSA = Posterior superior alveolar nerve

Fig. 10 Sensory innervation of the oral cavity is principally from the trigeminal nerve (V) while the glossopharyngeal nerve (IX) supplies the posterior third of the tongue. NB: Taste sensation in the anterior two-thirds of the tongue is provided by fibres of VII nerve origin passing through the lingual nerve.

Paralysis/motor disturbance

Within the oral cavity, motor disturbance is seen in the tongue (owing to damage to the function of the hypoglossal nerve) and the soft palate (owing to lesions affecting the vagus nerve). With hypoglossal nerve lesions, there is deviation of the tongue towards the affected side when attempting protrusion. There is also a problem with speech, with 'lingual' sounds such as 'l', 't' and 'd' affected.

Tooth problems

Tooth problems are, of course, the commonest problems facing the dentist. The context is usually pain or swelling. A standard method of examination helps in reaching a diagnosis. You should not simply hammer the suspect tooth with the mirror handle and take a radiograph as your method of assessment! Indeed, careful examination may establish a diagnosis and thus avoid any need for radiography or other special tests. Examination will involve:

- visual
- probing restorations
- assessing mobility
- periodontal probing
- thermal tests
- pressure tests.

Visual examination will reveal gross caries, the presence of restorations, signs of tooth wear and gingivitis. A probe will allow tactile assessment of restoration margins.

Mobility should be assessed manually. Periodontal probing should be carried out to assess pocketing, the presence of calculus/overhangs and, ultimately, bone loss.

A basic test of vitality should always be performed, using a cotton wool pledget soaked with ethyl chloride (cold stimulus) and sometimes heated gutta-percha (hot stimulus). While these are usually sufficient to reveal a hypersensitive tooth with pulpitis, an electrical pulp test can be used to assess vitality in some cases.

Pressure sensitivity should be assessed using direct finger pressure and, when this does not evoke a response, can be supplemented by percussion using a dental mirror handle. This will assess whether periodontitis is present or not. However, if a single cusp is tender to percussion, this may be indicative of cracked cusp syndrome.

2.4 Special investigations

Learning objectives

You should:
- understand what samples can be taken for tests, how to take and treat these materials and what tests are available
- know how to interpret the results that are returned
- know when imaging techniques would be informative and which type of imaging to choose.

Chairside laboratory investigations

Evidence-based laboratory medicine

Whenever special tests are undertaken, it is important to consider medicolegal issues, informed consent, appropriateness of the test and the evidence base for the use of any particular laboratory investigation. It is always necessary to have a differential clinical diagnosis in mind when requesting an investigation. Certain tests, such as those for human immunodeficiency virus (HIV) infection, require pre-test counselling and informed consent; such tests should be undertaken only by specialists in the field. When requesting a test, it is vital to possess the knowledge and skills so that the result can be acted upon appropriately. In some situations, for example suspected oral cancer, it may be wise to refer the patient directly to a specialist for a biopsy. Other important considerations when considering laboratory testing are:

- obtaining a representative/appropriate sample
- collecting in the right specimen container and fluid if appropriate
- completing the information required by the laboratory correctly
- having systems that avoid mixing up specimens; labelling the specimen container with patient details
- organising the correct packaging and transport to the laboratory
- reading reports and acting on them; filling in patient records
- interpretation: sensitivity and specificity.

Most laboratories can advise on current codes of practice relating to the above issues and may give reference ranges and advice, for example about a particular biopsy result. Sending pathological material through the post is potentially hazardous and current regulations must be followed.

It should be remembered that laboratory tests require considered interpretation in conjunction with the patient's history. Some tests have low sensitivities, for example certain cytology tests, and a negative result cannot be relied upon to exclude disease. The test may need to be repeated, or an alternative test with a higher sensitivity used. Other tests have low specificity and a positive result does not necessarily indicate that disease is present. Examples include low-titre autoantibodies, which may be detected in the serum but which can be of no clinical significance. The receiver–operator curve (ROC) for any laboratory test can be plotted to guide clinical use. Use of resources is also important, particularly when expensive reagents or complex procedures are required.

Microbiology

Diagnosis of infection and determination of sensitivity of the infectious agent to pharmacotherapeutic agents are the principal requirements for microbiology tests in dentistry.

Viruses. Most often a clinical diagnosis is adequate for acute or recurrent viral oral infections such as herpes simplex. A viral swab can be used to collect virus from fresh vesicles and must be forwarded in special transport medium to the virology laboratory. Other virus infections such as glandular fever can be detected by looking for a rising titre of antibodies in the patient's serum.

Bacteria. Bacterial infections in the oral cavity, jaws and salivary glands may be identified by forwarding a swab or specimen of pus to the laboratory, with a request for culture and antibiotic sensitivity.

Fungi. Candida sp. is the most common organism to cause oral fungal infection. Often clinical diagnosis is adequate; for example in denture-related stomatitis, the clinical history and appearance of the mucosa may be sufficient. Direct smears from the infected mucosa and the denture-fitting surface can be stained by the periodic acid-Schiff or Gram's method. The presence of typical pseudohyphae indicates candidal proliferation consistent with infection. Swabs or oral rinses can be used to discriminate the various *Candida* species and heavy growth suggests infection rather than carriage.

Aspiration biopsy

Fluid from suspected cysts can be collected with a standard gauge needle and syringe: radicular cysts contain brown shimmering fluid because of the presence of the cholesterol crystals, whereas odontogenic keratocysts contain pale greasy fluid, which may include keratotic squames. Infection after aspiration biopsy can be a problem and indeed the technique tends to be restricted to atypical cystic lesions where neoplasia is suspected. Fine needle aspiration biopsy (FNAB) can be used to obtain a sample of cells from a solid tumour and is a hospital procedure.

Incisional/excisional biopsy

Mucosal biopsy is one of the more common investigations used by dentists in primary and secondary care. Tissue is removed under local or general anaesthesia using sharp dissection to avoid crushing the specimen. It is fixed in at least 10 times its volume of 10% neutral buffered formalin or similar fixative. It is then forwarded to the histopathology or specialist oral and maxillofacial pathology laboratory.

Excisional biopsy. The entire lesion is removed and submitted for diagnosis. It is suitable for benign polyps, papillomas, mucocoeles, epulides and other small reactive lesions.

Incisional biopsy. A representative sample of a larger lesion is taken for diagnosis prior to treatment. This is a specialist procedure requiring some expertise and experience. It is used for generalised mucosal disorders such as lichen planus or for the diagnosis of other red and white patches. An important consideration is obtaining a sample from an appropriate area. Non-healing ulcers are often investigated by incisional biopsy; here it is important to include the margin of the ulcer with some normal tissue and to obtain a sufficiently large sample (normally 10 mm × 10 mm) to identify or exclude cancer. Sometimes fresh tissue is required for diagnosis, for instance in the vesiculobullous diseases where immunofluorescence is needed. Special arrangements must be made with the laboratory when such tests are planned.

Haematology

Patients presenting with oral manifestations of haematological disease are normally referred for specialist opinion. Full blood count and assay of haematinics is an important investigation for patients presenting with lingual papillary atrophy or recurrent oral ulceration, for example. Coagulation studies and platelet counts may be required when excessive bleeding is encountered. Patients on anticoagulant therapy should have their INR (international normalised ratio) checked before any surgical procedure is undertaken.

The Sickledex test may be used to screen for sickle cell anaemia prior to giving general anaesthesia in situations of urgency. The blood sample should be subjected to haemoglobin electrophoresis.

Haematological parameters of importance in dentistry are described in Table 3.

Biochemistry

Biochemical investigations are used principally in specialist clinics to investigate patients presenting with oral manifestations of systemic disease, for example estimation of alkaline phosphatase in Paget's disease of bone, and serum calcium to exclude hyperparathyroidism when a giant cell granuloma is diagnosed. Biochemical estimation of cyst fluid for protein content is sometimes undertaken as part of the diagnosis of odontogenic keratocyst.

Immunology

Advances in knowledge and methods in immunology have resulted in a large number of laboratory immunological investigations, available in specialist laboratories. Sometimes diagnostic arrays of tests are offered by the laboratory. Examples of tests in dentistry include detection of antibodies against extractable nuclear antigens, including SS-A and SS-B, for the diagnosis of Sjögren's syndrome and autoantibodies in vesiculo-bullous diseases.

Table 3 Important haematological values in dentistry

	Conventional units	SI units
Haemoglobin (Hb)		
Male	13.0–18.0 g/dl	8.1–11.2 mmol/l
Female	11.5–16.5 g/dl	7.4–9.9 mmol/l
Red cell count (RBC)		
Male	4.5–6.5 million/mm³	4.5–6.5×10^{12}/l
Female	3.8–5.8 million/mm³	3.8–5.8×10^{12}/l
Haematocrit (HCT)		
Male	40–54 ml/dl	0.40–0.54
Female	37–47 ml/dl	0.37–0.47
Mean cell volume, adults (MCV)	80–90 µm³	80–97 fl
Mean cell haemoglobin, adults (MCH)	27–32 pg/cell	27–32 pg/cell
Mean cell haemoglobin concentration, adults (MCHC)	31–36.5 g/dl	31–36.5 g/l
White cell count, adults (leucocytes; WBC)	4500–11 000/mm³	4.0–11.0×10^{9}/l
Neutrophils	2000–7500/mm³	2.0–7.5×10^{9}/l
Lymphocytes	1500–4000/mm³	1.5–4.0×10^{9}/l
Monocytes	200–1200/mm³	0.2–1.2×10^{9}/l
Eosinophils	40–400/mm³	0.04–0.40×10^{9}/l
Platelets, adults (PLT)		150–400×10^{9}/l
Erythrocyte sedimentation rate, adults (ESR)	0–8 mm/h	0–8 mm/h

Every laboratory has its own reference range which should be consulted when laboratory test results are received. The values are typical for adults; the ranges for full-term infants and children vary considerably.

HIV testing should only be undertaken by specialists and does not fall directly into the remit of dentistry. It requires informed patient consent and counselling. Dentists must be able to recognise the oral manifestations of immunodeficiency states and arrange proper referral.

Imaging

Imaging is an important special test in dentistry and oral and maxillofacial surgery. Because X-ray exposure carries a quantifiable risk (see Ch. 16), X-ray examinations should be selected according to specific selection (referral) criteria. Other imaging investigations not using ionising radiations (ultrasound and magnetic resonance imaging) have their place and should be used in preference to X-ray techniques (radiography and computed tomography) when they can provide the same or better diagnostic information. Selection criteria should be based upon the diagnostic efficacy of the technique for the disease process being examined. For example, approximal caries diagnosis is best aided by bitewing rather than other radiographs. There are a large number of imaging techniques available and these are summarised below. Details of the specific uses of these techniques are given where appropriate in subsequent chapters.

Conventional radiography

This is familiar to every dentist and student in the forms of bitewing, periapical, occlusal and panoramic radiography and these techniques are covered in more detail in the companion volume to this book (Dentistry II).

Other maxillofacial radiographs should be used in addition to the traditional 'dental' techniques when appropriate. While detailed prescription of radiographs depends on the particular needs of each patient, some general guidelines are useful and are given in Table 4.

Contrast investigations

Some radiological techniques use radio-opaque contrast media injected into parts of the body. In the maxillofacial region, they can be used to demonstrate fistulae and sinuses and in vascular studies (angiograms). However, they are most commonly used for sialography (Ch. 13). Arthrography of the TMJ (Ch. 15), although still used by some specialists, is of largely historical interest.

Computed tomography

Computed tomography (CT) is also known as CAT scanning (Fig. 11). It provides primarily *axial* cross-sectional images and uses X-rays. The computer calculates the X-ray absorption (and thus indirectly the density) of each unit volume (voxel) of tissue and then assembles the information into an image made up of many pixels (picture elements). Each pixel is given a grey-scale value according to its density (Hounsfield scale). Dense bone is white, most soft tissues are mid-grey, fat is dark grey and air is black. Metals are beyond the comprehension of the computer software, so dental fillings cause artefacts.

Clinical maxillofacial applications include:

- large maxillary cysts/benign tumours
- malignancy arising in the antrum
- soft tissue masses
- oral carcinoma.

Table 4 Guidelines of radiographic projections

Anatomical site to be examined	Radiographic projections
Anterior mandible	Periapical, oblique and true occlusal views
Body of mandible	Periapical, true occlusal, panoramic (or lateral oblique) views
Third molar region, angle and ramus of mandible	Periapical and true occlusal (third molar region only)
	Panoramic (or lateral oblique) view
	Postero-anterior (PA) view of mandible
Condyle temporomandibular joint	Panoramic (or lateral oblique) view
	Transcranial views (open/closed)
	Reverse Towne's view (modified PA projection)
Anterior maxilla	Periapical and oblique occlusal views
Posterior maxilla	Periapical, oblique occlusal, panoramic (or lateral oblique) views
Maxillary sinus	Periapical, oblique occlusal, panoramic (or lateral oblique) views
	Occipitomental view
	Intra-oral soft tissue view of parotid papilla region
Parotid gland (for calculi)	Localised PA/antero-posterior of face with cheek blown out
Submandibular gland (for calculi)	True occlusal of floor of mouth
	Modified oblique occlusal for submandibular gland

Images can be reconstructed in two or three dimensions. In maxillofacial work, reconstructions are invaluable for implantology and useful in major facial trauma and orthognathic surgical treatment planning.

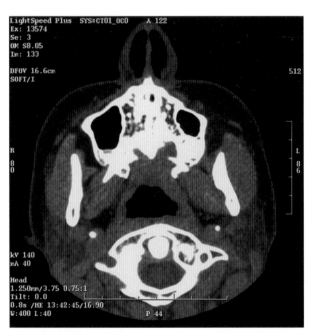

Fig. 11 A typical computed tomographic scan.

CT is associated with a relatively high dose of radiation. Generally, the thinner the sections (and the better the fine detail), the higher the dose.

Cone beam computed tomography

This technique (also known as digital volume tomography) has come to prominence in the last few years as a relatively low-cost method of producing cross-sectional images with lower radiation dose than conventional CT. The cone beam computed tomography (CBCT) equipment still uses X-rays, but uses a cone-shaped beam instead of the fan-shaped beam used in CT. This results in a volume of image data that can be used to provide images of equivalent quality in any desired plane. Voxel sizes are smaller than with CT, so give better image resolution. CBCT equipment is substantially cheaper than CT, so is a feasible purchase for dentists in large practices.

Diagnostic ultrasound

Ultrasound uses the principle that high-frequency (3.5–10 MHz) sound waves can pass through soft tissue but will be reflected back from tissue interfaces. The echoes can be detected to produce an image. The sound is transmitted and detected by the same hand-held *transducer*. Imaging is 'real-time'.

Clinical maxillofacial applications include: soft tissue lumps in the neck and the salivary glands.

Radioisotope imaging

Radioisotope imaging is also known as nuclear medicine (Fig. 12). The technique uses radioisotopes (usually gamma ray emitters) tagged on to pharmaceuticals, which are usually injected into the bloodstream. By choosing the radiopharmaceutical appropriately, particular organs or types of tissues will become radioactive.

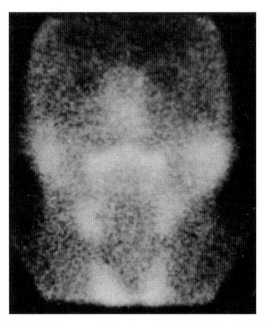

Fig. 12 Radioisotope scan of the salivary glands. Frontal view. Foci of activity are visible in the four major salivary glands, in the mouth and, at the bottom of the image, the thyroid gland.

The patient is placed in front of a gamma camera, which detects the emitted radiation to give an image of physiological activity. It is not an anatomical imaging modality.
Clinical maxillofacial applications include:

- salivary scanning (particularly in Sjögren's syndrome): uses sodium pertechnetate-99 m
- bone scanning (for bone tumours, metastatic disease, Paget's disease, arthritis and condylar hyperplasia): uses technetium-99 m-labelled methylene disphosphonate.

Magnetic resonance imaging

Magnetic resonance imaging is also known as MR, MRI or NMR. In this technique, patients are placed into an intense magnetic field, forcing their hydrogen nuclei (principally in water molecules) to align in the field. Radiofrequency waves are pulsed into the patient, the hydrogen nuclei 'wobble', producing an alteration in the magnetic field. This induces an electric current in coils placed around the patient. The computer is capable of reading this and, because different tissues contain different amounts of

---

The Dental Practice
1, High Street
Anytown

Dr A Smith
Consultant Oral and Maxillofacial Surgeon
Anytown General Hospital
Anytown

2 January 2008

Dear Dr Smith,

Re: Mr John Doe, 24 Green Lane, Anytown. Date of birth: 25.12.40 Tel: 0123 456789

I would be grateful if you would see this 60-year-old man. He presented today complaining of a 'growth' from a recent extraction socket in his upper jaw. He said that this had appeared after an extraction I carried out two weeks ago and was getting slowly bigger. He also complains of a numb feeling on the left cheek. I had extracted /6 two weeks ago at the request of the patient because it was loose.

Examination revealed a palpable left cervical lymph node. There was reduced sensation to touch on the left upper lip and cheek. Intra-orally there was a mass on the left maxillary alveolus in /6 region, about 2 by 1 cm. The mass has an irregular surface, feels indurated, bleeds easily on palpation and looks necrotic in places. I have taken a periapical radiograph, which shows some bone destruction at the site of the socket.

I am worried that this might be maxillary sinus malignancy and I would appreciate your urgent opinion and management.

Mr Doe has a history of mild hypertension for which he takes a bendrofluazide tablet (2.5 mg) in the morning. Otherwise there is no other medical history of note. He is a nervous patient generally and will probably be accompanied by his wife. Mr Doe is a non-smoker and drinks 7-8 units of alcohol per week. He can attend at any time.

Yours sincerely,

Mrs B Jones BDS

Fig. 13 An example of a referral letter.

hydrogen (in water), of producing an image that, superficially, is like a CT scan. However, imaging can be in any plane (axial, sagittal or coronal).

Clinical maxillofacial applications include:

- almost anything CT can do (but no ionising radiation)
- imaging of the TMJ.

Problems are twofold: the immense cost of MR and, second, patients with some metallic implants (intracranial vascular clips, cardiac pacemakers) are not eligible for the technique. Fixed orthodontic appliances may, depending on the material from which components are made, need to be removed before MR imaging.

2.5 Writing a referral letter

Learning objectives

You should:
- know when to refer a patient
- be able to write a competent referral letter
- know now to keep good records of the referral.

However good your diagnostic abilities are and however skilled you are as a clinician, there will come a time when you need to refer a patient on to a colleague. The letter should be thorough, providing the second clinician with a detailed history and the results of your examination. It is reprehensible to write a 'Dear Sir, please see and treat, yours sincerely' letter. The referral must include:

- name, address, date of birth of the patient
- description of the patient's problem/symptoms

- a history of the problem
- the results of your examination
- the results of any special tests you have performed
- your provisional diagnosis, if any
- the medical history
- any special factors, such as difficulty in attending
- all relevant radiographs or investigations.

The letter should be word-processed wherever possible, rather than hand-written, to ensure accuracy. A model letter is shown in Figure 13. It is important to remember that patients tend to open and read referral letters and that they become ultimately part of the hospital medical record. Such records are available to patients and their legal advisers. The example in Figure 13 demonstrates that the dentist acted promptly and exercised a high standard of care and consideration for the patient. A copy of the referral letter should be kept with the patient's records.

It is good practice to establish a working relationship between primary and secondary carers. In the situation described in Figure 13, when an oral cancer is suspected, it can be helpful for the primary care dentist to telephone the oral and maxillofacial department for advice. Sometimes an early appointment can be offered. A letter should still be forwarded, for the reasons given above. However, it is not helpful to telephone or send patients with non-urgent conditions to hospital with an expectation of being seen immediately. It is better for all concerned to write a letter and advise the patient of likely waiting times, often obtainable from hospital intranet links. Guidelines for referral have been produced by national and local authorities, such as the National Institute for Clinical Excellence (NICE) and the Royal Colleges. These should be consulted whenever possible, as inappropriate referral should be avoided.

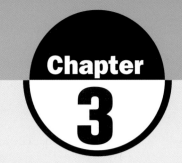
Medical aspects of patient care

Overview

This chapter discusses the assessment of a patient with a pre-existing medical condition that might affect dental treatment. Particular aspects are the effects that anaesthetic drugs might have on these conditions and the potential for drug interactions. Medical emergencies are described in terms of their signs and symptoms. The immediate first-line treatment is listed and subsequent management steps outlined. The technique for resuscitation of a patient is clearly described. Finally the methods of administration of drugs are described and their relative merits in dentistry.

3.1 Medical assessment

Learning objectives

You should:
- know how to obtain information on relevant medical problems
- be able to assess a patient's fitness for treatment
- know when a patient should be referred for treatment in a hospital setting.

Today, many patients with life-threatening disease survive as a result of advances in medical and surgical treatment and may present for dental treatment looking deceptively fit and well. The medical assessment:

- is important to establish the suitability of the patient to undergo dental treatment and may significantly affect the dental management
- may prompt examination for particular oral manifestations
- may be particularly relevant when a sedation technique or general anaesthesia (GA) is being considered
- may give prior warning of a possible medical emergency.

Medical history

As a full medical examination of the patient is generally not feasible or appropriate, the medical history should be comprehensive. This will include questions about previous serious illness and operations, present drug history and known allergies, and the possibility of pregnancy. Information may then be obtained concerning the individual systems by relevant questions depending on the age of the patient, the dental treatment necessary and the anticipated type of anaesthesia.

Questions should refer to known medical problems, past history and present general fitness.

Cardiovascular system

- Is there a history of heart valve surgery, rheumatic fever or murmurs, which might necessitate prophylactic antibiotic cover?
- Is the patient aware of any heart disease or hypertension?
- Does the patient suffer from palpitations, swelling of the ankles and dizziness?
- Can the patient lie flat without breathlessness?
- What is the patient's general fitness? For example, can the patient climb stairs without breathlessness or chest pain?

Respiratory system

- Does the patient have a cough or cold? If there is a cough, is this continuous or intermittent and is it productive?
- Does the patient suffer from bronchitis, emphysema or asthma?
- Is there shortness of breath or symptoms of wheeze or chest pain?
- If the patient is a smoker, how many cigarettes are smoked on average each day?

Gastrointestinal system

Questions concerning the gastrointestinal system may include:

- Does the patient have a good appetite and weight constancy?
- Is there history of jaundice, liver and kidney disease?
- How many units of alcohol does the patient consume on average each week?

The neurological system

- Does the patient suffer from fits or faints?
- Is there any sensory loss or motor weakness at any site?

The examiner should note the patient's balance, gait and the degree of general mobility.

Physical examination

Sufficient information can usually be obtained by obtaining a thorough history such that a physical examination is unnecessary outside the hospital setting. However, if a sedation technique is being considered, then it may be appropriate to undertake a limited examination as follows.

Observe the patient in general. Is the patient clinically well or are there any obvious generalised clinical signs such as cyanosis, pallor or jaundice? Is the patient unusually anxious? Are they talking continuously? Do they appear calm but have sweaty palms? Weigh the patient and also take note of any excessive fat under the chin, particularly in a retrognathic mandible as this may indicate a less than ideal airway.

Check the cardiovascular system. The radial pulse should be checked for rate, rhythm, volume and character. The arterial blood pressure may be measured using a sphygmomanometer on the upper arm of the patient while they are sitting. This limited examination is the minimum that should be carried out for adult patients for whom intravenous sedation is proposed.

Social history. Social factors also affect the patient's ability to cope with treatment. The patient's age, the distance they have to travel for treatment, and the availability of an escort if considering sedation or general anaesthesia should be determined.

Hospital setting

A full physical examination may be required in a hospital setting if patients require GA for surgical or extensive dental treatment. The appropriateness and extent will depend on the history. The aim is to establish the baseline condition of the patient and to identify any problems that may have an effect on the treatment or anaesthesia.

3.2 Dental relevance of the medical condition

. . . .

The cardiovascular system

Congenital and rheumatic heart disease

> **Learning objectives**
>
> You should:
> * know when to use antibiotic cover and suitable regimens
> * know the prerequirements for dental treatment in medical conditions in terms of control and stabilisation of the condition
> * know how to monitor such patients during treatment
> * understand how to deal with medical problems arising during treatment.

Valvular anomalies and damage may predispose to colonisation and subsequent potentially fatal infective endocarditis following a bacteraemia caused by dental treatments such as subgingival periodontal therapies or surgical procedures including dental extraction. This risk has been reduced in the past by providing antibiotic prophylaxis for such dental procedures (Box 3). A cardiologist should have confirmed the presence of valve damage. However, there is lack of consensus on the precise clinical conditions that indicate a need for antibiotic cover. Current guidelines should always be checked and institutional recommendations followed. Indeed, it has been suggested that the risk of endocarditis may actually be very small following dental treatment and therefore it would be sensible to restrict antibiotic prophylaxis for dental treatment to patients in whom the risk of developing endocarditis is the highest. The recommendations of one group (Working Party of the British Society for Antimicrobial Chemotherapy) suggested that high-risk patients were those that had a history of endocarditis, cardiac valve replacement surgery, or a surgically constructed systemic or pulmonary shunt or conduit. Good oral hygiene is the most important factor in reducing the risk of endocarditis in susceptible individuals and antibiotic cover may not be required at all.

Hypertension

The risk of stroke and myocardial infarction associated with GA is known to be increased when the diastolic pressure is persistently above 110 mmHg.

Local anaesthetic (LA) solutions containing adrenaline (epinephrine) may be used safely providing that aspirating syringes are used to reduce the incidence of intravascular injection (which may cause hypertension or arrhythmia, or trigger angina in susceptible patients).

Treatment

Blood pressure should be controlled before sedation/GA for elective treatment and patients should continue to take their antihypertensive drugs up to and on the day of sedation/GA.

Blood pressure should be monitored during treatment involving conscious sedation techniques.

Cardiac failure

Diuretics are the usual treatment. Cardiac failure should be controlled before sedation/GA.

Exercise tolerance gives useful information about the severity of the disease.

Arrhythmias

The patient may give a history of palpitations or have irregular pulse, but arrhythmias are only diagnosed accurately from an electrocardiogram.

Treatment

Arrhythmias should be controlled before sedation/GA, for example atrial fibrillation (Fig. 14) treated with digoxin.

Additional monitoring and supplemental oxygen therapy are required when using conscious sedation techniques.

Angina and myocardial infarction

About 5% of patients have a myocardial infarction during GA if they have already had a myocardial infarction in the past. The death rate of myocardial infarction associated with GA is 50%. GA is particularly dangerous for patients who have had an infarction in the previous 6 months.

Angina should be controlled before sedation/GA.

Box 3 Antibiotic protocol for prevention of endocarditis from dental procedures

Cardiac risk factors for antibiotic prophylaixis	Dental procedures requiring antibiotic prophylaxis	Antibiotic regimens for endocarditis prophylaxis
Previous infective endocarditis Cardiac valve replacement surgery, i.e. mechanical or biological prosthetic valves Surgically constructed systemic or pulmonary shunt or conduit	All dental procedures involving dento-gingival manipulation. Simple and complex dental treatment A simple dental examination with or without radiographs does *not* need antibiotic prophylaxis	Amoxicillin 3 g orally 1 hour before the dental procedure ≥ 5 < 10 years of age 1.5 g < 5 years of age 750 mg *If allergic to penicillin:* clindamycin 600 mg orally 1 hour before the dental procedure ≥ 5 < 10 years of age 300 mg < 5 years of age 150 mg *Patients allergic to penicillin and unable to swallow capsules:* a single dose of azithromycin 500 mg orally 1 hour before the dental procedure < 5 years of age 200 mg ≥ 5 < 10 years of age 300 mg

Intravenous regimens for dental treatment (when considered expedient)
A single IV dose of 1g amoxicillin (< 5 years of age 250 mg, ≥ 5 < 10 years of age 500 mg) given just before the procedure or at induction of anaesthesia.
If allergic to penicillin:
A single IV dose of 300 mg clindamycin (given over at least 10 minutes) is recommended.
(< 5 years of age 75 mg, ≥ 5 < 10 years of age 150 mg)
There is a continuing case for the use of preoperative mouth rinsing with chlorhexidine gluconate (10 ml for 1 minute).
Where a course of treatment involves several visits the antibiotic regimen should alternate between amoxicillin and clindamycin.

LA solutions containing adrenaline (epinephrine) may be used safely. Aspirating syringes are recommended to reduce the incidence of intravascular injection, which may theoretically lead to an increase in hypertension.

Treatment
Preoperative glyceryl trinitrate should be considered for patients with angina receiving treatment under LA.

Patients may be treated using conscious sedation techniques but require additional monitoring and should receive supplemental oxygen therapy.

The respiratory system
The upper airway
Abnormalities between the lips and the trachea such as swelling, trismus or tumours of the mouth or pharynx may compromise the airway and make intubation of GA difficult. Nasal obstruction may contraindicate dental treatment as the patient needs to breathe through their nose for many procedures. Certainly, upper respiratory tract infections would contraindicate dentistry performed under relative analgesia.

Chronic obstructive airways disease
Chronic obstructive airways disease (COAD) is defined as the presence of a productive cough for at least 3 months in 2 successive years. Figure 15 shows a chest radiograph of a patient with COAD. A frequent cause is smoking. The severity may be assessed from the patient's exercise tolerance, together with drug usage and the frequency of related hospital admissions.

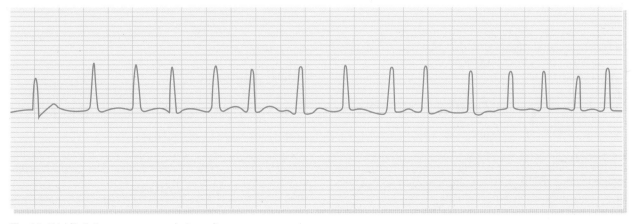

Fig. 14 Atrial fibrillation as seen on an electrocardiogram.

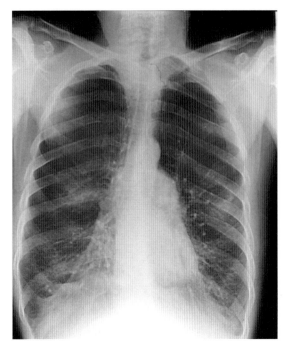

Fig. 15 Chest radiograph of patient with chronic obstructive airways disease.

LA may be used safely. The patient may be more comfortable in a semi-supine or upright position, as they can become increasingly breathless in the supine position.

Intravenous conscious sedation techniques are likely to further compromise respiratory function and should be undertaken in hospital. Similarly, GA involves risk of respiratory impairment.

Asthma

Frequency and severity of attacks gives an indication of the severity of the disease.

Asthma may occasionally be precipitated by anxiety or emotional stress. Patients with asthma are more likely to be allergic to drugs such as penicillin. Non-steroidal anti-inflammatory drugs (NSAIDs) should be prescribed only if the patient has taken the drug before on more than one occasion without a hypersensitivity reaction.

LA may be used safely.

Treatment

Conscious sedation techniques may be indicated in mild asthma to reduce anxiety and avoid an attack.

It is important to avoid GA drugs that release histamine such as atracurium and morphine.

Other respiratory diseases

Upper or lower respiratory tract infections. These do not contraindicate dental treatment under LA or conscious sedation although the nasal obstruction of the common cold may make treatment with an open mouth uncomfortable for the patient. Similarly, patients may find it difficult to inhale nitrous oxide. It is usually preferable to postpone treatment, especially if the patient is pyrexial. Elective GA treatment should be postponed because of the risk of causing much more serious infection as a consequence of a reduced immune response or intubation transferring microorganisms further into the respiratory tract.

Cystic fibrosis. The best time for sedation/GA for patients with cystic fibrosis should be discussed with the patient's physician. Sedation should be undertaken in hospital.

Pulmonary tuberculosis. If active and open, this is highly infective and dental treatment should be postponed.

Haematological disorders

Anaemia

Low haemoglobin levels owing to decreased red-cell mass imply a reduced oxygen-carrying capacity of the blood. There may be associated oral signs and symptoms such as sore mouth or angular stomatitis.

Elective sedation/GA treatment should be postponed until the anaemia has been treated by the patient's GP or specialist. Patients are at risk of hypoxia when respiratory depressant sedatives are administered and during induction and recovery of GA. Such a risk is more significant if the patient's oxygen-carrying capacity is already reduced.

Sickle-cell anaemia. Red cells sickle and cause infarcts or, rarely, haemolysis in sickle-cell anaemia. Sickling tests detect the specific haemoglobin form (HbS). Electrophoresis distinguishes homozygous (SS), heterozygous (AS) states and other haemoglobin variants. Sickle-cell crisis is precipitated by hypoxia, dehydration, pain and infection.

Leukaemia

The acute leukaemias pose problems of oral infections, gingival swelling and ulceration, anaemia, bleeding and immunocompromise. The chronic leukaemias pose similar problems to the acute leukaemias.

Elective dental treatment other than preventive should be postponed until a remission period.

Infections should be treated aggressively with antibiotics and antifungal agents. NSAIDs should be avoided because of the increased risk of gastrointestinal bleeding. Local anaesthetic blocks should be avoided. Patients may be anaemic, may have hepatitis B or C or HIV, or may be receiving corticosteroid treatment.

Lymphoma

Hodgkin's and non-Hodgkin's lymphomas may present as enlargement of the cervical lymph nodes. They pose problems of oral infections, anaemia, bleeding and immunocompromise in similar way to patients with leukaemia. Patients may also suffer cardiac disease and impaired respiratory function following mediastinal irradiation.

Bleeding disorders

Haemostasis consists of vessel constriction, platelet plug formation and the coagulation cascade. Defects of any of the components of haemostasis will be of significance in dentistry.

Patients should be investigated and managed in the hospital setting even for treatment under LA. The haematologist should be involved. Local anaesthetic blocks should be avoided.

Thrombocytopenia. Patients with platelet counts below 50×10^9/L will require platelet transfusion before any invasive dental treatment coagulation. One unit of platelets may raise the count by $10 \times 10^9/L$.

Specific coagulation defects. Coagulation factor replacement is required.

Emergency management of a bleeding patient. This may consist of giving fresh frozen plasma and vitamin K.

Anticoagulant therapy

Anticoagulants are used in the treatment of deep-vein thrombosis, pulmonary embolism, following heart valve replacement and for those with atrial fibrillation who are at risk of embolisation. Treatment for deep-vein thrombosis may last only 3 to 6 months but will continue for life for atrial fibrillation and for those with mechanical prosthetic heart valves. The anticoagulant of choice is warfarin which antagonises vitamin K. Warfarin takes 36 hours or longer to peak anticoagulant effect which is measured by prolonged prothrombin time (PT) and activated partial thromboplastin time (APTT). The international normalised ratio (INR) comparing the patients' PT with that of a control is increased with warfarinisation. An INR near 1 is normal and patients taking anticoagulants are usually in the range 2–4.

In the past, patients have had their warfarin dose adjusted to reduce the risk of bleeding during and after oral surgery but more recently the research evidence has indicated that this might not be necessary. The risk of thromboembolic event after withdrawal of warfarin outweighs the risk of bleeding after oral surgery. Patients within the normal range may not require any change to their warfarin dose at all for minor surgery but should be warned that there is an increased risk of bleeding after surgery. If possible a single extraction should be undertaken in the first instance with further extractions at subsequent visits to limit the extent of surgery. An international normalisation ratio (INR) measurement should be carried out within 24 hours of surgery and preferably on the day of surgery. Patients should receive appropriate verbal and written information about postoperative care and how to access assistance should there be any postoperative bleeding, as should any other patient. Local measures for haemostasis are likely to be adequate. Patients who do bleed should be transferred to hospital for haematological management including the administration of vitamin K by slow intravenous injection or fresh frozen plasma.

Patients undergoing more major surgery are likely to require reduction in their anticoagulation and this should be done in discussion with a haematologist who will advise. Similarly haematological collaboration is required even for minor surgery for patients whose anticoagulation is not stable.

Intramuscular injections should be avoided in all patients with a haemostasis disorder or on anticoagulants, and local anaesthetic regional nerve blocks should be avoided if possible and infiltration or intraligamentary injection techniques used instead. Metronidazole interacts with warfarin and should be avoided, as should erythromycin which has unpredictable effect. Amoxycillin interferes less with warfarin but patients should be warned to look out for bleeding. Apirin and to a lesser extent other NSAIDS should be avoided. The anticoagulant effect of warfarin is not usually affected by paracetamol.

Endocrine disease

Diabetes mellitus

Patients with diabetes mellitus are immunocompromised and require early vigorous treatment of infections. Where surgery is being performed patients may need antibiotic prophylaxis. It should be established whether the patient is controlled with diet alone, tablets or insulin injections. If the patient is not to be starved (LA or sedation), then treatment is arranged so as to interfere least with mealtimes, such as within 2 hours of breakfast, and the patient is instructed to take medications and food as normal.

Treatment

- The patient should be reasonably well controlled before sedation/GA. When the patient is starved prior to a GA they must have their oral hypoglycaemic drug or insulin adjusted. Non-insulin-dependent diabetes mellitus patients can usually withstand a short period of starvation but may need insulin if undergoing prolonged surgery. Their oral hypoglycaemic should be stopped the day before surgery.
- Patients with insulin-dependent diabetes mellitus should have their long-acting insulin omitted the night before surgery and blood glucose monitored 4 hourly and then 2 hourly. Insulin and glucose therapy is started using a variable-rate insulin infusion (soluble insulin 50 i.u. in 50 ml normal saline by syringe driver) and adjusted as required. The patient also receives carbohydrate. Alternatively the Alberti regime may be used if the patient is usually well controlled. This consists of an infusion of glucose 10% 500 ml; human-soluble insulin 10 i.u.; KCl 10 ml, over 5 hours via a dedicated cannula. The insulin and KCl concentrations are adjusted according to the results, aiming for a blood glucose of 6–10 mmol/L.
- Hypoglycaemia must be avoided as it may cause brain damage. Blood glucose should be measured regularly with BM-Stix or blood glucose tests because control is upset by surgery and anaesthesia.

Hypothyroidism and hyperthyroidism

Patients with hypothyroidism should avoid opioids, sedatives and GA. They are, therefore, best treated using LA unless well managed with thyroxine.

There is a serious risk of arrhythmias if an untreated hyperthyroid patient receives a GA.

Hypoparathyroidism and hyperparathyroidism

Hypoparathyroidism. This should be considered in patients presenting with facial paraesthesia or twitching. Other signs include delayed tooth eruption and enamel hypoplasia.

Hyperparathyroidism. This may cause oral signs, as described in Chapter 7. GA may be complicated by the risk of arrhythmias and sensitivity to muscle relaxants.

Hepatic disease

Hepatic disease can cause problems with production of fibrinogen and clotting factors (II, V, VII, VIII, IX, X, XI, XII, XIII) and drug metabolism. There is a cross-infection risk if viral hepatitis is present.

Clotting dysfunction. The diagnosis should be confirmed and the severity of problem (by arranging for a coagulation screen) prior to treatment and especially before surgery. Patients may need vitamin K or fresh frozen plasma to correct coagulation and, therefore, should be managed in hospital.

Drugs. Prescribing is a problem and many drugs should be used with caution or avoided completely in severe hepatic disease. Paracetamol, NSAIDs and sedatives are among these. Any drug prescribing should include reference to a drug formulary. It is difficult to predict the impairment of drug metabolism even when using liver function tests.

Cross-infection. Universal precautions for cross-infection control means that all patients, whether known high risk or not, should be managed in the same way to minimise the risk of transmission of infectious agents.

Renal disease

If there is renal disease, then drug doses should be reduced as drug excretion may be reduced and NSAIDs should be avoided. The severity of renal impairment is expressed as the glomerular filtration rate (GFR), which is usually measured by the creatinine clearance.

Fluid balance and sodium and potassium levels may be upset and platelet dysfunction (impaired production, impaired conversion of prothrombin to thrombin, and vasodilatation and poor platelet aggregation) may lead to a bleeding tendency.

Treatment

- Patients should receive dental treatment the day following dialysis when any heparin is no longer active but they are still at maximum benefit from the dialysis.
- Patients who have undergone renal transplantation will be receiving immunosuppressive drugs and will require an increase to their steroid dose prior to extensive treatment or GA. They may also require antibiotic prophylaxis.

Gastrointestinal disease

Peptic ulceration is a relatively common disease that can be exacerbated by NSAIDs. These drugs should not be prescribed for patients with such a history.

Bone disease

Bone diseases are discussed in Chapter 7.

Neurological disorders
Epilepsy
Treatment

- Patients should be maintained on anticonvulsant therapy.
- It may be advisable to undertake dental treatment using a mouth prop in patients with poorly controlled epilepsy.

Psychiatric disorders

Whenever a person's abnormal thoughts, feelings or sensory impressions cause objective or subjective harm that is more than transitory, a mental illness may be said to be present.

There are many classification systems, some more helpful than others, but the distinction between the brain and the mind often provides a philosophical difficulty for patients and maybe also for some dentists. Patients may accept a psychiatric diagnosis that is recognised to be the result of organic brain disease but less readily accept one of non-organic cause. There remains prejudice about conditions that relate to the mind.

Acute psychiatric illness is treated in general hospital units and the community and these patients may attend for dental care to the general dental practitioner or community or hospital dentist.

Organic pathology. Psychiatric disorders may lead to neglect of oral health. There may be potential for drug interaction between medications for illness and those used in dentistry, including conscious sedation and anaesthesia.

Psychological origin. Patients may present with dental, oral or facial physical symptoms that are of psychological cause. The dentist should exclude organic pathology, which may be responsible for the symptoms, by means of a careful history, thorough examination and appropriate special tests. The general dental practitioner may need to refer to a dental specialist to confirm the exclusion of organic pathology. The dentist or specialist who considers that the patient's symptoms may be of psychological origin should communicate with the patient's general medical practitioner, who may be aware of multiple and variable symptoms and should arrange for psychiatric assessment.

The psychoses

The psychoses may be organic where there is established biochemical, infective or structural brain disease, or functional where no such disease process can be demonstrated.

Organic psychoses may be described as acute (delirium) or chronic (dementia).

Functional psychoses may be divided into disorders of mood, manic depressive psychosis and disorders of thinking, and schizophrenia.

The neuroses

In the neuroses, there is no alteration of external reality but rather patients try to avoid some unacceptable aspect of themselves or of their internal reality.

Four main patterns are: anxiety neurosis and phobia, depressive neurosis, hysteria and obsessive compulsive neurosis.

Personality disorders

Unlike psychosis and neurosis, personality disorders are not an illness. They may be described as extreme personality types that handicap the individual and include the paranoid, schizoid, antisocial and obsessive–compulsive disorders. They often coexist or may predispose to psychiatric illness.

Other psychiatric disorders

These include addictions to alcohol or drugs, eating disorders and sexual dysfunction and deviation.

Medications

Most drugs have some side effects. Check for any drug interactions with drugs being used for dental treatment.

Routine medication. It is important that patients take their normal medication before dental treatment, including on the morning of a GA when these may be taken with a sip of water. Exceptions to this are:

- anticoagulants – discuss with haematology (warfarin needs 3 days to wear off)
- monoamine oxidase inhibitors (MAOIs) should be stopped 3 weeks before GA because of a risk of interaction with opioids which have sometimes been fatal.

Steroid drugs. Steroids reduce the ability of the adrenal cortex to respond to physical stress and additional steroids are required prior to extensive treatment or GA. This may be given as 100 mg intravenous (i.v.) hydrocortisone and hydrocortisone may need to be continued postoperatively after major surgery. There is some doubt as to whether such steroid cover is necessary for straightforward dental treatment and tooth extraction under local anaesthesia.

Contraceptive pill. Patients taking any oestrogen-containing oral contraceptive pill are known to be at increased risk of developing a deep-vein thrombosis and pulmonary embolism following GA, which is associated with reduced mobility in the postoperative period. To eliminate this risk, the pill should be stopped 1 month before the anaesthetic or, if emergency surgery is required, heparin should be given. These precautions are unnecessary when minor or intermediate surgery is undertaken. The progesterone-only oral contraceptive pill is associated with no increased risk and no precautions are necessary.

Allergies

The patient may be aware of existing reaction to a drug, which should then be avoided. Note that a true allergy is an immune-mediated response comprising one or all of skin rash, bronchospasm, flushing, hypotension, oedema and collapse; it is not fainting after local anaesthetic injection or gastrointestinal effects of NSAIDs. Patients may need to have the difference explained so that they are not denied the benefit of drugs to which they are not actually allergic.

Allergy to latex is now more common. It is important to avoid local anaesthetic cartridges that have a latex bung or stopper.

Pregnancy

It is preferable to avoid drug treatments during pregnancy, especially during the first trimester. Some dental treatments and especially surgical procedures may be better postponed until after the birth of the baby, otherwise the second trimester is best. If it is necessary to prescribe analgesia or antimicrobial drugs, paracetamol and codeine and penicillin, cephalosporins and erythromycin are probably the safest.

Treatment

- Elective treatment under sedation/GA is contraindicated because midazolam and anaesthetics may increase the risk of spontaneous abortion. In late pregnancy there is a risk of regurgitation with GA.
- Patients are likely to lose consciousness if placed in the supine position during the third trimester because venous return to the heart is compromised by the fetus. Position the patient on her left side to permit recovery.

3.3 Medical emergencies

Learning objectives

You should:
- have a logical approach to emergency management
- know the first-line treatment protocols
- understand the more comprehensive management undertaken by dentists with special training, paramedics or hospital staff
- understand when to transfer a patient to an accident and emergency department.

Medical emergencies require prompt assessment and action. There may not be time for a detailed assessment, but it is possible to buy time by using a basic protocol that simultaneously assesses and supports vital functions. Fortunately, serious medical emergencies in dental practice are not common, but that means that they are all the more likely to be alarming when they do occur. The ability to stay calm and manage the situation successfully depends on prior planning and rehearsal for such an event.

Emergency drugs and equipment

There are essential drugs and items of equipment that every dental practitioner should have available for use in an emergency. Some of these are based on providing simple and uncomplicated treatments while others necessitate providing early definitive treatment. Acute asthma and anaphylaxis are two examples of emergencies where simple first-aid measures are inadequate and definitive treatment should be started by the dentist while waiting for the ambulance service to transfer the patient to an accident and emergency (A&E) department. This essential treatment is described as *first-line treatment* in the following protocols. Some drugs are available in preloaded syringes for fast preparation (Fig. 16).

Some dentists by way of special interest and training may have the skills to provide more comprehensive definitive management and may wish to instigate this while waiting for the emergency services to transfer the patient. These dentists would wish to hold a larger range of drugs and equipment depending on their individual experience. Such treatment is described by the *Further management* sections in the following protocols.

Emergency conditions

Faint

Signs and symptoms

- May be preceded by nausea and closing in of visual fields

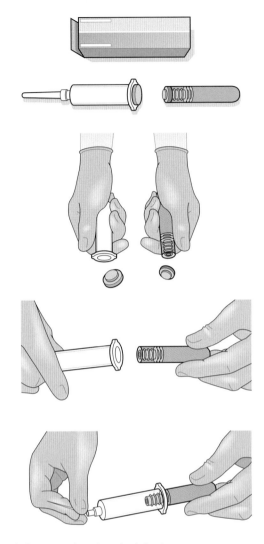

Fig. 16 Emergency drugs in preloaded syringes.

- Pallor and sweating
- Heart rate below 60 beats/min (bradycardia) during attack.

Clinical box   First-line treatment of faint

- Lay flat
- Give oxygen
- Check pulse at carotid
- Expect prompt recovery.

Cause

Pain or anxiety.

Principles of treatment

- Need to encourage oxygenated blood flow to brain as rapidly as possible
- May need to block vagal activity with atropine and allow heart rate to increase.

Further management

If the patient is slow to recover, consider other diagnosis or give 0.3–1 mg atropine i.v.

Hyperventilation
Signs and symptoms

- Light-headed
- Tingling in the extremities
- Muscle spasm may lead to characteristic finger position (carpo-pedal spasm).

Clinical box   First-line treatment of hyperventilation

- Reassure
- Ask patient to rebreathe from cupped hands or reservoir bag of inhalational sedation or general anaesthetic apparatus.

Causes

Anxiety.

Principles of treatment

- Reduce anxiety
- Over-breathing has blown off carbon dioxide, resulting in brain blood vessel vasoconstriction. Return carbon dioxide levels in blood to normal.

Postural hypotension
Signs and symptoms

- Light-headed
- Dizzy
- Loss of consciousness on returning to upright or standing position from supine position.

Clinical box   First-line treatment of postural hypotension

- Lay the patient flat and give oxygen
- Sit the patient up very slowly.

Causes

More likely to occur if the patient is taking beta-blockers, which reduce the capacity to compensate for normal cardiovascular postural changes.

Principles of treatment

Encourage oxygenated blood flow to brain.

Diabetic emergencies: hypoglycaemia
Signs and symptoms

- Shaking and trembling
- Sweating
- Hunger
- Headache and confusion.

> **Clinical box** First-line treatment of hypoglycaemia
>
> - If the patient is conscious, give sugar or glucose and a little water or glucose oral gel; repeated if necessary in 10 minutes
> - If the patient is unconscious, inject 1 mg (1 unit) glucagon by any route (subcutaneous, intramuscular or i.v.).

Cause

- Usually known diabetic
- Patient may have taken medication as normal but not eaten before dental visit.

Principles of treatment

Return blood glucose level to normal by giving glucose or by converting the patient's own glycogen to glucose by giving glucagon.

Further management

- Transfer the patient to A&E
- Give up to 50 ml 20% glucose i.v. infusion followed by 0.9% saline flush as the glucose damages the vein
- Expect prompt recovery and give sugary drinks once conscious.

Grand mal epileptic seizure

Signs and symptoms

- Sudden loss of consciousness associated with *tonic phase* in which there is sustained muscular contraction affecting all muscles, including respiratory and mastication
- Breathing may cease and the patient becomes cyanosed
- The tongue may be bitten and incontinence occur
- After about 30 seconds, a *clonic phase* supervenes, with violent jerking movements of limbs and trunk.

> **Clinical box** First-line treatment of epileptic seizure
>
> - Ensure patient is not at risk of injury during the convulsions but do not attempt to restrain convulsive movements
> - Make no attempt to put anything in mouth or between the teeth
> - After movements have subsided, place the patient in the recovery position and check airway
> - The patient may be confused after the fit: reassure and offer sympathy
> - After full recovery, send the patient home unless the seizure was atypical or prolonged or injury occurred.

Cause

- Usually the patient is a known epileptic
- Epilepsy may not be well controlled
- Seizure may be initiated by anxiety or by flickering light tube.

Principles of treatment

- Maintain oxygenated blood to brain
- Protect from physical harm
- Administer anticonvulsant.

Further management

Risk of brain damage is increased with length of attack; therefore, treatment should aim to terminate seizure as soon as possible.

If convulsive seizures continue for 15 minutes or longer or are repeated rapidly (status epilepticus):

- Transfer to A&E
- Remove dentures, insert Guedel or nasopharyngeal airway
- Give oxygen
- Give 10–20 mg i.v. diazepam (2.5 mg/30 s) as Diazemuls but beware of respiratory depression, or diazepam solution for rectal administration in hospital
- Check blood sugar to exclude hypoglycaemia as precipitant.

Hypoadrenalism

Signs and symptoms

- Pallor
- Confusion
- Rapid weak pulse.

> **Clinical box** First-line treatment for hypoadrenalism
>
> - Lay flat
> - Give oxygen
> - Give 200 mg hydrocortisone sodium succinate by slow i.v. injection.

Cause

Usually the patient is known to have Addison's disease or to be taking steroids long term and has forgotten to take the tablets.

Principles of management

- Give steroid replacement
- Determining and managing underlying cause once the crisis over.

Further management

- Transfer to A&E
- Fluids and further hydrocortisone, both i.v.
- Glucose may be needed if hypoglycaemic.

Acute asthma

Signs and symptoms

- Persistent shortness of breath poorly relieved by bronchodilators
- Restlessness and exhaustion

- Tachycardia greater than 110 beats/min and low peak expiratory flow
- Respirations may be so shallow in severe cases that wheezing is absent.

Clinical box   First-line treatment of acute asthmatic attack

- Excluded respiratory obstruction
- Sit the patient up
- Give oxygen
- Salbutamol (Ventolin) via a nebuliser (2.5–5 mg of 1 mg/ml nebuliser solution) or via a large-volume spacer (two puffs of a metered dose inhaler 10–20 times: one puff every 30 seconds up to 10 puffs for a child)
- Reassure and allow home if recovered.

Cause

Exposure to antigen but precipitated by many factors including anxiety.

Principles of treatment

- Oxygenation
- Bronchodilatation.

Further management

- If little response, transfer to A&E
- Hydrocortisone sodium succinate i.v.: adults 200 mg; child 100 mg
- Add ipratropium 0.5 mg to nebulised salbutamol
- Aminophylline slow i.v. injection of 250 mg in 10 ml over at least 20 minutes: monitor or keep finger on pulse during injection.

Caution in epilepsy: rapid injection of aminophylline may cause arrhythmias and convulsions.

Caution in patients already receiving theophylline: arrhythmias or convulsions may occur.

Anaphylactic shock

Signs and symptoms

- Paraesthesia, flushing and swelling of face, especially eyelids and lips (Fig. 17)
- Generalised urticaria, especially hands and feet
- Wheezing and difficulty in breathing
- Rapid weak pulse.

These may develop over 15 to 30 minutes following the oral administration of a drug or rapidly over a few minutes following i.v. drug administration.

Clinical box   First-line treatment of anaphylactic shock

- Lay patient flat and raise feet
- Give oxygen
- Give 0.5 ml epinephrine (adrenaline) 1 mg/ml (1 in 1000) intramuscular
- 0.25 ml for 6–12 years of age
- 0.12 ml for 6 months to 6 years of age
- Repeated every 10 min until improvement.

Principles of treatment

Requires prompt energetic treatment of

- Laryngeal oedema
- Bronchospasm
- Hypotension.

Further management

- Transfer to A&E
- Chlorphenamine (chlorpheniramine) 10 mg in 1 ml intramuscular or slow i.v. injection
- Hydrocortisone sodium succinate 200 mg by slow i.v. injection; valuable as action persists after that of epinephrine has worn off

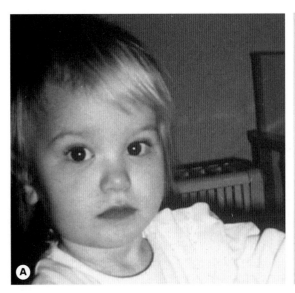 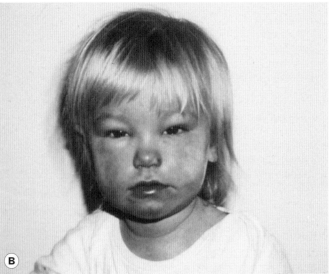

Fig. 17 Facial flushing and swelling, especially of eyelids and lips, in anaphylactic shock. **A,** child normally; **B,** after anaphylactic shock.

- Fluids i.v. (colloids) infused rapidly if shock not responding quickly to adrenaline
- Basic and advanced life support if cardiorespiratory arrest
- Endotracheal intubation or tracheostomy if required.

Stroke
Signs and symptoms

- Confusion followed by signs and symptoms of focal brain damage
- Hemiplegia or quadriplegia
- Sensory loss
- Dysphasia
- Locked-in syndrome (aware, but unable to respond).

Cause

Stroke results from either cerebral haemorrhage or cerebral ischaemia unrelated to dental treatment.

Principles of treatment

Maintain and transfer for further investigation.

Benzodiazepine overdose
Signs and symptoms

- Deeply sedated
- Severe respiratory depression.

Clinical box   First-line treatment

- Flumazenil (Annexate) 200 mg over 15 seconds as 100 mg/ml i.v. followed by 100 mg every 1 minute up to maximum of 1 mg
- Maintain airway with head tilt/chin lift
- Give oxygen.

Cause

Overdose can result from a large or a fast dose of benzodiazepine or can occur in a sensitive patient.

Principles of treatment

The action of the benzodiazepine is reversed with the specific antagonist.

Psychiatric emergencies
Signs and symptoms

Unusual/bizarre/agitated/violent behaviour.

Cause

Usually there is a known psychiatric illness.

Principles of treatment

Transfer to A&E.

Angina and myocardial infarction
Signs and symptoms

- Sudden onset of severe crushing pain across front of chest, which may radiate towards the shoulder and down the left arm or into the neck and jaw; pain from angina usually radiates down left arm
- Skin pale and clammy
- Shallow respirations
- Nausea
- Weak pulse and hypotension
- If the pain not relieved by glyceryl trinitrate (GTN) then cause is myocardial infarction rather than angina.

Clinical box   First-line treatment of angina and myocardial infarction

Allow patient to rest in position that feels most comfortable:
- In presence of breathlessness this is likely to be the sitting position, whereas syncopal patients will want to lie flat
- Often an intermediate position will be most appropriate.

Angina

Angina is relieved by rest and nitrates:
- Glyceryl trinitrate spray 400 mg metered dose (sprayed on oral mucosa or under tongue and mouth then closed)
- Give oxygen
- Allow home if attack is mild and the patient recovers rapidly.

Myocardial infarction

If a myocardial infarction is suspected:
- Give oxygen
- Aspirin tablet 300 mg chewed.

Cause

- Angina results from reduced coronary artery lumen diameter because of atheromatous plaques
- Myocardial infarction is usually the result of thrombosis in a coronary artery.

Principles of treatment

- Pain control
- Vasodilatation of blood vessels to reduce load on heart.

Further management for severe angina or myocardial infarction

- Transfer to A&E
- Diagnosis of myocardial infarction made on basis of two or three out of the history, ECG changes, and enzyme changes suggestive of myocardial infarction
- Diamorphine 5 mg (2.5 mg in older people) by slow i.v. injection (1 mg/min)
- Early thrombolytic therapy reduces mortality.

Cardiorespiratory arrest
Signs and symptoms

- Unconscious
- No breathing.

Cause

- Most cardiorespiratory arrests result from arrhythmias associated with acute myocardial infarction or chronic ischaemic heart disease
- The heart arrests in one of three rhythms (Fig. 18):
  - VF (ventricular fibrillation) or pulseless VT (ventricular tachycardia)
  - asystole
  - PEA (pulseless electrical activity) or EMD (electromechanical dissociation)
- VF is the most common cause.

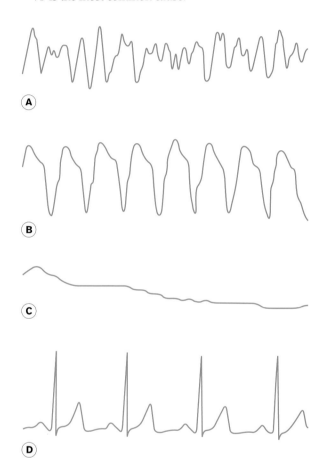

Fig. 18 Rhythms seen in cardiac arrest. **A,** ventricular fibrillation (VF); **B,** ventricular tachycardia (VT) and absent pulse; **C,** asystole; **D,** pulseless electrical activity (PEA). Initially there is normal QRS complex but this soon becomes more bizarre in appearance.

Principles of treatment

- Circulation failure for 4 minutes, or less if the patient is already hypoxaemic, will lead to irreversible brain damage
- Institute early basic life support (see clinical box below) as holding procedure until early advanced life support is available.

Further management

- Transfer to A&E
- Advanced life support.

Advanced life support for cardiac arrest

Advanced airway management techniques and specific treatment of the underlying cause of cardiac arrest constitute advanced life support (ALS).

Advanced airway management

- A self-inflating bag and mask with attached oxygen at 5–6 Lmin^{-1} permits ventilation with around 45% oxygen. However, it is preferable also to use a reservoir as oxygen can then be provided at around 90% with a flow rate turned up to 10 Lmin^{-1} (Fig. 24).
- The laryngeal mask airway (LMA), which seals around the larynx, is becoming popular as it provides more effective ventilation with a bag-valve system than with a face mask.
- The 'gold standard' of airway management is endotracheal intubation as it protects against contamination by regurgitated gastric contents and blood, allows suctioning of the respiratory tract, and drugs can be administered by this route. However, its use requires considerable training.
- A surgical airway intervention such as a needle cricothyroidotomy may be necessary if it is not possible to ventilate with bag-valve-mask or to intubate. This may be because of maxillofacial trauma or laryngeal obstruction. High-pressure oxygen is given via a cannula inserted into the trachea, although this is only a temporary measure lasting about 40 minutes until a theatre is prepared for formal tracheostomy.

Defibrillation

- Defibrillation is indicated in ventricular fibrillation and pulseless ventricular tachycardia, which are the commonest arrhythmias causing cardiac arrest and

---

Clinical box Adult basic life support for cardiorespiratory arrest

The following instructions are based on the UK Resuscitation Council guidelines for basic life support. The essential features are remembered by ABC: *a*irway, *b*reathing and *c*irculation.

Risks to the rescuer

- Before starting a resuscitation attempt, the rescuer must rapidly assess the risks: traffic, falling masonry, toxic fumes and other potential hazards relevant to the environment.
- Mucous membrane exposure to hepatitis B virus (HBV) and human immunodeficiency virus (HIV) is less of a risk than needlestick exposure, strongly suggesting that the chance of infection from mouth-to-mouth ventilation is negligible. Transmission of HIV during cardiopulmonary resuscitation (CPR) has never been reported. There are no human studies to address effectiveness of barrier devices during CPR but rescuers should take appropriate safety precautions where feasible, especially if the victim is known to have a serious infection such as tuberculosis.

Clinical box   Adult basic life support for cardiorespiratory arrest   Cont'd

Basic life support
- Initial patient assessment, airway maintenance, expired air ventilation and chest compression constitute basic life support (BLS) or CPR.
- BLS is a 'holding operation' maintaining ventilation and circulation until treatment of the underlying cause can be instigated.
- BLS implies that no equipment is used. Where a simple airway or face mask is used, this is described as 'basic life support with airway adjunct'.

Theory of chest compression
- The 'thoracic pump' theory proposes that chest compression, by increasing intrathoracic pressure, propels blood out of the thorax, forward flow occurring because veins at the thoracic inlet collapse while the arteries remain patent.
- Even when performed optimally, chest compressions do not achieve more than 30% of the normal cerebral perfusion.

Basic airway management
- Jaw thrust rather than chin lift is the method of choice for trauma victims (Fig. 19).
- An oropharyngeal airway such as a Guedel or nasopharyngeal airway may be used (Fig. 20).
- A face mask used for ventilation allows oxygen enrichment (Fig. 21).

Sequence of actions
1. Ensure safety of rescuer and victim (referred to below as 'he', for simplicity).
2. Check whether casualty is responsive by shaking by the shoulders and shouting, 'Are you alright?'
3A. If he responds by answering or moving:
    - Leave him in the position in which you find him (providing he is not in further danger), check his condition and get help if needed
    - Reassess him regularly.
3B. If he does *not* respond:
    - Shout for help
    - Open the airway by tilting the head and lifting the chin (Fig. 22).
4. Keeping the airway open; look, listen and feel for breathing for no more than 10 seconds.
5A. If he *is* breathing:
    - Turn him into the recovery position
    - Check for continued breathing
    - Send someone for help or call an ambulance.
5B. If he is *not* breathing normally:
    - Send someone to call an ambulance or if alone, leave the victim if necessary to call it yourself
    - Start chest compression (Fig. 23)
6A. Combine chest compression with rescue breaths:
    - After 30 compressions open the airway again
    - Pinch the soft part of the victim's nose
    - Give two breaths
    - Provide further 30 chest compressions
    - Continue with chest compressions and rescue breaths in a ratio of 30:2
6B. Chest-compressions-only CPR:
    - If not able to give rescue breaths
    - Chest compressions continuously at rate of 100/minute
7. Continue until successful, help arrives, or you become exhausted.

Going for assistance
- A lone rescuer will have to decide whether to start resuscitation or go for help first. If the cause of unconsciousness is likely to be trauma, drowning, or if the victim is an infant or a child, the rescuer should perform resuscitation for about 1 minute before going for help.
- If the victim is an adult and the cause of unconsciousness is not trauma or drowning, the rescuer should assume that the victim has a heart problem and go for help immediately it has been established that the victim is not breathing.

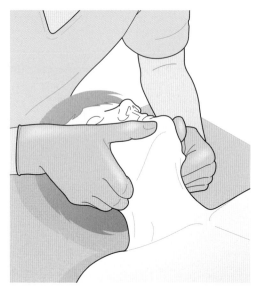

Fig. 19 The jaw thrust airway manoeuvre.

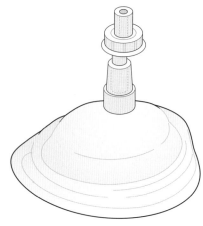

Fig. 21 Pocket face mask.

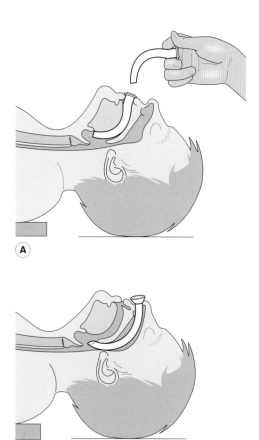

Fig. 20 The oropharyngeal (Guedal) and nasopharyngeal airway. Insertion via the mouth **(A)** and nose **(B)**.

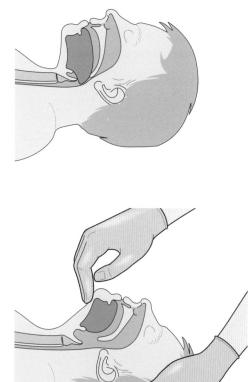

Fig. 22 Head tilt and chin lift airway manoeuvre.

the most treatable. There is overwhelming scientific evidence to support early defibrillation. The chances of successful defibrillation decline by about 7–10% with each minute of delay; therefore early management is vital (Fig. 25).

- Sudden cardiac arrest is a leading cause of death in Europe affecting 700 000 individuals a year. Many victims of arrest could survive if managed while in VF before deteriorating to asystole.
- Defibrillation depolarises most or all of the cardiac muscle simultaneously, allowing the natural pacemaking tissues to resume control of the heart.

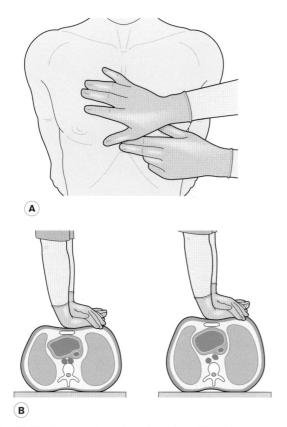

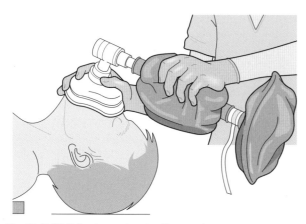

Fig. 23 Chest compressions: shown from above **(A)** and in cross-section **(B)**.

Fig. 24 Self-inflating bag and mask with reservoir.

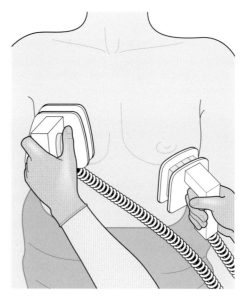

Fig. 25 Placement of defibrillator pads. One to the right of the sternum below the clavicle. The other in the mid-axillary line, level with the female breast but clear of breast tissue by placing sufficiently lateral. The mid-axillary pad should be placed with its long axis vertical to improve efficiency.

Three

- All defibrillators have two features in common: a power source capable of providing direct current, and a capacitor, which can be charged to a predetermined level and subsequently discharged through two electrodes placed on the casualty's chest.
- Defibrillators may be manual (the operator interprets the rhythm and decides if a shock is necessary), or automated (when the tasks of recognising the arrhythmia and preparing for defibrillation are automated). Automated external defibrillators (AEDs) are sophisticated, reliable computerised devices that use voice and visual prompts to guide lay rescuers and health-care professionals through safe defibrillation. All health-care professionals should consider the use of an AED to be an integral component of basic life support. A semi-automatic AED advises the need for a shock but this has to be delivered by the operator when prompted.

Defibrillation strategy
- VF and pulseless VT are treated with a single shock followed by immediate resumption of CPR. After two minutes of CPR, the rhythm is checked and a further shock is given if indicated.
- For biphasic defibrillators the recommended initial energy is 150–200 J. Second and subsequent shocks are given at 150–360 J.
- For monophasic defibrillators the recommended energy is 360 J for both initial and subsequent shocks.

Epinephrine (adrenaline)
- Epinephrine 1 mg i.v. is given if VF/VT persists after a second shock and is repeated every 3–5 minutes if persists.
- Epinephrine 1 mg i.v. is given as soon as intravenous access is achieved and repeated every 3–5 minutes in pulseless electrical activity or asystole.

There is no placebo-controlled trial to demonstrate that the routine use of any vasopressor at any stage during human cardiac arrest increases survival. There is insufficient current evidence to support or refute the routine use of any particular drug or sequence of drugs. Despite this, epinephrine is still recommended based on experimental data showing an increased myocardial and cerebral perfusion pressure during cardiac arrest.

3.4 Drug delivery

The administration of drugs may be required in dentistry to provide analgesia, antibiotic or steroid cover, a conscious sedation technique or to manage a medical collapse. The usual routes are oral (p.o.), intravenous (i.v.), intramuscular (i.m.) and subcutaneous (s.c.).

Learning objectives

You should:
- understand how to administer drugs by the various routes
- know the complications that can be associated with a particular method of administration.

Oral administration

Drugs taken by mouth are generally not absorbed until they reach the small intestine and this progress may be delayed if the drugs are taken after a meal. Usually about 75% of the drug is absorbed in 1–3 hours. Absorption is also affected by gastrointestinal motility, splanchnic blood flow, particle size of drug preparation and physiochemical factors. It may be important to observe a patient while they are taking a particular medication to ensure that it has been taken. Drugs may be taken with a limited volume of water prior to general anaesthesia but this should always be discussed with the anaesthetist.

Intravenous access

A variety of devices can be used to secure venous access. Hollow metal needles of the 'butterfly' variety easily become displaced, leading to extravasation of drugs and fluids administered through them. The cannula-over-needle device is more popular.

The veins most commonly used are the superficial peripheral veins in the upper limbs, which may appear very variable in their layout but certain common arrangements are found. The veins draining the fingers unite on the back of the hand to form three dorsum metacarpal veins. The cephalic vein is found along the radial border of the forearm, with the basilic vein passing up the ulnar border of the forearm. There is often a large vein in the middle of the ventral (anterior) aspect of the forearm, the median vein of the forearm. In the antecubital fossa, the cephalic vein on the lateral side and the basilic vein medially are joined by the median cubital or antecubital vein. Although the veins in this area are prominent and easily cannulated, there are many other adjacent vital structures that can be damaged (Fig. 26). These include the brachial artery, median nerve and the medial and lateral cutaneous nerves of the forearm.

Complications

There are a large number of early and late complications associated with venous cannulation. Fortunately, most of them are relatively minor.

Early complications
- Failed cannulation: usually as a result of pushing the needle completely through the vein; it is experience related

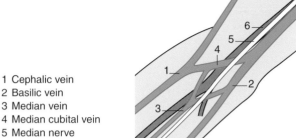

1 Cephalic vein
2 Basilic vein
3 Median vein
4 Median cubital vein
5 Median nerve
6 Brachial artery

Fig. 26 Cubital fossa and forearm anatomy.

- Haematomas
- Extravasation of fluid or drugs
- Damage to other local structures
- Shearing of the cannula
- Fracture of the needle.

Late complications
- Inflammation of the vein (thrombophlebitis)
- Inflammation of the surrounding skin (cellulitis).

Intramuscular route

The intramuscular route is used to deposit a drug into muscle. Absorption is faster than with the subcutaneous route because muscle is very vascular. However, systemic effect may take 15 to 30 minutes after injection to occur. This site is, therefore, not appropriate for drug delivery in cardiac arrest, although it is useful for other medical emergencies.

Intramuscular injections are generally given at one of five sites: mid-deltoid, gluteus medius, gluteus minimus, rectus femoris and vastus lateralis (Fig. 27). The muscles of the buttock offer a large injection site and are, therefore, frequently used for elective drug administration such as antibiotics and analgesics in the hospital situation. However, they have the lowest drug absorption rate. One of the main considerations in a medical emergency in dentistry is ease of access in a clothed patient and therefore the mid-deltoid site is preferable.

Complications

Sciatic nerve damage. This nerve arises from spinal nerves and is the largest nerve in the lower limb, supplying the entire limb except for the gluteal structures and the medial and anterior compartments of the thigh. Damage to this nerve is avoided by injecting into the upper and outer quadrant of the buttock (Fig. 28).

Intravascular injection. The superior gluteal artery enters the buttock and divides into a superficial branch, supplying the overlying gluteus maximus, and two deep branches, an upper and lower, which supply gluteus medius and minimus. The accompanying veins form an extensive plexus between the muscles. Failure to aspirate prior to injection could result in i.v. injection.

Leakage of drug into subcutaneous tissues.

Fracture of needle. This is unlikely to occur if one-third of the needle shaft is left exposed; it therefore depends on the correct assessment of muscle bulk and needle length.

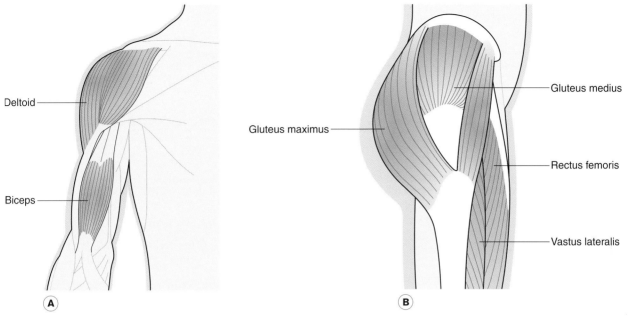

Fig. 27 Intramuscular injection sites in the arm (A) and buttocks (B).

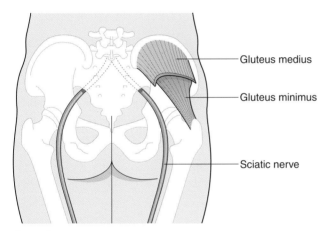

Fig. 28 Sciatic nerve anatomy.

Subcutaneous route

In subcutaneous injection, the drug is placed into the fat and connective tissues below the dermis but above the muscle layer. Absorption is more rapid from this layer than from the intradermal layer because of the increased capillary supply, though it is slower than absorption by the intramuscular route. This characteristic is desirable when a sustained drug effect is needed. Such factors as peripheral oedema, vasoconstriction and the presence of burns can slow absorption; therefore, subcutaneous injections should not be administered to patients with hypotension, oedema in the injection areas, severe skin lesions such as burns and psoriasis, or severe arterial occlusive disease in the affected extremity.

The lateral aspect of the upper arms and thighs, the abdomen below, above and lateral to the umbilicus, and the upper back are the sites of injection.

Only small volumes (0.5 to 1.5 ml) of soluble, well-diluted, non-irritating drugs should be given.

Complications

Intramuscular injection. This may occur with a faulty technique such that the needle tip enters deeper tissues.

Self-assessment: questions

Multiple choice questions

1. Intramuscular injections:
   a. Should not be given to patients with a bleeding disorder
   b. Are not appropriate for drug delivery in emergencies because of the slow absorption into the circulation by this route
   c. Produce the fastest absorption when a gluteal muscle is used because these muscles have the greatest blood flow of the muscles used
   d. Of hydrocortisone can be used to mimic cortisol secretion in patients on long-term treatment with corticosteroids who may suffer from adrenocortical suppression
   e. Of vitamin K may be used in hospital for acute haemorrhage caused by liver disease

2. Anaphylaxis:
   a. Is mediated by IgE antibodies, which cause release of histamine and other vasoactive mediators to be released
   b. Is most frequently caused by non-steroidal anti-inflammatory drugs (NSAIDs) in dentistry
   c. Treatment includes administration of intravenous fluids, using sodium chloride in the first instance
   d. First-line management should be the immediate transfer of the patient to a hospital accident department
   e. Is particularly associated with antibiotics, blood products, vaccines, aspirin and other NSAIDs, heparin and neuromuscular blocking agents

3. A pregnant woman:
   a. Who faints should be placed in the supine position
   b. With dental pain should be prescribed paracetamol rather than an NSAID
   c. Who suffers a fracture of her mandible should have reduction and fixation carried out using a conscious sedation technique and local anaesthesia rather than general anaesthesia
   d. May develop an aggravation of gingivitis or a pyogenic granuloma at the gingival margin
   e. Should not work in an environment where she might be exposed to nitrous oxide

4. Anaemia:
   a. Is said to be present in an adult male if the haemoglobin concentration is less than 13.5 g/dl (8.4 mmol/l) and in an adult female if less than 11.5 g/dl (7.4 mmol/l)
   b. Is most commonly caused by a shortened red cell lifespan
   c. Will result in elective surgery under general anaesthesia being cancelled if the haemoglobin concentration is less than 10 g/dl (6.2 mmol/l)
   d. Is not associated with oral ulceration
   e. Of the sickle cell type contraindicates dental treatment under general anaesthesia

5. A patient who suffers from angina:
   a. May be safely treated using intravenous sedation
   b. Is likely to be taking daily aspirin and, therefore, may be at risk of postoperative haemorrhage
   c. May be taking drugs that cause oral signs
   d. Suffers from a pressing chest pain that may radiate to the jaw and left arm and is not relieved by nitrates
   e. During dental treatment should be placed in the supine position and given oxygen immediately

Extended matching items

EMI 1. Theme: Medical emergency drugs

Options:

A Adrenaline (epinephrine) 1:1000 (1 mg/ml)
B Adrenaline (epinephrine) 1:10 000 (1 mg/10 ml)
C Glucagon
D Glucose
E Hydrocortisone
F Aspirin
G Atropine
H Glyceryl trinitrite (GTN) spray
I Fresh frozen plasma
J Salbutamol

Lead in: Select the most appropriate drug from the list above for each of the following cases. Each option can be used once, more than once or not at all.

1. A 60-year-old patient develops chest pain during the administration of local anaesthetic. His pain does not improve despite returning the patient to a semi-supine position and providing oxygen and glyceryl trinitrate spray.
2. A patient, not known to be diabetic, loses consciousness. He does not regain consciousness despite being put in a supine position and receiving oxygen via a therapy mask.
3. Just prior to the administration of nitrous oxide and oxygen inhalational sedation a 10-year-old girl becomes irritable and develops shortness of breath.
4. A 65-year-old patient about to have a tooth removed under local anaesthesia becomes confused and sweaty. She chose not to have her usual breakfast alongside her insulin injection as she believed that she should be starved before a tooth extraction.
5. A short time after receiving 3 g amoxicillin orally an 18-year-old man complains of feeling unwell. He then develops a red skin rash and describes some difficulty in getting his breath.

EMI 2. Theme: Cardiorespiratory arrest

Options:

A Chest-compression-only CPR at a rate of 100/minute
B Chest compression and rescue breaths in a ratio of 30:2
C Jaw thrust

D Head tilt and chin lift
E Five initial breaths before starting chest compressions
F Automated external defibrillator (AED)
G Manual defibrillator
H 1 mg epinephrine (adrenaline) IV
I 3 mg atropine IV
J 4 ml magnesium sulphate 50% solution IV

Lead in: Select the most appropriate management from the list above for each of the following cases. Each option can be used once, more than once or not at all.

1. A 20-year-old male suffers cardiorespiratory arrest shortly after arriving in the accident and emergency department with serious facial trauma.
2. A layperson is anxious about the possibility of infection when performing basic life support.
3. A collapsed patient makes infrequent noisy gasps.
4. The appearance of asystole is observed on the ECG rhythm strip during CPR.
5. A child suffers cardiorespiratory arrest.

Case history question

Mrs Walker is an energetic 68-year-old lady. She is fit and well apart from hypertension, which is well controlled with atenolol. Two large upper anterior composite fillings are unsightly and she has decided to go ahead with the crowns that you have advised. At the end of crown preparation treatment, you press the auto-return button of the dental chair to sit Mrs Walker up. She starts to say that she feels a little dizzy and then loses consciousness.

Discuss the management of this patient.

Viva questions

1. What do we mean by antibiotic prophylaxis?
2. How in general terms may a collapsed patient be diagnosed and managed?
3. How should a patient taking warfarin be managed prior to dental extractions?
4. What is a common cause of faint in dentistry? Describe the underlying mechanism of the collapse.
5. Discuss the management of a patient who is an insulin-dependent diabetic and presents with an acute dento-alveolar abscess.

Self-assessment: answers

Multiple choice answers

1. a. **True.** This would cause formation of a large haematoma. Similarly, an inferior alveolar nerve block injection could cause bleeding into the pterygomandibular space, which at this site could be particularly dangerous as the airway could be obstructed by the swelling. Infiltration type injections of local anaesthetic are much safer.

   b. **False.** Whilst not appropriate for drug administration in the management of cardiac arrest, the intramuscular route is suitable for many other medical emergencies. It is preferable to give epinephrine (adrenaline) by the intramuscular route in anaphylaxis, for example, rather than by the intravenous route, when arrhythmias may lead to cardiac arrest.

   c. **False.** The gluteal muscles have the lowest absorption rate of the muscles used for intramuscular injections but are appropriate for the administration of some drugs, such as morphine for postoperative analgesia. It would only be appropriate to use this injection site in hospital dentistry.

   d. **True.** Steroid cover attempts to replicate the normal rise in cortisol that occurs in stress in those patients that are unable to mount this response because of adrenocortical suppression. This may be accomplished by giving steroids orally or by intramuscular or intravenous injection; however, steroids are least well absorbed when given by the intramuscular route. There is some debate about what constitutes a significant physiological stress in dentistry. It is likely that conservative dentistry or minor surgery under local anaesthesia do not require steroid cover. However, more significant surgery or a general anaesthetic does constitute a significant stress and it is important that cover is provided. Adrenocortical suppression may be assumed if the patient is currently taking systemic steroids or has taken more than a 1-month course during the previous year. Hydrocortisone 100 mg may be required 6 hourly for 72 hours for major surgery under general anaesthesia.

   e. **False.** Liver disease can lead to bleeding disorders, as a consequence of reduced synthesis of clotting factors, reduced absorption of vitamin K and abnormalities of platelet function. Vitamin K is needed for the synthesis of factors II, VII, IX and X. Acute haemorrhage in a patient with liver disease may be treated with intravenous vitamin K or fresh frozen plasma. Intramuscular injections must be avoided as the patient has a coagulation problem and the injection into muscle will lead to a haematoma.

2. a. **True.** These mediators are released from mast cells and basophils, producing respiratory, circulatory, cutaneous and gastrointestinal effects. Increased vascular permeability and peripheral vasodilatation reduce venous return and cardiac output.

   b. **False.** The penicillin antibiotics are the most common cause of anaphylaxis in dentistry. NSAIDs such as ibuprofen are recognised as causing hypersensitivity, such as rashes, angio-oedema and bronchospasm, but anaphylaxis is rare compared with penicillin.

   c. **False.** The hypotension of anaphylaxis may well need management but it is preferable to use a plasma substitute. Sodium chloride will leave the vascular compartment much more rapidly than a macromolecular plasma substitute substance such as gelatin (Gelofusine or Haemaccel). It is, therefore, better to use a plasma substitute initially when attempting to maintain blood pressure in shock arising in conditions such as anaphylaxis.

   d. **False.** First-line treatment of anaphylaxis includes restoration of blood pressure by laying the patient flat, the administration of oxygen by therapy mask and epinephrine (adrenaline) by intramuscular injection. This treatment must be carried out by the dentist as soon as the diagnosis is made as death can occur within minutes. Thus treatment begins while awaiting the emergency services to transfer the patient.

   e. **True.** Anaphylactic reactions are particularly associated with all of these medicinal products.

3. a. **False.** Pressure on the inferior vena cava from the pregnant uterus can reduce venous return and cardiac output and cause the patient to collapse if placed supine during the third trimester. It is important, therefore, to provide dental treatment in a semi-supine position. Management of a faint requires the patient to be moved onto the left side to relieve the pressure on the vena cava.

   b. **True.** Most manufacturers advise avoiding NSAIDs during pregnancy. Drugs should be prescribed during pregnancy only if the expected benefit to the mother is thought to be greater than the risk to the fetus. All drugs should be avoided if possible during the first trimester.

   c. **False.** General anaesthesia is best avoided during pregnancy and elective treatment postponed. However, the nature of the emergency surgery may dictate that general anaesthesia has to be used, in which case this will be safest after the first trimester and before the last month. Conscious sedation techniques using nitrous oxide or an intravenous benzodiazepine such as midazolam are not without risk themselves.

   d. **True.** These conditions usually resolve after the birth of the baby.

   e. **True.** The literature relating to nitrous oxide exposure and risk to health professionals has been controversial. To date, there is no direct evidence of any causal relationship between chronic low-level exposure to nitrous oxide and potential biological effects. However, every attempt should be made to reduce the level of trace nitrous oxide to exposed health-care staff and women should avoid the setting during the first trimester.

4.
a. **True.** These concentrations are typical of the lower limits of normal for adult males and females.

b. **False.** The haemolytic anaemias (subdivided into inherited and acquired types) are not the most common. Iron-deficiency anaemia is the most common and may result from an inadequate diet or chronic blood loss through gastrointestinal or menstrual bleeding.

c. **True.** While a haemoglobin concentration of 10 g/dl is less than the lower normal limit, most anaesthetists use this figure to decide when elective surgery should be postponed.

d. **False.** Oral ulceration is amongst several oral changes that may be associated with anaemia. Others include glossitis, sore tongue, candidiasis and angular stomatitis, although it is important to remember that these conditions may have other causes.

e. **False.** Of the haemoglobinopathies, haemoglobin S is the most clinically significant. The S gene is carried by 10% of patients of African origin but is also seen in Italy, Greece, Arabia and Indian subcontinent. Homozygous patients usually have anaemia (6–10 g/dl). Heterozygotes are almost asymptomatic and sickling only occurs when oxygen tensions are low. The presence or absence of haemoglobin S should be determined before general anaesthesia in risk groups. General anaesthesia, while not absolutely contraindicated, will require special precautions and may even require exchange transfusion to raise the percentage of haemoglobin A.

5.
a. **True.** If angina is mild. A conscious sedation technique may be preferable in this situation if the patient is anxious as this will minimise the activity of the sympathetic nervous system and reduce the stress on the cardiovascular system. However, angina should be controlled before elective treatment. The clinician should only proceed with methods with which he or she feels competent. Generally, patients of the American Society of Anesthetists (ASA) physical status I (see Table 8, p. 51) are suitable for sedation and also some status II patients, although the latter may require referral to the hospital service.

b. **True.** Angina patients are usually prescribed aspirin (75 or 150 mg daily) to prevent future myocardial infarction, unless contraindicated by allergy, intolerance or active peptic ulceration. Low-dose aspirin antiplatelet therapy is of value in preventing arterial thrombosis and also protects against venous thromboembolism. The clinical significance of postoperative bleeding depends on the severity of the surgery. Some recent research indicates that low-dose aspirin may lengthen the bleeding time but only within normal limits. It has been reported that intraoperative bleeding is more common but postoperative haemorrhage is not.

c. **True.** Calcium channel blockers reduce myocardial contractility and may cause lichenoid reactions and gingival overgrowth.

d. **False.** Angina is typically an exercise-related pressing precordial chest pain, radiating to the jaw and left arm, but it is relieved by nitrates.

e. **False.** Many patients are more comfortable in an upright or semi-reclined position than supine. Intra-oral glyceryl trinitrate spray and oxygen should be administered.

Extended matching items answers
EMI 1

1. **F.** If a patient's chest pain does not respond to GTN sublingual spray and oxygen therapy, then it is likely that he or she is having a myocardial infarction rather than angina pectoralis. Early thrombolysis has been shown by systematic reviews to greatly improve the outcome from myocardial infarction. On transfer to accident and emergency care, the patient will receive thrombolytic therapy and oral aspirin will initiate this effect.

2. **G.** In the event of a non-pregnant patients' vasovagal syncope not responding within a few minutes to placement in the supine position and administration of oxygen, the clinician should consider alternative causes of the collapse. Hypoglycaemia is a possibility in this situation but some syncopes are more significant and occasionally require atropine to aid recovery. Not knowing that a patient is diabetic does not of course mean that the patient isn't diabetic. It is always worth rechecking the medical history with the patient or people that may have accompanied the patient.

3. **J.** A young patient having inhalational sedation may be assumed to be anxious about the dental treatment and so an expression of irritability may be related to this. It is possible that she is hyperventilating but this would be accompanied by light-headedness, but more likely if she is 'short of breath' then she has some bronchoconstriction. An asthma attack may be induced by anxiety and occur in this situation. Airway obstruction is unlikely as dental treatment has not started.

4. **C.** It sometimes happens that a patient wrongly believes that he or she should starve themselves before an anaesthetic even when this is to be local rather than general anaesthesia. If a patient suffering from Type I diabetes takes their insulin as usual but then omits food then hypoglycaemia will ensue. Glucagon should be the first option although there is the possibility that this will be ineffective in a patient who may have used up all reserves of glycogen stores during the night and they may require intravenous glucose on transfer to accident and emergency care.

5. **A.** The diagnosis of anaphylaxis is clear because of the combination of respiratory distress and the red rash and the association of these in time with the ingestion of a penicillin antibiotic. The more concentrated dose of epinephrine of the two listed is appropriate for the intramuscular injection route of administration.

EMI 2

1. **C.** The jaw thrust is an alternative manoeuvre to head tilt and chin lift for opening the airway useful when there is a potential neck injury. The index and other fingers are placed behind the angle of the mandible and steady pressure is applied to lift the mandible and obstruction by the tongue.
2. **A.** Whilst the risk to the rescuer is remote some lay people may be unwilling to carry out mouth-to-mouth ventilation. In this situation the rescuer should give chest compressions only.
3. **B.** Agonal gasps are present in up to 40% of cardiac arrest victims. They are an indication to start CPR immediately and should not be confused with normal breathing.
4. **I.** There is no conclusive evidence that atropine is of value in asystole cardiac arrest but asystole carries a grave prognosis and there are anecdotal accounts of success after giving atropine. Atropine antagonises the action of the parasympathetic neurotransmitter acetylcholine at muscarinic receptors. It blocks the effect of the vagus nerve on both the sinoatrial (SA) node and the atrioventricular (AV) node.
5. **E.** For ease of teaching and retention laypeople should be taught that the adult sequence may also be used for children who are not responsive and not breathing. It is far better that the adult sequence is used rather than nothing because of unfounded fear of causing harm. However, minor modifications to the sequence make it more suitable for children. Five initial breaths before starting chest compressions are helpful. Also, if alone to perform CPR for one minute before going for help. Compress the chest by approximately one-third of its depth and use only two fingers for an infant under 1 year.

Case history answer

The patient should be placed in the supine position again and her airways, breathing and circulation (ABC) checked. Resuscitate as appropriate. If the patient is unconscious but breathing and has a circulation, then provide oxygen therapy and move into the recovery position. If the patient has fainted, then a prompt recovery could be expected. Knowledge of the patient's medication might suggest a diagnosis of postural hypotension, and the patient should recover spontaneously within a minute or so. Atenolol is a β-adrenoceptor blocking drug commonly prescribed for hypertension. As the heart and peripheral vasculature are less responsive to the sympathetic reflex on changing to an upright posture, the dental chair should be moved slowly to allow the patient time to compensate.

Viva answers

1. Antibiotics may be used to treat bacterial infections or to prevent infections occurring, when treatment is described as prophylactic. Antibiotic prophylaxis may be used in three situations:
   a. to prevent postoperative infection in a healthy patient undergoing invasive treatment such as major surgery or even when a wisdom tooth is surgically removed
   b. to prevent an immunocompromised patient developing a postoperative infection following a straightforward treatment such as dental extraction
   c. to prevent a serious infection occurring following a bacteraemia such as patients at risk of subacute bacterial endocarditis although no longer considered necessary.
2. When confronted with a collapsed patient, the diagnosis may not be instantly apparent. However, the ABC (airways, breathing and circulation) of resuscitation is the mainstay of primary assessment and treatment. This should always be the first step. Once confirmation of satisfactory airway, breathing and circulation has been obtained, further assessment may provide a working diagnosis that permits appropriate emergency treatment. Conditions such as acute asthma, anaphylaxis and hypoglycaemia may be identified at this stage. Further evaluation will lead to a definitive diagnosis and care.
3. Anticoagulants are used in the treatment of deep-vein thrombosis, following heart valve replacement and atrial fibrillation. Anticoagulant activity is monitored using a prothrombin time test, and is expressed as the international normalised ratio (INR) by comparing it with a control and adjusting for laboratory variation. An INR near 1 is normal and patients taking anticoagulants are usually in the range 2–4. Patients have in the past had their INR brought down to 2.5 or less before dental extractions. However, current evidence suggests that no change need be made as long as the INR is within normal range. There is evidence of rebound thromboses caused by reducing warfarin dosage. There is no doubt that the INR should be reduced for major surgery. However, drug dosage *must only* be adjusted on the advice of the haematologist. Occasionally, rather than reducing the warfarin dose prior to treatment, the haematologist may recommend replacing the warfarin with heparin. This is usually for patients with less stable coagulation status.
4. Anxiety is the usual cause. There is an increase in sympathetic activity and release of adrenaline, which causes an increase in heart rate and force of contraction, vasodilatation of blood vessels in skeletal muscle and vasoconstriction in skin, in preparation for fight or flight. Venous return to the heart is reduced because of blood pooling in skeletal muscles not being used for fight or flight and cannot sustain cardiac filling. This triggers a reflex vagal activity that causes bradycardia. The massive drop in blood pressure results in reduced blood flow to the brain and loss of consciousness.

5. An infection such as a dental abscess is more likely to result in a rapidly spreading cellulitis in a diabetic patient. Also, such an infection can disrupt diabetic control. With these two factors in mind, a thorough history and examination should be undertaken and aggressive treatment started promptly.

Dental history and examination. This will indicate the cause of the abscess and the potential route of spread. Any likely involvement of tissue spaces about the airway is obviously important. Trismus, cervical lymphadenopathy, pyrexia or tachycardia indicate that the patient should be referred for hospital admission and management. The priority, as in other patients, is drainage; this may be via the root canal or by extraction of the associated tooth. These may be undertaken in the primary care setting in early infections and if the patient is well. There may also be the need to incise and drain an associated intra-oral or extra-oral swelling. The latter will be undertaken in hospital under general anaesthesia. Intravenous antibiotics such as penicillin together with metronidazole, fluids to rehydrate the patient, analgesics and an antipyretic drug may all be required. The stress of illness tends to increase the basal requirements of insulin and it is important to check the blood frequently.

Preoperative management. This should be meticulous and according to an agreed policy between the diabetes care team, surgeons, anaesthetists and ward staff. This may mean stopping the regular insulin and giving a continuous infusion of balanced amounts of glucose, potassium and insulin, which will both maintain satisfactory glycaemic control (5–10 mmol/l) and prevent hypokalaemia. This regimen is continued until the patient is able to eat and drink normally. Alternatively, insulin may be given as a variable rate infusion, providing more flexibility.

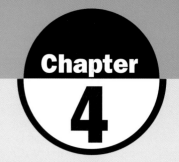

Chapter 4

Control of pain and anxiety

Overview

This chapter deals with pain; it describes the types of pain and their significance and the methods available to the dentist for the control of pain and anxiety.

Systemic analgesic protocols are outlined and related to the types of procedure for which they are suitable. Considerations of dosing schedules and preoperative and postoperative regimens are discussed. Local anaesthetic drugs in common use are described together with their mechanisms of action. Drug dosages, including maximum safe doses, are covered as are the types of complication that can arise from the use of local anaesthetics. The use of vasoconstrictors with a local anaesthetic is also explained.

The role of conscious sedation is outlined with both the indications and contraindications. Nitrous oxide and the benzodiazepines are described. Various sedation techniques are outlined together with the methods for monitoring patients during and after sedation.

The assessment of patients for general anaesthetic is covered together with the possible investigations to establish suitability and the medical conditions that can complicate general anaesthesia. Preoperative preparation of patients for general anaesthesia is described.

4.1 Systemic analgesia

Learning objectives

You should:
- understand the types of pain and how pain is initiated and transmitted
- know suitable pain relief regimens to recommend patients for systemic pain relief
- understand how to use pain relief at all stages of treatment.

Nociception and pain

Nociception. Nociception has been defined as the process of detection and signalling the presence of a noxious stimulus.

Detection involves the activation of specialised sensory transducers, nociceptors, attached to Aδ and C fibres.

Pain. The International Association for the Study of Pain (IASP) has endorsed a definition of pain as an 'unpleasant sensory and emotional experience associated with actual or potential damage, or described in terms of such damage'. Pain involves a motivational-affective component as well as a sensory-discriminative dimension and can occur without nociception.

The pain system

Not all noxious stimuli that activate nociceptors are necessarily experienced as pain. While the sensations we call pain, pricking, burning, aching or stinging may have an urgent and primitive quality, they can be modulated. For example, in situations of crisis or emergency, or even when an individual's attention is simply elsewhere, noxious inputs may trigger much less pain sensation than would otherwise be expected. It is observed that fear for survival in a war situation may suppress the pain of an inflicted injury until the individual is away from the immediate danger of the front line. Equally, anxiety about undergoing elective surgery may intensify the postoperative pain experience.

The variability of human pain suggests that there are neural mechanisms that modulate transmission in pain pathways and modify the individual's emotional experience of pain. The transmission of pain is, therefore, no longer viewed as a static process using exclusive pathways from peripheral tissues through the spinal cord to the brain but rather as messages arising from the interplay between neuronal systems, both excitatory and inhibitory, at many levels of the central nervous system (CNS).

Acute pain

Acute pain has been described as pain of recent onset and probable limited duration. It usually has a causal relationship to injury or disease. Patients' report of pain stops long before healing has been completed. Pain following injury or surgery would be typical of this type of pain.

Chronic pain

Chronic pain is frequently defined as pain lasting for long periods of time; however, it is not the duration of pain that distinguishes it from acute pain but rather the inability of the body to restore its physiological functions to normal homeostatic levels. Chronic pain commonly persists beyond the time of healing of an injury and its intensity usually bears no relation to the extent of tissue damage, indeed there may be no clearly identifiable cause.

Inflammatory and neuropathic pain

Clinical pain may be inflammatory or neuropathic in origin; the former refers to pain associated with peripheral tissue damage, such as that produced during surgery, and the latter refers to pain resulting from nervous system dysfunction, such as is seen in postherpetic neuralgia or trigeminal neuralgia (Ch. 14).

Both inflammatory and neuropathic pains are characterised by changes in sensitivity, notably a reduction in the intensity of the stimuli necessary to initiate pain, so that stimuli that would never normally produce pain begin to do so; this is called **allodynia**. There is also an exaggerated responsiveness to noxious stimuli, termed **hyperalgesia**.

Pain control

Several publications including reports by the Royal College of Surgeons and College of Anaesthetists have shown that relief of pain following surgery in the UK has been suboptimal. Reasons include inadequate recognition or evaluation of pain and prescription of inappropriate drugs and inadequate doses.

Dental pain and pain after surgery

Systemic pain relief can be related to the type of procedure, to the level of pain and to the needs of the particular patient (Table 5). Non-steroidal anti-inflammatory drugs (NSAIDs) are contraindicated in:

- age over 75 years
- hypersensitivity to aspirin or any other NSAID
- pregnancy/breast feeding
- history of gastrointestinal bleed.

Dosing schedules

Analgesic drugs should be given at regular times according to their half-life and at high enough doses to ensure therapeutic plasma levels. Adequate doses of analgesics should not be withheld because of misconceptions and fears on the part of the prescriber. It is wrong to believe that pain is the inevitable consequence of surgery or that the use of opioids for acute pain in hospital will lead to addiction.

Men and women require the same analgesic doses for pain relief, although older patients may require smaller doses.

Pre-emptive analgesia

Sustained pain causes the pain system to become sensitised and this has the effect of amplifying the pain experience significantly. Prevention of pain rather than treating pain is, therefore, important and theoretically could reduce the analgesic requirements after surgery. However, the evidence for the clinical advantage of giving an analgesic before pain as opposed to giving the same analgesic after pain is still unconvincing. Despite the debate about pre-emption, it is worth giving systemic analgesics before the local anaesthetic (LA) has worn off or an LA during general anaesthesia (GA) to prevent pain in the early postoperative phase, even though this may not reduce the later analgesic requirements.

Table 5 Systemic pain relief after dental and surgical procedures

Typical pain level	Type of procedure	Protocol
Mild to moderate	Forceps extraction	Two 500 mg paracetamol tablets every 6 hours as necessary up to a maximum of eight tablets in 24 hours
Moderate to severe	Surgical removal of tooth involving bone removal	Ibuprofen 400 mg four times a day regularly. If inadequate: Paracetamol (500 mg)/codeine (30 mg) combination tablets, two every 4 hours as necessary up to a maximum of eight tablets in 24 hours. When NSAIDs contraindicated: Paracetamol (500 mg)/codeine (30 mg) combination tablets, two every 4 hours regularly up to a maximum of 4 g paracetamol in 24 hours
Moderate to severe for inpatient	More difficult surgical removal of teeth or osteotomy	Morphine by intravenous titration or intermittent intramuscular injection

These protocols are based on evidence from postoperative pain systematic reviews. The *British National Formulary* and other sources contain more extensive lists of analgesics.

Preoperative patient preparation

Most patients are anxious about postoperative pain. Relieving this anxiety by explaining how postoperative pain will be dealt with has been shown to reduce the postoperative pain experienced.

Patient-controlled analgesia

Usually intravenous (i.v.) morphine is used via an infusion pump, with a lock to limit dose for safety. Patients given this control over their own pain relief usually use smaller doses than would have been prescribed.

Route of drug administration

The oral route is preferable but tablets, capsules or oral suspension should be chosen as appropriate for age and the nature of the treatment. Alternative routes such as intramuscular, i.v. and rectal may be appropriate in hospital.

Pain and the mind

It is well established that pain and depression are related, although the reasons for the association remain unclear. This has led to the unfortunate situation in the past when the dentist or other clinician, who could not find an obvious cause of the patient's pain, believed that the reported pain was imaginary. It is now understood that if a patient reports pain then that pain is real. It is also now understood that any emotional disturbance in a patient with pain is more likely to be a consequence than a cause of the pain and it is dangerous to ascribe pain routinely to psychological causation. Traditional concepts focused either on medical or psychological explanations for pain, but the boundaries between these are being eroded as psychogenic cause is found to have a biochemical 'physical' basis.

4.2 Local anaesthesia

You should:
- understand how local anaesthetics work
- know the potency, speed of onset and duration of action of common agents
- be aware of reasons for failure of anaesthesia and complications that can occur
- know the safe dosages of common local anaesthetic drugs.

The correct selection of pain control technique for patients requiring dental treatment is important for safe and successful practice. As with other aspects of clinical dentistry, this clinical decision making is based on knowledge and experience. Generally patients for treatment under local anaesthesia will be managed by the dentist in a primary care setting, whereas those requiring a GA will be referred to hospital. However, there may be a few patients requiring local anaesthesia whose medical history dictates that they are treated in hospital. Patients requiring conscious sedation techniques are treated in both the primary care and hospital setting.

By common usage, the localised loss of pain sensation is referred to as 'local anaesthesia', rather than local analgesia, which would be more accurate. The word 'anaesthesia' implies loss of all sensation including touch, pressure, temperature and pain.

Mechanism of action

LA agents reversibly block nerve conduction and belong to the chemical groups of amino-esters or amino-amides.

Amino-esters

Procaine was produced in 1905 and in use for more than 40 years. It is still available.

Amino-amides

Lidocaine (lignocaine) was produced in 1944 and superseded procaine because of its pharmacological advantages. It is the most widely used LA in dentistry and also has topical anaesthetic properties.

Mepivacaine is similar to lidocaine but is used less in dentistry.

Prilocaine is similar to lidocaine. It has low systemic toxicity.

Bupivacaine and levobupivacaine are used where long duration of action is important.

Articaine is the most recent introduction. It is classified as an amide although it has both an amide and an ester link.

Potency

Procaine is the least potent. Prilocaine is three times more potent than procaine and lidocaine is four times more potent than procaine. The potency of articaine is one and a half times that of lidocaine.

Speed of onset

Agents with high lipid solubility act more quickly. Procaine takes longer than prilocaine and lidocaine, which take about the same time (within 2 minutes for infiltration injections and 3–5 minutes for inferior alveolar nerve blocks).

Duration of action

Duration of action depends on the diffusion capacity of the anaesthetic agent and the rate of its elimination. Bupivacaine is an extremely soluble LA with a long duration of action (6–8 hours); it is useful for postoperative pain relief. Levobupivacaine is an isomer of bupivacaine; it has similar analgesic properties to bupivacaine but is less cardiotoxic.

Metabolism and excretion

Amino-esters are metabolised in plasma by the enzyme pseudocholinesterase. Amino-amides are metabolised in the liver. Excretion occurs via the kidney.

Failure of anaesthesia

Failure of anaesthesia can occur for a number of reasons:

- Inadequate dose administered: the full contents of a dental cartridge (1.8–2.2 ml) are required to obtain a reliable mandibular block according to minimum-dose calculations (Fig. 29)
- Inaccurate injection technique: inadvertent injection of solution into a vein or muscle will result in inadequate anaesthesia
- Biological variation: duration of anaesthesia may vary widely between individuals
- Anatomical variation: can lead to ineffective anaesthesia (e.g. of an inferior dental block when an aberrant mandibular foramen occurs).

Complications

General complications

There are three typical types of complication.

Psychogenic. Fainting is the most common such complication.

Toxic. Overdose with LA may lead to light-headedness, sedation, circumoral paraesthesia and twitching. More serious overdose can result in convulsions, loss of consciousness, respiratory depression and cardiovascular collapse. Accidental i.v. injection may lead to excessively high plasma concentration. Prilocaine has low toxicity, similar to lidocaine, but if used in high doses may cause methaemoglobinaemia.

Allergic. Approximately two milion dental local anaesthetic injections are administered daily around the world. Reports of allergic reactions are extremely rare. In the past, they may have been associated with the preservative (methylparaben) that was included in the cartridge. If a

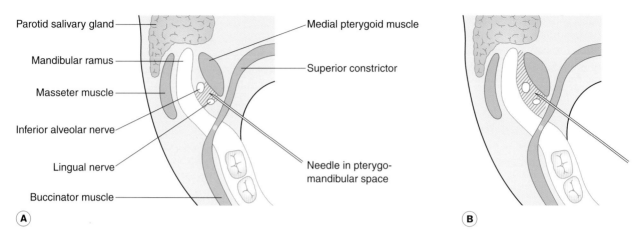

Fig. 29 Diagram of pterygomandibular space illustrating the need to inject an adequate dose of local anaesthetic for a reliable block of inferior alveolar and lingual nerve conduction. **A,** The area covered by 1 ml of local anaesthetic, which is not sufficient to block conduction. **B,** A full cartridge of local anaesthetic is necessary to block the inferior alveolar and lingual nerve conduction.

patient gives a history compatible with an allergic reaction (rash, swelling or bronchospasm), rather than psychogenic reaction or the consequences of i.v. injection (tachycardia), then they should be referred for allergy testing. Hypersensitivity reactions occur mainly with the ester-type local anaesthetics such as benzocaine, cocaine and procaine.

Local complications

Soft-tissue trauma. Too rapid an injection or injection of too large a volume may tear soft tissues.

Nerve trauma. A nerve may be lacerated by a needle or stretched and traumatised by injection of solution into the neural sheath. Prolonged paraesthesia will result.

Intravascular injection. Injections into a vein may result in a haematoma and/or the systemic effects of local anaesthesia or vasoconstrictor. Injection into an artery causes vasoconstriction and ischaemia of the tissue area of supply.

Complications of inferior alveolar nerve block

- Injection into the medial pterygoid muscle may result in trismus as well as ineffective anaesthesia.
- Deep injection into the parotid salivary gland may result in blockade of the facial nerve and temporary facial muscle paralysis.
- The patient may experience an 'electric shock' type of sensation if the needle touches the inferior alveolar nerve and the injection should only start after withdrawing the needle 1 mm; otherwise direct damage resulting in long-term paraesthesia may result.

Types of local anaesthetic drugs

Topical local anaesthetics

Topical LAs may be used on intra-oral mucous membranes prior to intra-oral injections of LA or to reduce discomfort of minor procedures. They may also be applied to the skin prior to venepuncture.

Intra-oral. Lidocaine (4%) is available as an ointment or gel. There are also spray formulations (10% lidocaine) available for intra-oral use.

Skin. Lidocaine 2.5% and prilocaine 2.5% (EMLA) or 4% tetracaine (amethocaine) (AMETOP gel). EMLA (eutectic mixture of LA) is contraindicated in infants under 1 year and AMETOP is not recommended in infants under 1 month.

Application method. The LA is applied to the skin and covered with a dressing. The dressing and gel is removed before venepuncture 60 minutes (EMLA) or 30 minutes (AMETOP) later. Systemic absorption is low from skin but topical LAs should never be applied to wounds or mucous membranes, where absorption is rapid.

Vasoconstrictors

Most LAs (except cocaine) cause blood vessel dilatation and, therefore, a vasoconstrictor is added to diminish local blood flow and slow absorption of the LA. In practice, LAs still enter the systemic circulation quite rapidly but vasoconstrictors are useful to accelerate the onset, lengthen the duration and increase the depth of anaesthesia. They also reduce the local haemorrhage, which can be very helpful during surgical procedures. However, vasoconstrictors should never be used for infiltration of the ears, fingers, toes or penis as ischaemic necrosis may result. The concentration used is higher in dentistry than in medicine, particularly in the UK.

Epinephrine (adrenaline)

- Natural catecholamine
- Constricts arterioles in skin and mucosa
- Increases cardiac output by raising stroke volume and heart rate, but this effect is difficult to accomplish with the doses in dental cartridges.

Felypressin (octapressin)

- Synthetic analogue of naturally occurring vasopressin
- Constricts venous outflow and, therefore, is less effective in haemorrhage control than adrenaline (epinephrine)
- Contraindicated in pregnancy as it is similar to oxytocin and there is a possibility of uterus contraction, although the dose is actually very small compared with the dose of oxytocin used by obstetricians to induce labour.

Prilocaine with felypressin is often recommended for use in patients with ischaemic heart disease rather than lidocaine with adrenaline (epinephrine), but there is no evidence that it is any safer. The latter is a more effective LA.

Common drugs in dentistry

Lidocaine (lignocaine)

Lidocaine is an effective LA and consequently the most commonly used in dentistry in the UK. It is available in dental cartridges as a plain 2% solution or with adrenaline (epinephrine) added in a concentration of 1:80 000. An adrenaline (epinephrine) concentration of 1:100 000 is more common in the rest of the world.

Prilocaine

Prilocaine is available as a 4% plain solution or as a 3% solution with 0.02 IU/ml felypressin. The latter is the usual alternative to lidocaine with adrenaline (epinephrine) in the UK. If a vasoconstrictor must be avoided, then plain 4% prilocaine is more effective than plain 2% lidocaine.

Articaine

Articaine is available as a 4% solution with either 1:100 000 or 1:200 000 adrenaline (epinephrine).

Bupivacaine

Bupivacaine is available as 0.25%, 0.5% and 0.75% solutions in ampoules but not dental cartridges. The two lower concentrations are available plain or with 1:200 000 adrenaline (epinephrine). Bupivacaine has a slow onset of anaesthesia but then provides pulpal anaesthesia for about 2 hours and soft-tissue anaesthesia for about 8 hours.

Drug dose for safety

Estimation of a safe dose must take into account:

- potency
- rate of absorption and excretion
- vascularity in area of administration
- patient's age, weight, physique and clinical condition.

The maximum recommended doses are given in Table 6.

4.3 Conscious sedation

Learning objectives

You should:
- be able to assess a patient for suitability for conscious sedation and know the dental and medical contraindications
- know the sedation techniques available
- know the characteristics and use of nitrous oxide and the benzodiazepines.

Some patients are anxious about routine dental treatment, while others, who may be able to cope with uncomplicated treatment, may be distressed by more unpleasant procedures such as minor oral surgery with local anaesthesia alone. Management approaches vary according to the

Table 6 Maximum recommended doses of local anaesthetics

Preparation	Maximum dose in healthy adult	Child (20 kg)
2% Lidocaine	4.4 mg/kg up to 300 mg (7 cartridges)	2 cartridges
3% Prilocaine	6.0 mg/kg up to 400 mg (6 cartridges)	1.8 cartridges
4% Prilocaine	6.0 mg/kg up to 400 mg (4.5 cartridges)	1.4 cartridges
4% Articaine	7.0 mg/kg up to 440 mg (5 cartridges)	1.5 cartridges

1 cartridge contains 2.2 ml.

severity of the anxiety, the age of the patient, the degree of cooperation and the medical history. Psychological approaches have been widely used and range from informal and common-sense methods to formal relaxation training and hypnosis. These techniques are safe, free from side-effects and give the patient a sense of control.

An increasing number of patients are managed with conscious sedation techniques in combination with a LA but the more severely anxious and uncooperative may require treatment under a GA. As patient awareness of the risks of anaesthesia and the availability of sedation has increased, so the demand and popularity of conscious sedation for dentistry has increased. The control of pain and anxiety is fundamental to the practice of dentistry.

The aim of a sedation technique is to keep the patient conscious and cooperative but in a state of complete tranquillity. Ideally, the patient should have the sensations of warmth, confidence and a pleasant degree of dissociation from the realities of the situation. Sedation with drugs is not a replacement for, but rather an adjunct to, a caring and sympathetic attitude towards the patient. Conscious sedation may be defined as state of depression of the central nervous system produced by a drug or drugs, enabling treatment to be carried out, and during which communication is maintained such that a patient will respond to command throughout the period of sedation. The techniques used should carry a margin of safety wide enough to render unintended loss of consciousness unlikely.

Routes of administration. Sedative drugs may be administered by a variety of routes, for example via the lungs, via the gastrointestinal tract (orally or rectally), intranasally, by intramuscular injection or directly into the circulation by intravenous injection. The most popular in the UK are the inhalational, oral and i.v. routes.

Risk avoidance. When using sedation techniques, it is important to avoid risks and the dentist should only proceed with methods with which he or she feels competent, in an environment that is adequately equipped and with staff that are appropriately trained. There should always be a second person present who is trained in the care of sedated patients. Whilst UK Dental Schools provide undergraduate students with the necessary knowledge and skills to enable them to provide conscious sedation to patients, the British General Dental Council currently recommends additional postgraduate training. It is essential that dentists and their staff working in these fields are familiar with the appropriate regulations according to their country of practice.

All dental treatment facilities must have appropriate equipment and drugs for resuscitation at hand and the dentist and his or her team must have the skills to use them in an emergency whether providing conscious sedation techniques or treatment under local anaesthesia alone.

Assessment for conscious sedation

Indications

Psychological indications

Anxiety may be the most obvious and common reason for prescribing conscious sedation rather than an LA but it is important to confirm this by discussion rather than accept a request for sedation from a patient who may not be aware of its implications or of treatment alternatives. It may be necessary to justify the selection and patient preference alone is not sufficient reason. Extremely anxious patients may require GA for their dental management.

Dental indications

Moderately difficult or prolonged procedures such as dental implant surgery may be an indication for sedation. Some patients who are happy to undergo routine dental treatment with a LA alone may require sedation to accept oral surgery procedures. Anxiety-induced gagging is often very successfully managed with sedation. Extensive dental treatment or surgery may require GA.

Medical indications

Systemic disorders such as mild angina, controlled hypertension or controlled anxiety-induced asthma may be an indication for the use of sedation as this minimises the psychological response to stress and so will reduce the activity of the sympathetic nervous system. This may avoid, or at least reduce, the likelihood of an angina or asthma attack or of raising the systemic blood pressure. Those with cardiorespiratory disease should receive supplemental oxygen.

In disorders such as spasticity, multiple sclerosis or parkinsonism, where a patient may be eager to cooperate but physically unable to do so, benzodiazepine sedation may be of use because of its muscle relaxant properties. Similarly, patients with controlled epilepsy may benefit from the anticonvulsant property of benzodiazepines.

Contraindications

Psychological and social contraindications

It is better to admit defeat and arrange for treatment under a GA than to attempt sedation of a totally uncooperative patient. Successful sedation requires a patient to have sufficient intellect, insight and cooperation. Psychologically immature individuals unmanageable with LA alone may exhibit disinhibited or childish behaviour when sedated and so a GA may be preferable.

Patients who are unable to provide a responsible adult (over 16 years) to accompany them, escort them home and remain with them for the rest of the day are not suitable for treatment with intravenous sedation or GA.

Dental contraindications

Prolonged or difficult oral surgery is a contraindication to treatment under any form of sedation as this may stretch both the patient and operator beyond their limits of endurance. It must also be remembered that sedation techniques do not reduce surgical morbidity. Planned GA may be preferable.

Medical contraindications

Allergy. Allergy to sedatives or anaesthetics is obviously an absolute contraindication to the use of these drugs, but such allergies are rare.

Systemic disease. Severe forms of systemic disease such as a recent myocardial infarct or poorly controlled or severe hypertension or angina may be obvious contraindications for sedation for GA, but even hay fever or the common cold may contraindicate inhalational sedation if there is nasal obstruction.

Respiratory disease. Chronic obstructive or restrictive airways diseases such as bronchitis, emphysema or bronchiectasis are contraindications. Such patients are particularly sensitive to the respiratory depression associated with benzodiazepines and anaesthetic drugs. Also, patients whose respiration is driven by a low partial pressure of oxygen rather than their partial pressure of carbon dioxide are likely to have their hypoxic drive removed by the relatively high concentration of oxygen administered during inhalational sedation. Patients with impaired cardiac function as well as those with chronic obstructive airways disease may be subject to hypoxic drive.

Pregnancy. Women who are, or may be, pregnant should preferably not be sedated or given a GA. Nitrous oxide inactivates vitamin B_{12}, inhibits DNA formation and may be teratogenic. Its use in elective situations is, therefore, contraindicated, particularly during the first trimester when cell differentiation is occurring. Nitrous oxide may be used safely, however, during late pregnancy and indeed is frequently used for pain relief during childbirth. Animal experiments have not indicated any teratogenic risk with midazolam, but evaluation in human pregnancy has not been undertaken and it would, therefore, be unwise to use it unless considered essential. High doses of benzodiazepines in the last trimester of pregnancy have been reported to produce irregularities of the fetal heart rate, hypotonia, poor sucking and hypothermia in the neonate. Midazolam should not, therefore, be used during the last trimester. Caution must be exercised when using intravenous sedation for breast-feeding mothers. If using midazolam, it is reasonable to ask the mother not to breast feed for 8 hours after the sedation and use synthetic or pre-expressed milk during this time.

Liver and kidney disease. Since benzodiazepines are metabolised by the liver and excreted by the kidneys, diseases affecting these organs may interfere with recovery. Alcoholics may have some degree of liver damage and should, therefore, be sedated with caution.

Muscle disease. Myasthenia gravis and other muscle-weakening or muscle-wasting diseases are an absolute contraindication to the use of benzodiazepines because of the risk of serious respiratory depression.

Obesity. Obese patients often have poor airway control and may also have difficult veins to canulate.

Psychiatric disorders. Patients with severe psychiatric or personality disorders may also be unsuitable for sedation as disinhibiting effects have been observed. Patients taking CNS depressants, such as potent analgesics, tranquillisers or sleeping tablets, may be unpredictably sensitive to or tolerant of sedation. The possibility of severe respiratory or cardiovascular depression should be considered when using benzodiazepines.

Patients who are using non-prescribed drugs may have increased tolerance and, if self-injecting, may have difficult venous access.

Drug interactions. The sedative effect of midazolam may be potentiated in patients receiving erythromycin, particularly if the sedative is administered orally, so caution should be exercised. There are other possible drug interactions with the benzodiazepines of varying clinical significance (Table 7) and patients taking such medications may be better managed in the hospital environment.

Physical status. Generally, patients of physical status I (on the American Society of Anesthetists (ASA) grading system, Table 8) are suitable for sedation and also some status II patients, although the latter may require referral to a more experienced anaesthetist.

Table 7 Drug interactions with benzodiazepine

Drug	Interaction
Alcohol	Enhanced sedative effect
Opioid analgesics	Enhanced sedative effect
Antibacterials	Erythromycin inhibits metabolism of midazolam; isoniazid inhibits metabolism of diazepam; rifampicin increases metabolism of diazepam
Antihistamines	Enhanced sedative effect
Antihypertensives	Enhanced hypotensive effect; enhanced sedative effect with alpha-blockers
Antipsychotics	Enhanced sedative effect
Dopaminergics	Benzodiazepines occasionally antagonise the effect of levodopa
Ulcer-healing drugs	Cimetidine inhibits the metabolism of benzodiazepines

Table 8 The American Society of Anesthesiologists, classification of physical status

Class	Physical status
I	No organic or psychiatric disturbance
II	Mild-to-moderate systemic disturbance
III	Severe systemic disturbance
IV	Life-threatening severe systemic disturbance
V	Moribund patient unlikely to survive

Sedative drugs

The drugs used for dental sedation are required to produce the rapid onset of a relaxed state for the period of the dentistry but then wear off rapidly so that the patient can return to a normal life. Such requirements for potent but short-acting drugs has led to the use of:

- nitrous oxide and oxygen administered by inhalation
- benzodiazepine drugs administered i.v.

The barbiturates, which were introduced in the 1930s, are no longer used as they depress respiration, interact with other drugs such as anticoagulants and increase the perception of pain. The opioids, which have been used for thousands of years, have similarly been superseded by the benzodiazepines for i.v. sedation. The 'Jorgensen technique' of i.v. administration of pentobarbital, pethidine and hyoscine, which was popular for many years, has lost favour since the development of the benzodiazepines with their high therapeutic index and wide safety margin.

The General Dental Council of the UK advises using the simplest technique necessary to enable treatment to be carried out and suggests that this will usually be by means of a single drug in the case of i.v. sedation. Outside the UK, there is no such restriction on clinical practice and it is worth noting that, particularly in the USA, a wide range of sedative techniques continues to be used in dentistry. The definition of 'sedation' varies around the world, with consequent confusion in communication. Deep sedation as well as conscious sedation, for example, is used for dentistry in the USA, but in the UK deep sedation would be understood to be GA.

Nitrous oxide

Nitrous oxide is a sweet-smelling, non-irritant, colourless gas that can produce analgesia, anxiolysis and anaesthesia. As an analgesic, a 25% concentration of nitrous oxide in oxygen has been compared favourably with morphine; however, while it is a potent analgesic, it is a weak anaesthetic (minimum alveolar concentration (MAC) 105 vol%). It does not cause measurable respiratory depression when administered with oxygen alone but may augment the respiratory depressant effect of opiates. The effects of nitrous oxide can be rapidly reversed when necessary. Nitrous oxide is relatively insoluble, having a blood gas solubility of 0.47 at 37 °C, but is 15 times more soluble than oxygen. If a gas is totally insoluble in blood, then none is taken up and the alveolar concentration will rise and will soon equal the inspired concentration. If gas has low solubility, like nitrous oxide, then only small quantities will be carried and the alveolar concentration will again rise rapidly. Since alveolar concentration determines the tension in arterial circulation, the tension will also rise rapidly, even though only a small volume of nitrous oxide is present in blood. As the blood passes through the tissues, the nitrous oxide is given up readily and because of the rich cerebral blood supply; the tension of the gas within the brain also rises rapidly and onset of clinical action is quickly apparent. Likewise the rate of recovery is equally rapid once the delivery of nitrous oxide ceases. Conversely, gases with a high blood solubility require longer periods of time for the onset of action to develop.

Elimination

Nitrous oxide is eliminated unchanged from the body, mostly via the lungs, the majority being exhaled within 3–15 minutes after termination of sedation. About 1% is eliminated more slowly (24 hours) via the lungs and skin.

Undesirable effects

Nitrous oxide is usually regarded as a non-toxic anaesthetic agent, provided that it is administered with sufficient oxygen, but it does have some undesirable effects.

Vitamin B$_{12}$ metabolism. Nitrous oxide depresses vitamin B$_{12}$ metabolism and prolonged exposure may lead to impaired bone marrow function, resulting in megaloblastic anaemia. All reported cases, however, have involved exposure for more than 24 hours. Of greater significance is a neuropathic vitamin B$_{12}$ deficiency, which may result in neurological damage from repeated short-term exposure.

Teratogenicity. A study in the 1970s suggested an increase in spontaneous abortion and congenital anomalies in female dentists and assistants heavily exposed to nitrous oxide (greater than 9 hours per week) and this led to recommendations of exposure limits for staff and scavenging of waste gas. Multiple attempts to reproduce these research results have failed and a world-wide review of literature in the 1990s concluded that there was no scientific basis for the previously established thresholds (25 ppm in the USA and 50 ppm in the UK). The scavenging of waste gas to decrease the pollution of the surgery air is of course of benefit to prevent the sedation of the staff.

Nausea or vomiting. Both are occasionally seen after the administration of nitrous oxide. As the gas is not known to affect the vomiting centre, this is more likely a result of other causes such as patient predisposition or hypoxia.

Increased pressure in gas-containing body spaces. The low solubility of nitrous oxide, which permits its rapid transfer from alveoli across endothelium to blood and vice versa, also permits rapid transfer into other air-filled body cavities. Nitrous oxide equilibrates with blood, tissue and gas-containing spaces more rapidly than nitrogen diffuses out into alveolar air, and there is a 35-fold difference in the blood/gas partition coefficients of the two gases. Consequently, for every molecule of nitrogen removed from air spaces, 35 molecules of nitrous oxide will pass in and there will be an increase in volume of a compliant space and increase in pressure of a non-compliant space. Nitrous oxide may diffuse from the intestinal wall into the abdominal cavity and cause a slight increase in abdominal girth, but this is of no clinical significance. More seriously, an increase in pressure may occur in the middle ear or sinuses should they be obstructed and this may result in pain.

Benzodiazepines

The first benzodiazepine, chlordiazepoxide, was synthesised at Hoffmann-La-Roche Inc. in the USA in 1956. It became available as an anxiolytic in 1960.

Mechanism of action

Benzodiazepines are also muscle relaxant and anticonvulsant. With the discovery of gamma-aminobutyric acid (GABA), the major inhibitory neurotransmitter in the CNS, and the development of sophisticated techniques for the localisation of receptors, the cellular and molecular mechanisms of action of the benzodiazepines were unravelled. It is now established that these drugs exert their pharmacological effects by facilitating the transmission of GABA in the CNS through interaction with a benzodiazepine–GABA receptor complex. The latter was discovered in 1977.

The GABA receptors, which are tetrameric proteins in the cell membranes, act as highly selective chloride channels and when activated allow negative chloride ions to enter the cell, which then becomes inhibited. The chloride channel is continually opening and closing and there is a constant flux of chloride ions. An agonist accelerates the process of ion flux. The following range of possible drug actions based on the benzodiazepine–GABA receptor complex are possible:

- agonist, e.g. midazolam
- partial agonist
- antagonist, e.g. flumazenil
- partial inverse agonist
- inverse agonist, e.g. betacarbolines.

Undesirable effects

Benzodiazepines have a very wide safety margin and a high therapeutic index but nonetheless do have some unwanted side-effects.

Respiratory depression. The benzodiazepines are mild respiratory depressants and although this effect is usually insignificant in normal patients, rapid i.v. injection of benzodiazepines can sometimes cause profound respiratory depression or even apnoea. Respiratory depression is greatly increased if benzodiazepines are given together with opioids. This is a synergistic effect rather than additive effect; therefore, if both drugs are combined, only about one-quarter of the dose of each drug is required to cause the same effect as the full dose of each drug administered alone. Unless extreme care is taken, such a combination is likely to cause anaesthesia or respiratory arrest and is, therefore, not recommended.

The elderly. In some elderly patients, benzodiazepines have caused hyperactivity, anxiety and agitation rather than sedation because the neurotransmitter profile of individuals is subject to age changes. These unwanted effects have been reversed with flumazenil.

Elimination

All benzodiazepines are metabolised by the liver and excreted via the kidneys. The metabolism of midazolam involves the hydroxylation by hepatic microsomal oxidative mechanisms to a few metabolites. Very little intact drug is excreted unchanged in the urine.

Diazepam

Diazepam (Valium) has a half-life of 20–50 hours and also has active metabolites (e.g. desmethyldiazepam) that have even longer half-lives and may cause a delayed sedative effect. Full recovery may take 48–72 hours.

Diazepam, producing less amnesia than midazolam, may be beneficial in weaning patients off pharmacological sedation and is available in an organic preparation as Diazemuls, which is much less irritant on injection than Valium. Diazepam for injection is insoluble in water and is supplied in propylene glycol, which is irritant to endothelium. This can lead to thrombophlebitis. Accidental intra-arterial injection in the antecubital fossa has been known to cause such severe arteriole spasm that the ensuing ischaemia has resulted in the loss of digits.

Midazolam

Midazolam has a shorter half-life than diazepam; in normal subjects, it is 1.5–3 hours. It is, therefore, much more appropriate for dental sedation. It also has active metabolites (e.g. 1-hydroxymethylmidazolam glucuronide), but the elimination half-life of these is so short that they are of no significance in clinical practice and recovery is usually complete in 8 hours. Midazolam also offers the advantages of deeper sedation, more potent anterograde amnesia and less irritation on injection; it is, therefore, the current drug of choice for i.v. sedation. It is water soluble, hence the minimal local irritation on injection, but becomes highly lipophilic at physiological pH and enters the brain rapidly.

Temazepam

An alternative to diazepam for oral use is temazepam (Normison), which has a short half-life and no active metabolites.

Sedation techniques

The sedation technique required will vary according to a particular patient's needs. One patient may require oral sedation alone, while another may require oral premedication followed by i.v. sedation. Individual susceptibility to sedative agents varies widely, and a suitable dosage regimen has to be established for each patient. Written informed consent to treatment under sedation must be obtained prior to treatment.

Oral sedation

Oral sedation in child dental patients is useful but the effects are sometimes unpredictable and individual dose requirements vary considerably. Sometimes children become hostile with oral sedation. In adult patients, oral sedation may also be an effective way of managing anxiety and nitrazepam, diazepam and temazepam are the most popular in the UK. The preoperative and postoperative instructions that are given to patients having i.v. sedation also apply to those having oral sedation (Fig. 30).

Nitrazepam has a prolonged action and may, therefore, give rise to residual effects the following day. Diazepam also has a long half-life but does not interfere with dream sleep to the same extent. Temazepam has the shortest half-life and is, therefore, preferred. It may be given in a dose of 10–30 mg for adults and is very effective at the larger dose, producing a degree of sedation similar to that seen with the i.v. technique.

BEFORE YOUR APPOINTMENT

1. Your may eat and drink up to two hours before your appointment, but this last meal should be a light one.
2. Bring with you an adult friend or relative (over 18) who will be responsible for caring for you afterwards. You are asked to make your own arrangements for transport home after your treatment and this should be in a car or in a taxi.
3. Take your routine medicines at the usual times and discuss any medicines you are taking, before your sedation starts.
4. Please inform us if you think that you may be pregnant.

AFTER YOUR TREATMENT

Although you may think that you have recovered quite quickly, the effects of your sedation may not have worn off entirely for the rest of the day. It is important that until the next day you:

1. Do not take alcohol in any form.
2. Do not drive any vehicle, or operate any machinery, or go out alone.
3. Do not take important decisions, such as buying expensive items or signing important documents.

Fig. 30 Typical instructions for patients undergoing intravenous sedation.

Individual susceptibility has already been mentioned and this is particularly a problem with oral sedation, as is the optimal timing of the dose owing to the variability of gastric absorption. By comparison, inhalational and i.v. sedative techniques allow individual titration of drug doses by the dentist at the time of treatment. Oral sedation involves estimating the required drug dosage and this is sometimes difficult. It does not permit individual titration of a drug against a clinical response. It is usually prescribed for administration about 1–1.5 hours before dental treatment is due to start. Oral sedation may also be used the night before treatment to permit sleep in an anxious patient who may otherwise not sleep. Temazepam is available as tablets, capsules or oral solution. It is worth remembering when prescribing that, while the capsules provide excellent absorption, capsules are currently a popular drug of abuse, the contents being used for self-injection in combination with other drugs. There is also the risk of the patient having sexual fantasies, as there is with the i.v. benzodiazepine technique.

Inhalation sedation

Inhalation sedation is suitable for children and adults alike but as it is particularly successful when the administration of gases is accompanied by hypnotic suggestion in the form of confident reassurance and encouragement, it is especially successful with children. This group of patients often exhibit anxiety transposed from their parents' own fear of dentistry. It is a very simple and safe technique and allows for rapid sedation and equally rapid reversal. Special equipment is required to administer nitrous oxide and oxygen at precise concentrations and flow rates (Fig. 31). This equipment must be unable to provide less than 30% oxygen. A special nasal breathing mask is needed and should be provided with scavenging to reduce the nitrous oxide pollution of the surgery. Disposable nasal masks

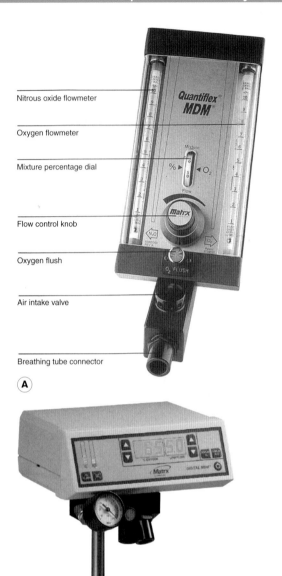

Nitrous oxide flowmeter

Oxygen flowmeter

Mixture percentage dial

Flow control knob

Oxygen flush

Air intake valve

Breathing tube connector

Fig. 31 A, a typical flow meter to administer nitrous oxide and oxygen inhalation sedation; **B,** a digital version of the inhalational sedation apparatus.

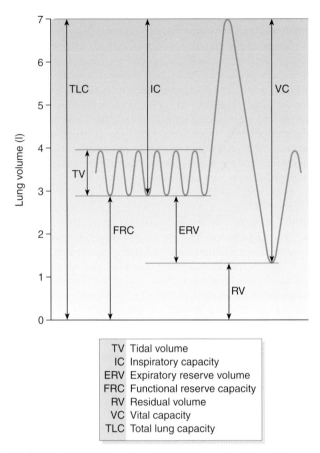

TV	Tidal volume
IC	Inspiratory capacity
ERV	Expiratory reserve volume
FRC	Functional reserve capacity
RV	Residual volume
VC	Vital capacity
TLC	Total lung capacity

Fig. 32 Physiological lung volumes. Tidal volume can be increased by taking a deeper breath in or out, using the inspiratory capacity or expiratory reserve volume, respectively. The volume of air breathed out after the largest possible inspiration followed by the largest expiration is the vital capacity.

with strawberry or other pleasant impregnated odours are available to enhance the acceptability of masks.

Nitrous oxide is administered by titration, such that the drug is delivered in increments and the patient response monitored until the desired level of sedation is achieved. Titration allows precise control of the level of sedation. A 10% nitrous oxide and 90% oxygen mixture is administered initially for a period of about 3 minutes and then the concentration of nitrous oxide is increased if necessary in increments of 5% every 2–3 minutes until the desired level of sedation is achieved and up to a maximum of 70% nitrous oxide. The patient is discouraged from talking so that the nitrous oxide is not diluted by mouth breathing. The gas flow rate is adjusted by the sedationist to maintain the patient's pulmonary ventilation, which is a product of the tidal volume (Fig. 32) and the respiratory rate.

Although individual susceptibility varies, a plane of sedation and analgesia has been described with concentrations of 5–25% nitrous oxide, at which the patient may experience tingling in the hands and feet. This is accompanied by marked relaxation, anxiolysis and elevation of the pain threshold. At concentrations of 20–55% nitrous oxide, a deeper plane of dissociation occurs, and sedation and analgesia is experienced. This is frequently accompanied by a general tingling of the body and the patient may experience a slight humming or buzzing in the ears. A plane of total analgesia is described with concentrations of 50–70%. However, since consciousness may be lost at concentrations as low as 50%, it is prudent to decrease the level of sedation if a patient is thought to be entering this plane, and some would limit the maximum concentration for administration of nitrous oxide to 50%. While described as the plane of total analgesia, the analgesia is not sufficient to permit dental extractions to be performed. The laryngeal reflex becomes partially impaired and verbal contact starts to be lost. The ability to maintain an open mouth independently is lost. It is, therefore, essential not to use a mouth prop during inhalation sedation so that this plane is readily recognised.

The patient should be advised of the sensations to be expected prior to their experience of them and, as there is some individual variation of the nitrous oxide concentrations that induce the above planes, it is useful if the patient indicates when they occur. The patient may be reassured that they can lighten the level of their sedation at any time by breathing through their mouth. At the completion of treatment, 100% oxygen should be administered to the patient to prevent diffusion hypoxia and also to reduce the pollution of the local air with exhaled nitrous oxide. If too high a concentration of nitrous oxide is administered to a patient, they may enter the excitement plane of anaesthesia, become agitated and complain of palpitations. Complete psychomotor recovery is usually expected 22 minutes after exposure to 30% nitrous oxide for 40 minutes.

Intravenous sedation

The i.v. route is very effective and benzodiazepines provide excellent patient sedation, but the technique requires a higher level of training than does the inhalational sedation technique. The patient should be in the supine position for sedation.

Dosage

Midazolam for i.v. injection is available as 10 mg/2 ml or 10 mg/5 ml. In most circumstances, the latter is more convenient as titration is easier. Over 30 seconds, 2 mg midazolam is administered via an indwelling cannula with the patient in the supine position. If, after 2 minutes, sedation is not adequate, incremental doses of 0.5–1 mg are given until the desired sedation end-point is achieved. Adequate sedation is demonstrated by drowsiness and slurred speech but response to commands will be maintained. Drooping of the eyelid half-way across the pupil (Verrill's sign), frequently observed with diazepam, is *not* usually seen with midazolam. The usual dose range is 2.5–7.5 mg total dose. The drug manufacturers suggest a dose of approximately 0.07 mg/kg body weight. The final dose is, however, determined by titration against response and not by calculation. The elderly are more sensitive to the effects of benzodiazepines, and as little as 1–2 mg midazolam in total may be adequate. Patients weighing less than 45 kg require a reduced initial dose.

Venous access

It is important to have continuous venous access during i.v. sedation as the midazolam is administered incrementally and it also enables swift administration of resuscitation drugs should the need arise. An indwelling flexible teflon cannula is less likely to 'cut-out' of a vein than an indwelling steel needle. The two most convenient sites for venepuncture are the antecubital fossa and the dorsum of the hand. The latter offers the advantages of a flat, stable, immobile surface with very little risk of damage to structures such as nerves or arteries. Veins slip easily from beneath the needle and should be fixed by gentle traction of the overlying skin, achieved by finger and thumb pressure beside the underlying vessel. Start the venepuncture at the junction of tributaries, if evident, as the veins will be relatively fixed (Fig. 33). A normal saline flush may be used to ensure patency and correct placement before any drug is administered. The cannula should remain in place until recovery is complete and the patient goes home.

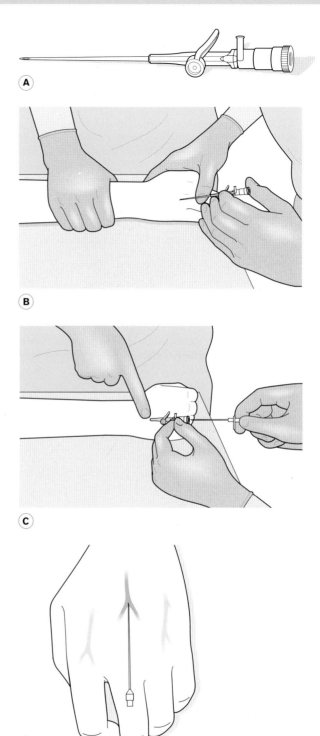

Fig. 33 Intravenous cannulation of the dorsum of the hand. **A,** The cannula. **B, C,** The cannulation procedure. **D,** Using the junction of tributaries, if this is evident, may help to stabilise veins.

Amnesia

Midazolam produces good sedation and profound amnesia such that the patient cannot recall anything for a 20 minute period following the induction of sedation. Occasionally, this period is much longer and patients are unable to remember how they got home when questioned later.

The duration and quality of amnesia are difficult to predict. It is for this reason that it is essential to provide instructions and advice in a written form to the patient having sedation and in advance of the appointment (Fig. 30). Hallucinations, some of a sexual nature, are another effect of benzodiazepine sedation and, although uncommon, may be of profound significance if the dentist, male or female, is unchaperoned and unable to counter possible claims of assault. This cannot occur if the dentist always has a second person present during treatment under i.v. sedation to assist with the monitoring of the patient and also to be ready to assist with the management of any emergency that might arise. It is important to avoid putting oneself at risk by being alone with the patient during the recovery phase. It is sensible to ask the patient's escort to join them at this point.

Analgesia

Benzodiazepine sedation may affect a patient's perception of pain but does not offer any clinically useful analgesia, and an LA must, therefore, be used where appropriate. A mouth prop is usually necessary because of the muscle relaxation after i.v. sedation. The patient should be kept under supervision until at least 1 hour has elapsed from the time of the last incremental injection. They should always be accompanied home by a responsible adult who can then stay with them. They should be warned not to drive or operate machinery for 8 hours and to be accessible to their escort for the rest of the day (e.g. do not lock bathroom doors).

Preoperative starvation

The question of whether a patient should be starved or not prior to i.v. sedation is a controversial one. Some operators believe that all patients should be starved from solid food for 4 hours and clear fluids for 2 hours preoperatively (as for a GA) because, while the risk of laryngeal reflex impairment is small, the consequences may be grave should there be regurgitation of stomach contents and lung aspiration. Others believe that obtundment of the laryngeal reflex is so unlikely to occur during the conscious sedation techniques required for dentistry that it is unnecessary to starve all patients, particularly when the treatment being carried out is likely to prevent an early return to food and drink and the patient may consequently remain starved for a considerable period of time. Certainly most operators currently prefer patients to abstain from alcohol for 24 hours prior to sedation and request that the last meal before sedation should be a light non-fatty one. It is reasonable to starve patients from food and drink for 2 hours only prior to treatment. Some sedationists starve their patients as for a GA and infuse crystalloid solutions for rehydration purposes, but this would be unusual in the UK.

Monitoring sedated patients

Monitoring depth of sedation and the patients physiological variables is done clinically and electromechanically.

Sedation. The level of sedation and consciousness must be monitored clinically by the dentist and the assistant. The patient should be relaxed, cooperative and responsive to verbal contact. Adequately sedated patients are sometimes described as exhibiting an expressionless face, as their facial muscles relax. The psychomotor ability of patients becomes impaired and this may be witnessed by asking a patient to bring a finger to his or her nose. It will be observed that the movement is slow and inaccurate.

Respiration. The rate and depth of chest and abdominal movements should be monitored. Any signs of cyanosis should be noted and acted upon. Respiratory depression and even respiratory arrest have occurred with midazolam, especially in elderly patients, those with pre-existing respiratory insufficiency and particularly if excessive or too rapidly injected doses are administered. During inhalation sedation, the movement of the reservoir bag is a useful guide to respiratory rate and depth.

Oxygenation. For i.v. sedation, the use of a pulse oximeter is essential. This non-invasive monitor can provide rapid and accurate recording of arterial oxygen saturation and pulse rate, and therefore provides an invaluable check of the respiratory and cardiovascular function. Pulse oximetry is able to detect changes in oxygenation earlier than one can by clinical observation. The saturation of haemoglobin is calculated by measuring absorption of different wavelengths of haemoglobin and deoxyhaemoglobin. It is worth remembering that should the patient be anaemic (i.e. have less than about 10 g/dl (6.3 mmol/l) haemoglobin) the little haemoglobin present may be very well oxygenated even though the oxygen-carrying capacity of the blood is much compromised. Pulse oximetry is not necessary during inhalation sedation unless the patient has cardio-respiratory compromise.

Heart rate. Continuous electrocardiographic monitoring is not normally required as it provides no indication of the adequacy of the circulation and may lull the observer into a false sense of security. However, it may be a useful adjunct to oximetry in patients with cardiovascular risk factors and should be used if more than one drug is used for i.v. sedation. It is more likely to be used in the hospital environment.

Recovery. If patients are to be moved to a separate area for recovery, they should not be left alone but rather their escort should be asked to join them. Pulse oximetry should be continued during the recovery period and the area should be adequately equipped for resuscitation.

The patient's escort should remain with them for the rest of the day.

4.4 General anaesthesia

● ●

Learning objectives

You should:
- understand how local anaesthetics work
- know the potency, speed of onset and duration of action of common agents
- be aware of reasons for failure of anaesthesia and complications that can occur
- know the safe dosages of common local anaesthetic drugs.

GA can be used either in a day case or an inpatient setting (Table 9).

Table 9 Day case or inpatient general anaesthesia

Criterion	Day case	Inpatient
Type of surgery	Minor	Intermediate or major
Patient's health	Completely fit and well or minor well-controlled medical condition	Pre-existing medical condition, but also completely well
Premedication	Not usually given as may delay recovery	Usually used

Patient assessment

Social history

Age. It is generally agreed that elderly patients are subject to increased risks of anaesthesia and surgery. They are more likely to have diseases of cardiovascular or respiratory systems and multiple drug treatment. There is an increase in the risk of postoperative dementia.

Smoking. Smoking causes damage to blood vessels of peripheral, coronary and cerebral circulations, carcinoma of lung and chronic bronchitis. Cigarette smoke contains carbon monoxide, which may reduce the oxygen carried by haemoglobin by 25%. Patients should stop smoking for at least 12 hours before anaesthesia as this leads to an increase in arterial oxygen. The effects of smoking on the respiratory tract leads to a sixfold increase in postoperative respiratory infection and ideally patients should stop smoking for 6 weeks before anaesthesia to reduce this risk.

Alcohol. Regular intake of alcohol leads to a reduction of liver enzymes and tolerance to anaesthetic drugs. Excessive alcohol intake leads to liver and heart damage and withdrawal leads to tremor and hallucinations (i.e. delirium tremens).

Home circumstances. The availability of an escort to accompany the patient home and stay with them for the rest of the day is essential for day case anaesthesia.

Drug abuse. There may be drug interactions and inadequate venous access in the i.v. drug abuser. There is also an increased risk of the patient having an infectious disease such as human immunodeficiency virus (HIV) or hepatitis B virus.

Hereditary problems

Porphyria. An inherited group of disorders in which there are errors in the synthesis of haem, resulting in the excessive production of porphyrins causing illness. An acute attack may be triggered by some drugs such as barbiturates in addition to alcohol and some antibiotics resulting in colicky abdominal pain with vomiting or constipation, proteinuria, peripheral neuritis, paralysis, hyponatraemia and hypokalaemia.

Malignant hyperpyrexia. Malignant hyperpyrexia or malignant hyperthermia (MH) is an inherited disorder showing marked increase in metabolic rate triggered by some drugs such as suxamethonium (succinylcholine) and any volatile agent. The body temperature may rise at more that 2°C per hour. The specific treatment is with dantrolene, and the patient should be cooled with body surface exposure, cooling blankets, and cool irrigation fluids. There is a high mortality (40%).

Scoline (suxamethonium) apnoea. A few people metabolise suxamethonium very slowly so that its duration of action is several hours rather than 5 minutes. A patient will then require ventilation until the effect of this muscle relaxant has worn off. Confirmation is by plasma cholinesterase assay to determine genotype.

Previous anaesthetic history

It is important to ask about any previous problems with allergies, difficult intubation or awareness during GA.

Physical examination

The appropriateness and extent of a physical examination will be determined by the history. In addition to the usual examination, examination of the teeth and mouth opening and neck mobility will give indication of ease of tracheal intubation. Also, a small mandible and soft-tissue fullness of the neck may indicate a compromised airway (Fig. 34).

Special investigations

The clinical history and examination are the best method of screening for disease, and routine tests in those who are apparently healthy on clinical examination are usually of little use and a waste of money. The indications for special investigations before dental treatment or surgery under GA are given below together with a note of those for whom the tests would be unnecessary.

Haemoglobin concentration

Indications are:

- history of blood loss or trauma
- anticipated blood loss > 10% total blood volume
- cardiorespiratory disease
- female patients
- male patient > 65 years of age
- haematological disorder.

Unnecessary for healthy male patients <65 years and children having minor surgery.

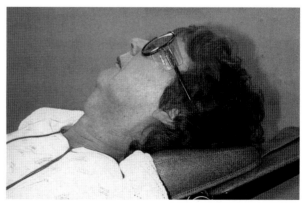

Fig. 34 Compromised airway in patient at rest because of small mandible and soft tissues of the neck.

Urinalysis

Indications are:

- may reveal undiagnosed diabetic
- may reveal presence of renal disease or urinary tract infection.

This is an inexpensive, simple investigation.

Sickle test

Indications are:

- Afro-Caribbeans or mixed-race Afro-Caribbeans for whom sickle status is unknown
- potential hypoxia, dehydration, acidosis or pain if anaesthesia provokes sickle crisis.

Unnecesssary if status is already known.

Urea and electrolyte (U&E) concentrations

Indications are:

- diuretic treatment
- hypertension
- heart or renal failure
- diabetes.
- patients > 65 years of age.

Unnecessary for most patients having minor surgery.

Blood glucose concentration

Indication is:

- diabetic patients.

Unnecessary for any other patients.

Liver function tests (LFTs)

Liver function tests include screening for clotting status. Indications are:

- surgery rather than anaesthesia
- liver disease
- alcoholism
- previous hepatitis.

Unnecessary in other patients.

Clotting studies

Indications are:

- known bleeding disorder or coagulopathy
- anticoagulant therapy
- recent transfusion
- unexplained blood loss
- liver disorder
- renal failure.

Unnecessary for all other patients.

Chest X-ray

Indications are:

- clinical signs of acute heart and lung disease
- malignancy.

Unnecessary in patients with uncomplicated angina, asthma and chronic obstructive airways disease.

Cervical spine X-ray

Indication is:

- rheumatoid arthritis with unstable neck (requires flexion and extension views).

Unnecessary in other patients.

Electrocardiogram (ECG)

Indications are:

- known arrhythmias, angina, history of myocardial infarction
- hypertension
- heart failure
- males > 40 and females > 50 years of age, as increased risk of ischaemic heart disease
- electrolyte imbalance
- diabetes
- renal disease.

Unnecessary in other patients and those who have had a recent electrocardiogram.

Pulmonary function tests

Indications are:

- very severe asthma with limited exercise tolerance
- assessment of lung disease: sophisticated tests of pulmonary function are no more useful than simple tests such as vital capacity and forced expiratory volume (FEV_1)
- need for intermittent positive pressure ventilation (IPPV) in the postoperative period: blood gas analysis is the most sensitive method of predicting this requirement.

Weight

The patient's weight is needed for the calculation of drug doses.

Obese patients have increased risk of postoperative complications (e.g. deep-vein thrombosis (DVT), chest infection).

Risk assessment

Is the patient in optimum physical condition for anaesthesia? Are the anticipated benefits of surgery greater than the anaesthetic and surgical risks produced by the medical condition? The most significant diseases for morbidity assessment are cardiovascular: heart failure, heart valve disease or recent myocardial infarction.

Predictors of risk are:

- clinical assessment: ASA greater than class III
- cardiac disease
- respiratory disease
- pulmonary abnormalities, confirmed by chest X-ray
- electrocardiogram abnormalities
- length and extent of surgery.

Grading of physical status

The ASA classification of physical status facilitates communication and patient comparison. Patients are allocated to a class between I and V depending on the severity of their general medical condition, I being the least severe and V the most severe (Table 8, p. 51).

Cardiovascular disease

The risk of postoperative reinfarction is related to the time interval between the first myocardial infarction and surgery. An interval of 6 months or less is associated with the highest incidence of reinfarction.

Hypertension

A diastolic pressure of 110 mmHg or more has increased risk of postoperative myocardial infarction.

Respiratory disease

Patients at risk of developing postoperative respiratory complications (chest infection) include smokers, those with pre-existing lung disease, and the obese.

Age

It is generally agreed that the elderly are subject to increased risks of anaesthesia and surgery. This is mainly because of increased cardiovascular and respiratory disease in the elderly.

Preoperative therapy

Having taken a history and carried out a physical examination, some preoperative preparation may be required before carrying out anaesthesia. Some preparation may be done on the inpatient ward:

- preoperative antibiotics as prophylaxis against subacute bacterial endocarditis
- chest physiotherapy and antibiotics for chest infection
- diabetic management: follow hospital protocol
  - diet-controlled diabetes: measure blood sugar; patients rarely require treatment
  - oral treatment: measure blood sugar, omit treatment 12–24 hours before surgery
  - insulin-dependent: measure blood sugar, give 5% glucose infusion with insulin.

Some conditions may require postponing surgery and referral to other specialities:

- uncontrolled/worsening angina, palpitations: cardiology referral
- hypertension: general practitioner for stabilisation and arrange surgery for 6 weeks
- uncontrolled chest disease: respiratory physician.

This decision should be taken in conjunction with the anaesthetist.

Preoperative medication

Premedication may be prescribed to:

- reduce anxiety
- reduce postoperative pain
- reduce postoperative nausea and vomiting
- produce amnesia
- reduce stomach acidity in pregnancy or hiatus hernia
- reduce vagal tone in those prone to bradycardia
- reduce secretions.

Drugs used for premedication include:

- benzodiazepines: diazepam, temazepam
- opioid analgesics: morphine, pethidine, papaveretum
- NSAIDs: diclofenac (Voltarol)
- antiemetics: metoclopramide, prochlorperazine
- antacid: histamine H_2 antagonist
- antivagal drug: atropine
- anticholinergic agents: atropine, hyoscine (scopolamine).

Preoperative starvation

Patients are starved before a GA to reduce the likelihood of regurgitation of stomach contents followed by aspiration into lungs. Traditionally, patients are starved from liquids and solid foods from midnight for elective morning surgery or from 7 a.m. for elective afternoon surgery. There is now evidence that clear fluids (e.g. cup of tea) up to 2 hours before surgery is safe.

Patients going into hospital for day surgery are given a set of instructions (Fig. 35).

Emergency surgery. The period of starvation depends on risk of aspiration versus risk of not carrying out surgery. There is a delay in gastric emptying if pain or trauma occur or if opioid analgesics are used.

---

1. Do not have anything to eat or to drink from midnight of the night before your operation. This includes early morning drinks.
2. Please bring with you a responsible friend or relative (over 18 years), who may then return later to accompany you home. You will not be allowed home on public transport or in a taxi alone. You must make your own arrangements to be collected and accompanied from hospital.
3. If you have a cold or are unwell near the time of your attendance, please telephone the hospital.
4. It is advisable not to consume alcohol or smoke for 24 hours prior to your operation.
5. Leave all jewellery at home.
6. Remove all nail varnish and heavy make-up.

Although you will be in hospital for one day only, you may feel slightly unwell for a day or two and, if so, you should remain in bed. It would also be wise to avoid making any social or other arrangements for a few days after your operation; you may even need to remain off work for a similar period.

Fig. 35 Typical instructions given to a patient who will undergo morning day case surgery under general anaesthesia.

General anaesthesia technique

Conduct of a general anaesthetic

Induction

Standard monitoring is placed with the patient in the supine position. Oxygen is administered and then anaesthesia is induced with a short-acting agent, such as propofol, via the intravenous route, or more rarely by inhalation of an anaesthetic agent such as sevoflurane. The latter may be used for children or adults with a fear of needles. A short-acting muscle relaxant is then administered to relax the vocal cords and enable tracheal intubation. The cuff around the tube is inflated and an oropharyngeal pack is placed to further protect the airway from blood and debris from the mouth when oral surgery is undertaken. The tube is secured with tape and the eyes are protected, usually by taping closed. Respiration is maintained by intermittent positive pressure ventilation. For very short procedures the patient may not be intubated and a laryngeal mask may be used instead with the patient breathing spontaneously.

Maintenance

Other lines such as arterial or central venous lines may be inserted. A nasogastric tube, temperature probe and urinary catheter if appropriate are sited. Anaesthesia is maintained with an inhalation agent such as isoflurane or sevoflurane. Alternatively it may be maintained with propofol using a total intravenous anaesthesia (TIVA) technique. The patient also receives oxygen (33%) and nitrous oxide (66%) and is monitored. Muscle relaxation is continued and the patient ventilated unless the patient is to breathe spontaneously with the airway maintained by a laryngeal mask for a very short procedure. The patient is positioned appropriately for the surgical procedure on the operating table and the head and limbs are protected with padding at pressure points or where nerves may be in danger of compression. Hyperextension or over-rotation of the neck and limbs are avoided. Intermittent compression devices are placed around the calves for long procedures or where there are other increased risks of deep-vein thrombosis.

Recovery

The anaesthetic and muscle relaxant drugs are stopped or reversed. Emergence from anaesthesia can be expected 2–3 minutes after stopping sevoflurane or desflurane. The surgeon removes the oropharyngeal pack and clears the mouth and oropharynx of blood and debris with a large-bore suction tube. Extubation is a critical moment and may be done as the patient awakes or with the patient in the lateral position and still deeply anaesthetised. Oxygen is administered via a therapy mask and the patient monitored.

Monitoring during anaesthesia

In addition to the clinical observation and pulse oximetry used during conscious sedation, additional electromechanical monitoring is required during anaesthesia. Arterial blood pressure, electrocardiography (ECG) and capnography are mandatory.

Cardiovascular system

Standard lead II positions using three electrodes are used for ECG monitoring during anaesthesia and provide information on the cardiac rate and rhythm. Pulse oximetry provides information on peripheral blood haemoglobin oxygen saturation. Arterial blood pressure can be measured manually with a stethoscope and sphygmomanometer or with automated oscillometry or directly and provides information on cardiac output and peripheral resistance. To measure blood pressure directly, an arterial cannula is placed in a peripheral artery such as the radial artery at the wrist. Central venous pressure may also be measured with a catheter via an arm vein, internal jugular or subclavian with its tip in the superior vena cava. The patient may also have a urinary catheter placed so that urine output can be measured hourly.

Respiratory system

Anaesthetic machines continuously measure airway pressure as part of the alarm system should the pressure fall because the circuit becomes detached from the patient. Capnography measures expired carbon dioxide by sampling gas and comparing with a reference. Confirmation of the correct placement of a tracheal tube is provided by detection of carbon dioxide in the expired gas.

Neuromuscular junction

Assessment of neuromuscular blockade provides an indication of onset and recovery from muscle relaxant drugs.

Body temperature

General anaesthesia inhibits temperature maintenance in patients and so temperature measurement is important. Also, the temperature of the theatre and fluids for replacement should be considered alongside exposure of large areas of the patient's body surface. Temperature probes may be inserted into the nasopharynx, oesophagus or rectum.

Depth of anaesthesia

Bispectral index (BIS) is used in some countries to measure the depth of anaesthesia. This is done non-invasively by recording EEG via forehead electrodes.

Self-assessment: questions

Multiple choice questions

1. Adequate analgesia:
   a. After oral surgery is most appropriately provided by a non-steroidal anti-inflammatory analgesic (NSAID)
   b. After maxillofacial injury, is best provided by opioids
   c. Provided by paracetamol may cause liver damage
   d. Provided by opioids may cause respiratory depression
   e. In terminal disease should be provided when necessary rather than continuously to avoid tolerance

2. Dental local anaesthetics:
   a. Cross the placenta during pregnancy
   b. May result in an immune reaction in patients allergic to latex
   c. May be administered via the periodontal ligament
   d. Include ethyl chloride
   e. Applied topically prevent the pain on injection for inferior alveolar nerve blocks

3. The vasoconstrictor adrenaline (epinephrine) added to local anaesthetic:
   a. Should not be used in hyperthyroid patients
   b. Is contraindicated for use in patients with ischaemic heart disease
   c. May be dangerous if used for a patient who is abusing cocaine
   d. Is less safe than felypressin for use in patients with heart disease
   e. Interacts with tricyclic antidepressants, resulting in hypertension

4. When using an intravenous sedative technique with midazolam:
   a. Airway protection is not appropriate
   b. Reversal may be accomplished with a bolus injection of 500 mg flumazenil
   c. The patient should be monitored with a pulse oximeter that is set to alarm should the oxygen saturation fall below 80%
   d. Supplemental oxygen therapy is not necessary for all patients
   e. Slight changes in blood pressure occur

5. Nitrous oxide when used for inhalational sedation:
   a. May cause hypoxia
   b. Is stored in metal cylinders in both liquid and gaseous states
   c. Must always be administered with oxygen
   d. Allows for the most rapid recovery of all current sedation techniques
   e. Provides good anxiolysis but no analgesia

Extended matching items

EMI 1. Theme: Local anaesthesia

Options:

A 9 cartridges (2.2 ml) lidocaine
B 7 cartridges (2.2 ml) lidocaine
C 6 ml of 0.5% bupivicaine
D 8 cartridges (2.2 ml) articaine
E Allergic reaction
F Intravascular injection
G Vaso-vagal attack
H Medial pterygoid muscle haematoma
I Posterior superior dental block
J Infra-orbital nerve block

Lead in: Select the most appropriate answer from the list above for each of the following cases. Each option can be used once, more than once or not at all.

1. A healthy adult male requires the removal of multiple teeth using local anaesthesia. He is given the maximum safe dose of local anaesthetic solution at the first treatment session to reduce the number of visits and because he has pain from several of the teeth.
2. A 55-year-old patient tells her new dentist that she is allergic to local anaesthetic following a previous incident when she felt very unwell, experienced palpitations and required oxygen.
3. A 20-year-old patient returns to the practice 10 days following the removal of the lower second molar, complaining that he is unable to open his mouth widely.
4. A patient requires endodontic surgery to the upper first premolar under local anaesthesia.
5. A patient has injections of a local anaesthetic whilst under general anaesthesia for the surgical removal of both mandibular wisdom teeth. These have been administered by the surgeon to improve the postoperative pain experience for the patient.

EMI 2. Theme: Analgesia

Options:

A Unselective NSAIDs
B COX-2 NSAIDs (coxibs)
C Morphine
D Fentanyl
E Pethidine
F Naloxone
G Tramadol
H Methadone
I Tricyclic antidepressant drugs
J Paracetamol

Lead in: Select the most appropriate answer from the list above for each of the following cases. Each option can be used once, more than once or not at all.

1. This group of analgesics are excellent for mild to moderate postoperative oral surgery pain but 20–40% patients may develop symptomless gastric erosions.

2. The risk of fatal haemorrhage is increased fivefold when this group of analgesics is used in patients over the age of 75 years.

3. This drug is available for administration by the oral, subcutaneous, intramuscular, intravenous and rectal routes. It is the drug of first choice for severe postoperative pain for in-patients.

4. This drug acts centrally, inhibiting brain cyclo-oxygenase and nitric oxide synthase. This central inhibition of CNS cyclo-oxygenase reduces the production of prostaglandins but is not antipyretic and has no peripheral anti-inflammatory effect.

5. More than 10 g/day of this drug may be toxic but the recommended therapeutic dose is very unlikely to cause toxicity.

Case history questions

Case history 1

A referral from an orthodontist requests the extraction of four first premolar teeth from a 14-year-old girl who is a resident at a local boarding school. She has a well cared for mouth and has had very little dentistry carried our previously. There is no relevant medical history.

Discuss your management.

Case history 2

A 22-year-old male attends for pain relief from an acute dental abscess. He has a history of using intravenous heroin and is currently taking methadone as part of his treatment for opioid dependence. On examination, he has multiple grossly carious teeth that require removal. He is anxious about the prospect of receiving dental treatment of any sort.

1. What treatment plan would be sensible?

2. How should this patient receive sedation/analgesia?

Self-assessment: answers

Multiple choice answers

1. a. **True.** As surgery causes inflammatory pain, then it is beneficial to use an analgesic that is also anti-inflammatory. NSAIDs act principally by inhibiting prostaglandin production by the enzyme cyclooxygenase in peripheral tissues but also in part in the central nervous system. There is a mismatch between the anti-inflammatory potency of these drugs and their analgesic activity, and many are relatively more selective for the constitutive form of cyclooxygenase, COX-1, than for the form of the enzyme that is induced in inflammation, COX-2. It is believed that COX-1 predominates in the stomach, yielding protective prostaglandins, and COX-2 is induced in inflammation, giving rise to pain and swelling, hence the development of COX-2 inhibitors as potentially gastro-safe NSAIDs.

   b. **False.** Maxillofacial trauma may be associated with head injury and opioids may interfere with neurological observations that are required. Codeine does not cause a problem and may be safely used.

   c. **False.** Paracetamol is one of the most widely used of all drugs and with proper use seldom causes adverse events or reports of serious side-effects. Therapeutic doses of paracetamol are, therefore, unlikely to cause liver damage and indeed paracetamol is commonly used for analgesia and fever in alcoholic patients. However, single doses of more than ten times the recommended dose are potentially toxic and can result in hepatic cellular injury.

   d. **False.** Opioids used for patients who are not in pain, or in doses larger than necessary to control pain, can depress respiration. However, opioids at doses used to provide adequate analgesia do not cause respiratory depression.

   e. **False.** The aim of pain management in terminal disease is for continuous pain relief, and this is best achieved by regular rather than when required administration of analgesia. Tolerance may develop but should not deter from providing effective pain relief.

2. a. **True.** Local anaesthetics cross the placenta by passive diffusion but are generally not harmful unless excessive amounts are administered. The drug of choice is lidocaine with adrenaline (epinephrine). Local anaesthetics also enter breast milk.

   b. **True.** The local anaesthetic itself contains no latex but the bung inside the cartridge may contain latex and this may be sufficient to provoke an allergic reaction.

   c. **True.** Intraligamentary or periodontal ligament anaesthesia is most often used as a supplementary method to conventional injection techniques. The solution is injected slowly under high pressure using a specially designed syringe. The technique may cause the tooth to be tender to percussion, which is a consideration when used for conservative dentistry but not when removing the tooth.

   d. **True.** Ethyl chloride is supplied as a liquid in a glass container. It is sprayed onto the oral mucosa where it evaporates, cooling the surface sufficiently to cause freezing and consequent anaesthesia. This technique has been traditionally used to anaesthetise mucosa over an abscess prior to its incision to permit drainage. The method is technique sensitive and less popular now. Ethyl chloride is also used on cotton wool pledgets to investigate the vitality of teeth.

   e. **False.** Topically applied local anaesthetics such as lidocaine produce anaesthesia of the oral mucosa to a depth of about 2–3 mm, which is not sufficient to prevent the pain of needle penetration through deeper tissues during an inferior alveolar nerve block.

3. a. **True.** Adrenaline (epinephrine) could precipitate a thyroid crisis in a hyperthyroid patient. However, there is no problem in patients who are taking thyroid replacement therapy.

   b. **False.** It is important to prevent large increases in heart rate in patients with ischaemic heart disease as this may precipitate cardiac ischaemic pain (i.e. angina) or a myocardial infarction. However, adrenaline (epinephrine) in a dental cartridge of local anaesthesia is not absolutely contraindicated. An aspirating technique should always be used for all patients, whether they suffer from ischaemic heart disease or not, and this will reduce the likelihood of inadvertently injecting adrenaline (epinephrine) intravenously. The maximum dose should be limited to about three cartridges, particularly if the heart disease is not well controlled. The patient should be managed with as much care as possible to ensure that they remain relaxed during the treatment. It is sometimes sensible to sedate these patients to ensure that they do not become physiologically stressed, although this should be undertaken in a hospital setting. Inhalational sedation is particularly useful for this group of patients. Adrenaline (epinephrine) should be avoided in patients with refractory arrhythmias and in those who have had a recent myocardial infarction, when plain 4% prilocaine is recommended.

   c. **True.** A patient who has used cocaine in the 24 hours before receiving a dental local anaesthetic containing adrenaline (epinephrine) is at risk of greatly increased adrenergic responses. The tachycardia may be significant enough to lead to a cardiac arrhythmia such as ventricular tachycardia.

d. **False.** High doses of felypressin may result in vasoconstriction of the coronary vessels and precipitate ischaemic cardiac pain. The maximum dose should be limited to about three cartridges in patients with ischaemic heart disease.

e. **False.** Tricyclic antidepressants prevent the presynaptic reuptake of noradrenaline (norepinephrine) and 5-HT (serotonin) and work by potentiating the effects of these neurotransmitters. Theoretically, exaggerated adrenergic effects such as hypertension could result when patients also receive adrenaline (epinephrine) in a dental injection. However, there is no evidence that this occurs in practice.

4. a. **False.** When excessive water, blood or debris are anticipated to collect in the mouth, then it may be advisable to protect the oropharynx with, for example, a butterfly sponge with a tie extra-orally. When carrying out oral surgery such as the removal of wisdom teeth, it is not possible to place a barrier behind the surgical area without triggering a pharyngeal gag reflex. Adequate high-velocity aspiration must always be available whether or not a physical barrier is employed.

b. **False.** Should reversal with flumazenil be necessary, an initial dose of 200 mg should be administered intravenously over 15 seconds. If the desired level of consciousness is not obtained within 60 seconds, further doses of 100 mg may be injected every minute as necessary up to a maximum total dose of 1 mg. The usual dose required is 300–600 mg. The dose of flumazenil should be titrated against the individual response and it may be preferable to maintain a degree of sedation during the early postoperative period rather than bring about complete arousal, particularly in very anxious patients or those with coronary artery disease.

c. **False.** It should be remembered that because of the nature of the affinity of oxygen for haemoglobin, the relationship between the partial pressure of oxygen in blood and haemoglobin saturated is represented by a sigmoid rather than linear graph (Fig. 36). This means that at the upper end of the curve, a reduction of 2% in the oxygen saturation of haemoglobin represents a fall in the partial pressure of oxygen of about 15%. In other words, small changes in haemoglobin saturation represent large changes in the partial pressure of oxygen. However, the partial pressure of oxygen has to fall to 10 kPa (75 mm in figure) before the amount of oxygen carried in the blood falls noticeably. Below an oxygen saturation of 90%, the oxygen carriage of the blood falls off drastically and correction of the fall is required to prevent hypoxia occurring. This may be achieved by asking the patient to take larger breaths or by lifting the chin to improve the airway. However, should these measures fail, then one should consider administering supplemental oxygen or reversing the sedation. Some consider

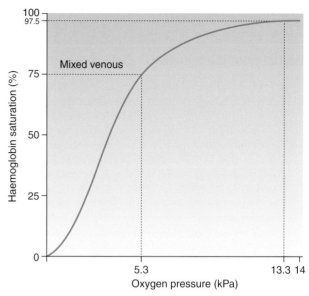

Fig. 36 The haemoglobin dissociation curve.

an oxygen saturation of 94% an indication of impending clinical hypoxia. Haemoglobin provides an effective oxygen reserve such that about 75% of the haemoglobin of mixed venous blood is saturated with oxygen.

d. **True.** It has been suggested in some reports that all patients sedated intravenously should have supplemental oxygen administered. While this may be helpful in some situations, such as sedation of elderly patients for endoscopy, it is not necessary for all dental patients, the majority of whom are young, fit and healthy, and where hypoxic episodes are best prevented by careful technique rather than universal oxygen administration.

e. **True.** Changes in cardiovascular parameters brought about by midazolam are slight but can induce a decrease in mean arterial pressure, cardiac output, stroke volume and systemic vascular resistance. It is useful to have a baseline measure of systemic arterial blood pressure with which to compare any later measurement that may be required in a sensitive patient or in an overdose situation. It is also an important part of the preoperative assessment. Arterial blood pressure may be measured indirectly by using a sphygmomanometer. Semi-automatic electrical sphygmomanometers are now readily available and inexpensive. These have a small piezo-crystal, which is positioned over the artery to detect arterial pulsations.

5. a. **True.** Immediately following the administration of high concentrations of nitrous oxide, a diffusion hypoxia may occur, as both nitrogen and nitrous oxide occupy space in the alveolar gas at the expense of oxygen. This may be harmful and so should be prevented by the administration of 100% oxygen to the patient for a few minutes following treatment.

b. **True.** Nitrous oxide is compressed and up to four-fifths of the contents of a full cylinder is in the liquid state, so the valves must be elevated above the horizontal. The amount of nitrous oxide present in a cylinder can only be determined by weighing, as the gas pressure above the level of the liquid remains constant as long as any liquid remains.

c. **True.** All inhalational machines must be fitted with a fail-safe system so that, should the oxygen supply be cut off or the oxygen cylinder become empty, the nitrous oxide alone will automatically cut out, making it impossible to deliver nitrous oxide alone to the patient and render them hypoxic. Machines are also designed so that they cannot deliver less than 30% oxygen.

d. **True.** Recovery is normally complete within 30 minutes of discontinuation of nitrous oxide and patients can then leave without an escort.

e. **False.** Nitrous oxide provides good analgesia such that the pain on injection of local anaesthesia can be prevented completely. This is particularly useful for children.

Extended matching items answers

EMI 1

1. **B.** Seven cartridges (2.2 ml) of lidocaine is the maximum recommended dose of local anaesthetic for a healthy adult.

2. **F.** The most likely explanation of the previous incident would be an intravascular injection of local anaesthetic containing epinephrine. The symptoms do not resemble those of an allergic reaction and palpitations do not suggest a vaso-vagal attack or faint during which there is a bradycardia.

3. **H.** This limited mouth opening is likely to have resulted from inflammation in muscles of mastication associated with a haematoma following an inferior alveolar nerve block. Patients experiencing this complication need antibiotics if diagnosed early, so there would be no benefit in this case. Explanation of the problem and reassurance is important.

4. **J.** An upper first premolar may be anaesthetised using a buccal infiltration and greater palatine block with local anaesthetic solution. Alternatively an infra-orbital block and greater palatine block may be used.

5. **C.** Bupivacaine has a long duration of action and is therefore the most appropriate for postoperative pain control.

EMI 2

1. **A.** Also, 10–30% patients taking unselective NSAIDs have gastroduodenal ulceration but clinical events are less common. For this reason, the COX-2 NSAIDs were developed with the intention of selectively inhibiting COX-2 only and affording mucosal protection.

2. **A** or **B.** Advancing age is an independent risk factor for the development of gastrointestinal complications of NSAIDS and fatal haemorrhage. Renal complications are also more common.

3. **C.** Morphine is the standard opioid analgesic for severe pain after surgery and for cancer pain and neuropathic pain that is poorly responsive to conventional analgesics.

4. **J.** The central inhibition of CNS cyclo-oxygenase reduces the production of prostaglandins and therefore the central sensitisation that results from inflammation.

5. **J.** In normal use paracetamol is very safe. Toxicity is very unlikely with the recommended doses of 4–6 g/day, although some people will be more susceptible to toxicity than others.

Case history answers

Case history 1

Reasonable cooperation for dental extractions could be expected of a 14-year-old child. However, if there are four to undertake and the patient has had little previous experience of dentistry, then she may find it difficult to cope with. If proceeding using local anaesthesia alone, then two treatment appointments would be reasonable. It would be advantageous to use inhalational sedation to ensure that undertaking this surgical treatment does not damage her confidence in dentistry. The sedation would ensure comfort of the local anaesthetic injections, particularly as two palatal infiltrations will be required during the course of treatment. Whether she has sedation or not, the issue of consent is complicated by the fact that her parents may not attend with her as she is resident at school perhaps some distance from her home. It is important that her parents are informed that she requires the removal of four teeth, understand the reasons for the treatment and that they provide their permission to go ahead.

Case history 2

1. Neglect of oral health and other health issues is not unexpected in a patient who has an opioid dependence. If he requires multiple extractions and potential surgical removal of some of these, and is anxious about any sort of dental treatment, then it would be appropriate to arrange for these procedures to be undertaken at one treatment session using general anaesthesia. The patient is likely to attend only when in pain and such a plan to remove all unrestorable teeth will reduce his suffering in the future. Attempts should be made to educate the patient to the advantages of oral care, and he should be offered the opportunity to receive restorative treatment.

2. The use of a sedation technique may facilitate the latter. Intravenous induction of general anaesthesia may be complicated by difficult venous access as may the use of sedation using an intravenous agent. Inhalational sedation can be a good choice in this situation.

Infection and inflammation of the teeth and jaws

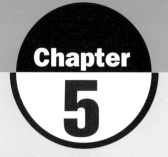

Overview

The common clinical problems in dentistry are related to infections and inflammation. The most prevalent dental diseases, dental caries and the periodontal diseases, are not included here. However, the sequelae of these diseases are frequently infection and inflammation of the bone. This chapter deals with these, along with other associated conditions of importance to the dentist.

5.1 Pulpitis

Learning objectives

You should:
- recognise the symptoms and management of acute and chronic pulpitis
- understand the pathological changes involved in pulpitis.

Pulpitis is inflammation of the pulp of a tooth and, in its acute form, is one of the most frequent emergencies facing the dentist. In general there is a poor correlation between the patient's clinical symptoms and the findings when the pulp is examined histologically. The division of pulpitis into the acute and chronic forms documented below is based predominantly on clinical symptoms. It should be remembered that the pathological processes occurring in pulpitis may be completely asymptomatic.

Acute pulpitis

Clinical features

Severe, sharp pain or throbbing pain is usually of several minutes (10–15) duration. The pain is poorly localised and often radiates away from the site of origin, but it only crosses the midline when anterior teeth are involved. The pain is precipitated particularly by heat, but also sometimes by cold and sweet stimuli. The symptoms are often relieved by analgesics.

Radiology

No specific features (see chronic pulpitis, below).

Pathology

The pulp may show only hyperaemia but may show both fluid and leukocyte emigration in more severe disease. A coronal pulp abscess may form. Sometimes acute pulpitis is superimposed on long-standing chronic pulpitis. Microbial factors are important in this respect.

Management

Clinical management depends on whether the pulpitis is deemed to be reversible or irreversible. This distinction encompasses a consideration of symptoms, findings on examination and the results of sensitivity testing and radiographic examination. For example, in some cases removal of caries may bring about resolution of symptoms while in others endodontic therapy or extraction of the affected tooth may be the most appropriate treatment.

Chronic pulpitis
Clinical features

A dull throbbing pain arises spontaneously and lasts for several hours. A tooth is likely to be heavily restored, grossly carious or have a history of trauma.

Radiology

There are no radiological signs associated with chronic pulpitis per se apart from the detection of the cause, most commonly caries. However, an uncommon finding is internal resorption. This typically appears as a localised enlargement of the pulp chamber or root canal (Fig. 37).

Pathology

The pulp is infiltrated by variable numbers of chronic inflammatory cells, particularly lymphocytes and their derivatives and macrophages (Fig. 38). Fibrosis may occur and an acute phase with fluid and leukocyte emigration may occur. The chronic inflammatory process may spread into the periapical tissues. In internal resorption, osteoclasts line the internal surface of the dentine, which becomes scalloped in outline.

Management

Endodontic therapy or extraction of the affected tooth. Pulpectomy will, obviously, also arrest internal resorption, as any cells capable of producing resorption will have been removed.

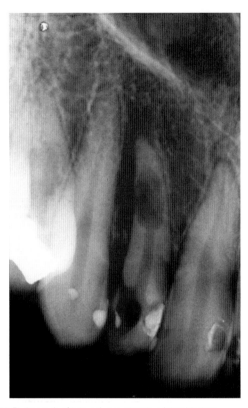

Fig. 37 Radiograph of internal resorption in a lateral incisor.

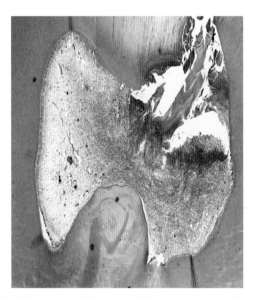

Fig. 38 Histopathology of chronic pulpitis as seen in a section through the pulp.

Pathological mechanisms in acute and chronic pulpitis

Using pulpitis arising in response to caries as our example, the earliest changes in the pulp are observed beneath the carious lesion. A chronic inflammatory infiltrate is seen beneath the odontoblast layer. As the carious lesion develops and bacteria advance towards the pulp, the classic features of acute inflammation are seen with vasodilatation and

the development of an inflammatory exudate. As oedema increases, the fact that the pulp is contained within a solid-walled compartment, the pulp chamber, makes expansion impossible. The rise in pressure results in the collapse of the local microcirculation, leading to hypoxia and necrosis. Abscess formation may occur involving the whole or part of the pulp. In low-grade chronic pulpitis, the odontoblasts respond to irritation from the advancing carious lesion by producing reactionary dentine and this function offers some protection to the pulp.

An uncommon finding, occurring in deciduous teeth or permanent molars with open apices, is the **pulp polyp**. This lesion develops in grossly carious teeth where a substantial portion of the pulp has been exposed. Granulation tissue forms that protrudes into the carious cavity in the form of a red or pink (if epithelialised) fleshy polyp.

5.2 Periapical inflammation

Learning objectives

You should:
* know how to diagnose periapical inflammation
* understand the management of acute and chronic periodontitis.

A necrotic pulp, with or without the presence of infection, will provoke an inflammatory response in the periapical periodontal ligament. Diagnosis of periapical inflammation is made by interpretation of a combination of symptoms and clinical and radiological signs.

Acute periapical periodontitis

Clinical features

The classic symptom is of a dull throbbing ache, usually well localised to a heavily restored or grossly diseased tooth. It may be difficult for the patient to determine whether an upper or lower tooth is affected as the pain is experienced particularly when the teeth are occluded. However, the affected tooth is painful to touch. The tooth should be non-responsive to sensitivity tests (as the periapical inflammation is usually provoked by a dead and/or infected pulp) although, particularly with multirooted teeth, some response may still be elicited, as well as tenderness on percussion.

Acute periapical periodontitis may also occur after trauma or endodontic treatment to a tooth. In such cases, the history should lead to the diagnosis.

Radiology

The basic radiological sign accompanying acute inflammation around the apex of a tooth is localised bone destruction. Where there is little or no previous chronic inflammation, this will appear as loss of the lamina dura (Fig. 39). Where the periapical periodontal ligament was previously widened or a granuloma was present, acute inflammation will appear as a poorly defined radiolucency, termed a **rarefying osteitis** (Fig. 40).

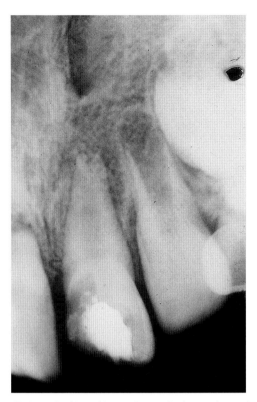

Fig. 39 Radiograph of loss of lamina dura on the fractured central incisor.

Pathology

Acute periapical periodontitis may arise de novo or develop against a background of pre-existing chronic periapical periodontitis (see below). In the former, the periodontal ligament is infiltrated by neutrophil leukocytes and macrophages while in the latter they accumulate within a periapical granuloma. In both cases, suppuration may occur, leading to the development of a periapical abscess.

Management

Endodontic therapy or extraction of the affected tooth is required. In cases of post-traumatic acute periapical periodontitis, the inflammation may resolve with splinting and time.

Chronic periapical periodontitis (periapical granuloma)

Clinical features

There may be few or no symptoms.

Radiology

The initial sign is widening of the periodontal ligament space with preservation of the radio-opaque lamina dura (Fig. 41). This naturally progresses with time to form a rounded periapical radiolucency with a well-defined margin – a granuloma (Fig. 42). Ultimately, this may undergo cystic change (radicular cyst; see Ch. 10). Differentiation between a large granuloma and a small radicular cyst is not possible on purely radiological grounds, but lesions greater than 1 cm diameter are often assumed to be cysts until histopathological diagnosis is established.

Fig. 40 Radiograph of rarefying osteitis associated with the lower right central incisor.

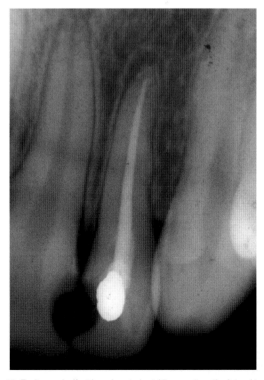

Fig. 41 Radiograph of widened periodontal ligament on the lateral incisor with intact lamina dura.

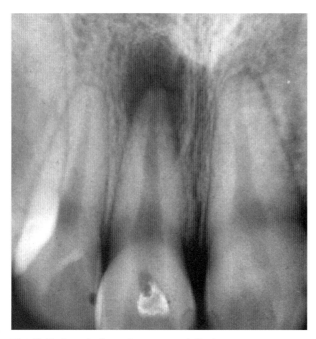

Fig. 42 Radiograph of granuloma on a central incisor.

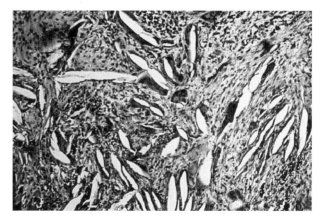

Fig. 44 Histopathological section of apical granuloma showing cholesterol clefts.

A further radiological sign frequently seen in chronic periapical periodontitis is sclerosing (or condensing) osteitis (Fig. 43). This appears as a fairly diffuse radio-opacity, usually around the periphery of a widened periodontal ligament or a periapical granuloma.

Pathology

Chronic periapical periodontitis is characterised by the formation of granulation tissue derived from the periodontal ligament, the periapical granuloma, surrounding the apex of a tooth (Fig. 44). Chronic inflammatory cells infiltrate the granuloma in variable numbers. Often plasma cells predominate because of multiple antigenic stimulations from pulpal infection. Foamy macrophages, cholesterol clefts often rimmed by multinucleate giant cells, and deposits

of haemosiderin are also frequent findings. Remnants of Hertwig's root sheath, the cell rests of Malassez, may proliferate as a result of release of inflammatory mediators. Neutrophil infiltration within this epithelium may be one factor leading to cavitation and formation of a radicular cyst (Ch. 10).

Management

Endodontic therapy or extraction of the affected tooth is required. Should the lesion persist following orthograde endodontic therapy, apicectomy should be considered (Box 4).

Box 4 Apicectomy surgical procedure

The procedure is also known as apical surgery or surgical endodontics.

1. A mucoperiostal flap is raised (Fig. 45).
2. Bone is removed over the buccal aspect of the tooth root in the area of the apex and associated pathology using an irrigated round surgical bur. The bone is thin and careful superficial sweeping movements are necessary to avoid removing tooth root tissue.
3. Pathological soft tissue about the root apex is removed with curettes and sent for histopathological examination.
4. At least 3 mm of the root apex should be removed using an irrigated fissure bur. The cut is made as close as possible to 90° to the long axis of the root to reduce the number of exposed dentinal tubules (Fig. 46).
5. A cavity is prepared in the root end using a small round bur or, better, an ultrasonically powered tip.
6. The cavity is isolated and packed with a biologically compatible material such as mineral trioxide aggregate, super EBA, glass ionomer, composite resin with a dentine bonding agent or reinforced zinc oxide-eugenol. Any excess material is removed and the area is irrigated to check this. Amalgam is no longer recommended.
7. The soft tissues are closed with a suture material such as vicryl.

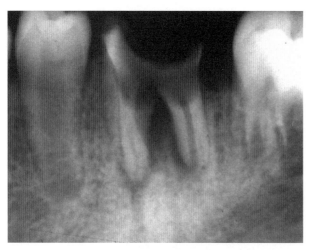

Fig. 43 Radiograph of condensing (sclerosing) osteitis relating to the grossly carious molar. The vertical radiolucent line is a vascular channel.

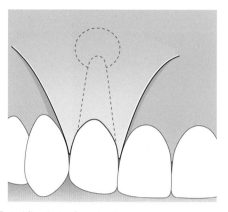

Fig. 45 Typical flap design for apicectomy.

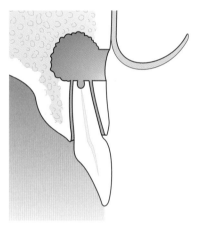

Fig. 46 Apicectomy of tooth and retrograde restoration.

Pathoses associated with periapical inflammation

Hypercementosis

Hypercementosis is usually identified on radiography. Affected roots of teeth become bulbous because of accretion of cementum (Fig. 47). The cause may be unidentifiable, but it is frequently associated with teeth affected by periodontal disease or periapical inflammation (hence its inclusion here). It is also seen in Paget's disease (Ch. 7), when multiple teeth are often affected. No treatment is indicated for hypercementosis per se, but its recognition is obviously important if extractions are planned.

External resorption

Resorption of the root surface, particularly apically, is occasionally seen on teeth with periapical inflammation, although there are a number of other known causes (e.g. trauma, iatrogenic (orthodontic), re-implanted teeth, adjacent cysts/tumours). Successful treatment of the periapical lesion by endodontic therapy often arrests the resorption.

5.3 Pericoronal inflammation

Learning objective

You should:
- be able to diagnose and manage pericoronal inflammation.

Five

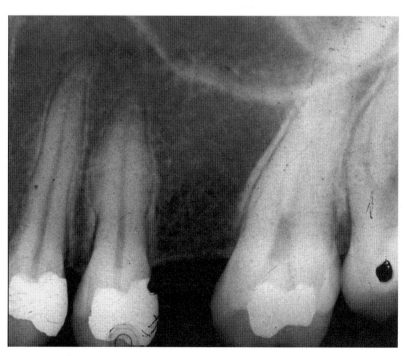

Fig. 47 Radiograph of hypercementosis affecting the premolar tooth.

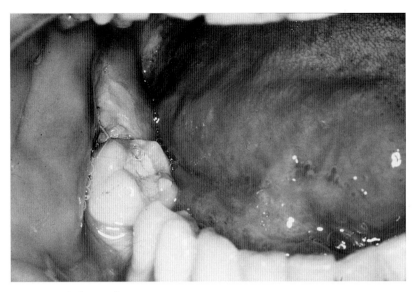

Fig. 48 Clinical photograph of pericoronitis (intra-oral).

When a tooth is partially erupted, the pericoronal space is connected to the oral cavity. Accumulation of food debris and plaque, along with mechanical trauma from mastication and trauma from an opposing tooth, favour the development of infection. Lower third molars are most frequently affected. Acute and chronic pericoronitis can both occur.

Clinical features

Early symptoms are of pain and swelling localised to the operculum (gum flap) overlying the crown of the tooth (Fig. 48). In more severe cases the patient may complain of limitation of mouth opening and facial swelling.

On examination, there may be extra-oral swelling and lymphadenopathy. Trismus may be present. Intraoral examination will reveal a swollen, tender operculum overlying the tooth. In chronic pericoronitis, pus may be seen exuding from beneath the operculum. A frequent finding with lower third molars is evidence of trauma from an opposing, often over-erupted, upper tooth. Spread of infection may occur to deeper tissues (see below).

Radiology

Apart from the appearance of a partially erupted, possibly impacted, tooth (Ch. 6), there are few radiological signs of pericoronitis. Soft-tissue swelling of the operculum may be identifiable and an over-erupted opposing tooth may be more easily seen radiologically than clinically when trismus is severe. The only specific radiological signs that are seen, in long-standing chronic pericoronitis, are an enlargement of the pericoronal space and a sclerosing osteitis in the bone immediately adjacent to the pericoronal space (Fig. 49).

Management

Irrigation beneath the operculum with saline or 0.2% chlorhexidine solution cleans and reduces infection.

Grinding the cusps (or extraction) of any opposing tooth will prevent further trauma. Where there is lymphadenopathy or severe trismus, antibiotic therapy is usually given. Advise the patient to use frequent hot salt mouthwashes and to maintain oral hygiene as best as they can (chlorhexidine mouthwash is sometimes prescribed as an aid to hygiene when normal hygiene procedures are difficult). Review is necessary to assess the partially erupted tooth and to determine its long-term management.

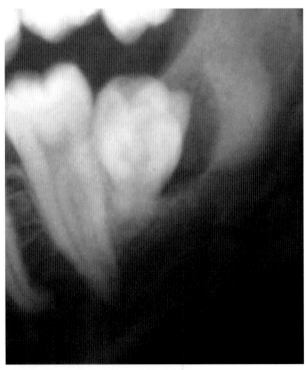

Fig. 49 Radiograph showing sclerosing osteitis around the follicle of the third molar. The patient had chronic pericoronitis.

5.4 Soft-tissue infections of the face

Infection sited at a tooth

Acute alveolar abscess

A common dental emergency facing the dentist is a patient with an acute alveolar abscess. There are a number of possible conditions that may lead to an abscess, including:

- periapical periodontitis
- periodontal disease
- pericoronitis
- infection of a cyst of the jaws.

Epidermoid (sebaceous) cysts in the facial skin may become infected and be confused with infections of dental origin, according to their site, although a punctum marking the blocked keratinous outflow may be obvious.

Clinical features

There is severe pain that is not well localised, although the affected tooth is painful to touch when the abscess follows periapical periodontitis. The tooth is non-responsive to sensitivity tests and a history of trauma to a tooth may be implicated. More commonly, the tooth is carious on examination. Without treatment, the infection spreads through bone and periosteum producing a soft fluctuant swelling, which may be present in the buccal sulcus or occasionally in the palate. As soon as the abscess spreads out of bone and into soft tissues, there is a reduction in the pain experienced.

An abscess following periodontal disease is likely to result in a mobile tooth that is tender to percussion. The tooth may remain responsive to sensitivity tests and any swelling is often nearer the gingival margin rather overlying the periapical region. Pus may exude from the gingival margin.

Trismus and cervical lymphadenopathy are signs of local spread of infection. Pyrexia and tachycardia are signs of systemic toxicity.

Radiology

While the acute abscess may be very obvious clinically, radiological signs vary enormously depending upon the pre-existing pathosis. An abscess may develop from a tooth with no previous chronic periapical lesion; here the most that may be visible is a loss of periapical lamina dura. Where a periapical granuloma or radicular cyst was present beforehand, the well-defined margin of the radiolucency tends to be lost. Such an ill-defined periapical radiolucency would be described as a rarefying osteitis.

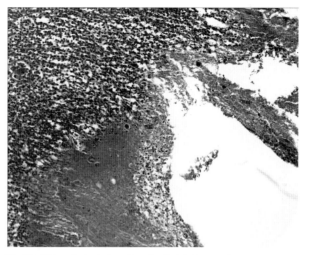

Fig. 50 Histopathological section of a dental abscess showing pyogenic membrane and necrosis lower centre of picture.

Pathology

An abscess may be defined as a pathological cavity filled with pus and lined by a pyogenic membrane (Fig. 50). The latter classically consists of granulation tissue but in a rapidly expanding lesion it may simply be a rim of inflammatory cells. The soft tissue surrounding an alveolar abscess may become swollen as a result of the inflammatory exudation and reactive to bacterial products, which have diffused from the abscess.

Management

The principle of treatment is to establish drainage of pus. In the case of a periapical abscess, this may be accomplished via the root canal after opening this up through the crown of the tooth with an air-rotor drill. This does not require local anaesthesia as the tooth is non-responsive to sensitivity tests, although it is important not to apply pressure to the tooth (as it may be exquisitely tender to percussion) by cutting tooth tissue slowly with a sharp bur. Alternatively, the tooth is extracted to gain adequate drainage. This may be undertaken under regional local anaesthesia, with or without conscious sedation, or using general anaesthesia.

Spread of infection to facial tissues

Lymphatic spread of infection

The lymphatic system is frequently involved in infections and gives an indication as to the pattern of spread. Enlargement and tenderness of nodes, described as **lymphadenitis**, is common, although inflammation of the lymphatic vessels, described as **lymphangitis**, may occur and can be seen as thin red streaks through the skin. The lymphatic drainage of the head and neck is described in more detail in Chapter 2.

Spread of infection through tissue spaces

In addition to spread through the lymphatic system, infection in the soft tissues of the face also spreads along fascial and muscle planes. These potential tissue spaces usually contain loose connective tissue and can be described anatomically (Fig. 51).

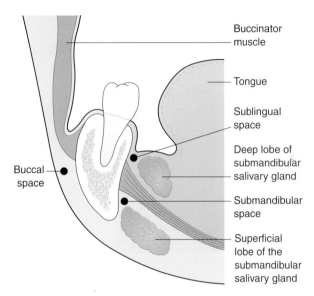

Fig. 51 Potential tissue spaces about the floor of the mouth.

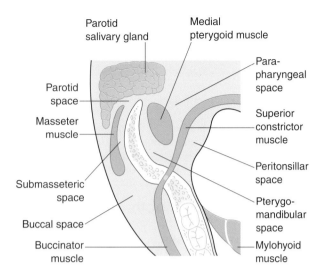

Fig. 53 Potential tissue spaces about the posterior mandible.

Floor-of-mouth tissue spaces

The mylohyoid muscle divides the sublingual and submandibular spaces although they are continuous around its posterior free edge (Fig. 52). The submental space is situated below the chin and between the anterior bellies of the digastric muscles. There are no restrictions on the spread of infection between the two submandibular spaces and the submental space; consequently, it can spread across the neck below the inferior border of the mandible.

Other tissue spaces of importance

Buccal spaces. These are located in the cheek on the lateral side of buccinator muscle. Submasseteric tissue spaces lie between the masseter muscle and the ramus of the mandible. The pterygomandibular spaces lie between the medial surface of the mandible and the medial pterygoid muscle (Fig. 53). The infratemporal space is the upper part of the pterygomandibular space and closely related to the upper

molar teeth. The parotid space lies behind the ramus of the mandible and about the parotid gland.

Pharyngeal tissue spaces. Of these, the parapharyngeal spaces are the most important in terms of spread of infection from the teeth and jaws. These spaces lie lateral to the pharynx and are continuous with the retropharyngeal space, to where infection may spread. The retropharyngeal space lies behind the pharynx and in front of the prevertebral fascia. The peritonsillar space lies around the palatine tonsil between the pillars of the fauces.

Hard palate area. There is no true tissue space in the hard palate because the mucosa is so tightly bound down to periosteum, but infection can strip away some of this and permit formation of an abscess.

Types of facial infection
Maxillary infections

The spread of periapical infection may be predicted by the relationship of the buccinator muscle attachment to the teeth. Infection from molar teeth usually spreads buccally or labially into the sulcus but may spread above the muscle into the superficial tissues of the cheek, where it can spread over a wide area with little to contain it. Infection frequently spreads to the palate from lateral incisors because of the palatal inclination of the root. Occasionally, infection may also spread palatally from a palatal root of a molar or premolar. The canine root is long and infection may spread superficially to the side of the nose rather than intra-orally.

Mandibular infections

Periapical infection may similarly spread according to muscle attachments. Infection from incisors usually spreads labially into the sulcus but may spread to the chin between the two bellies of the mentalis muscle. Infection from the canine may spread into superficial tissues because the root is long. Premolars and molars show spread of infection into the buccal sulcus leading to intra-oral or extra-oral spread according to the relation to the attachment of buccinator. Similarly, second mandibular molar teeth

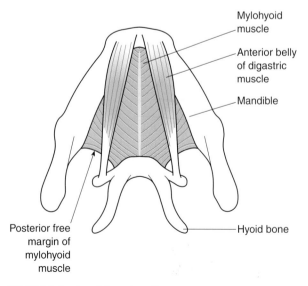

Fig. 52 Inferior view of floor of mouth.

have more lingually placed roots and may, therefore, result in either sublingual or submandibular spread depending on the relative position of the mylohyoid muscle.

Cellulitis

Cellulitis is a spreading infection of connective tissue typical of streptococcal organisms. It spreads through the tissue spaces as described above and usually results from virulent and invasive organisms. The clinical features are those of a painful, diffuse, brawny swelling. The overlying skin is red, tense and shiny. There is usually an associated trismus, cervical lymphadenopathy, malaise and pyrexia. The swelling is the result of oedema rather than pus and may be extensive when it involves lax tissues such as in the superficial mid-face about the eyes. Cellulitis usually develops quickly, over the course of hours, and may follow an inadequately managed or ignored local dental infection.

If the infection spreads to involve the floor of mouth and pharyngeal spaces, then the airway can be compromised. Initially, the floor of the mouth will be raised and the patient will have difficulty in swallowing saliva; this pools and may be observed running from the patient's mouth. This sign indicates the need for urgent management. Cellulitis involving the tissue spaces on both sides of the floor of mouth is described as **Ludwig's angina.**

Cavernous sinus thrombosis

Rarely infection in the tissues of the face may spread intracranially via the interconnecting venous system. This is more likely with the upper face via the facial vein to the cavernous sinus. While rare, cavernous sinus thrombosis is life threatening.

Management of infections about the face

A clinical and radiographic examination of the mouth should be carried out to identify potential causes such as carious or partly erupted teeth or retained roots.

The patient may need to be admitted to hospital if they are unwell or there are signs of airway compromise. A differential white-cell count may indicate an increase in neutrophils. A blood glucose investigation may be carried out to exclude an underlying undiagnosed diabetes mellitus. Blood cultures should be performed if there is a spiking pyrexia or rigors. Intravenous antibiotics such as penicillin together with metronidazole should then be started, as well as fluids to rehydrate the patient, analgesics and an antipyretic. Erythromycin or clindamycin may be appropriate if the patient is allergic to penicillin.

Drainage

Drainage should be established by opening or extracting the tooth or management as appropriate, such as for pericoronitis as described above. If there is an associated fluctuant swelling, then this may be incised and drained. This can be undertaken with ethyl chloride topical anaesthesia, local anaesthesia (carefully injected into overlying mucosa and not into the abscess) or general anaesthesia as appropriate.

Drainage should not be delayed if the patient does not show signs of improvement. This may need to be under general anaesthesia if it is anticipated that local anaesthesia would be ineffective because of exquisite tenderness of the tooth or the extent of the swelling. The causative carious or impacted tooth or retained root should be removed at the same time. If trismus is a feature, intubation of the trachea will be difficult and the patient's airway will be at risk on induction of anaesthesia. Such patients may need to undergo fibreoptic-assisted intubation while awake or sedated, prior to induction of anaesthesia.

Drainage of tissue spaces may require extra-oral skin incision, blunt dissection to open abscess locules and insertion of a drain such as a Yates to permit continued drainage for 24–48 hours (Fig. 54). Pus is sent to the microbiology laboratory for investigation of antibiotic sensitivity. When draining a cellulitis, little pus will be found, but tissue fluid will be released. In the case of Ludwig's angina, incisions

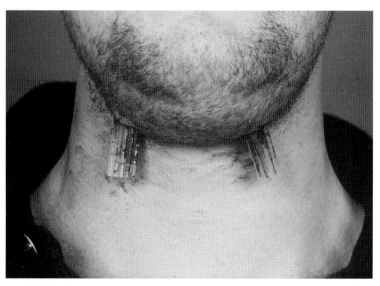

Fig. 54 Postoperative photograph showing drains in right and left submandibular spaces.

are made bilaterally to drain the submandibular spaces via an extra-oral approach, and the sublingual spaces via an intra-oral approach. The mortality of Ludwig's angina has reduced from 75% before the advent of antibiotic use to 5%. A drain may be placed through the skin to protrude intra-orally. If the airway is at risk, the patient will remain intubated postoperatively and return to the intensive care unit for ventilation.

Chronic infection

Acute infections may become chronic if treatment is inadequate. A persistent sinus may form, permitting intermittent discharge of pus. This may be intra-oral or extra-oral. The chronic infection may revert to an acute situation should the discharge be interrupted in any way.

5.5 Other infections and inflammations

Actinomycosis
Clinical features

Infection with *Actinomyces* species, most commonly *A. israelii*, may involve the cervicofacial and abdominal regions as well as skin and the lungs. The cervicofacial region is, however, the most commonly affected and acute infection here may be indistinguishable from an acute dentoalveolar abscess. There may be a history of trauma. Multiple discharging sinuses are a classic sign of chronic actinomyocosis infection.

Pathology

Actinomycosis is characterised by the presence of masses of the filamentous anaerobic bacteria visible in sections stained with haemotoxylin and eosin but more readily distinguished on Gram staining (Gram positive) (Fig. 55). These masses may be partially calcified and visible to the naked eye as bright yellow ('sulphur') granules. Diagnosis is made on clinical grounds accompanied by Gram staining, culture and sensitivity testing performed on a sample of pus. This is of particular importance as it is unusual for *Actinomyces* species to be the only bacteria present. Within the tissues, the masses of bacteria lie in areas of suppuration surrounded by acute inflammatory cells. The adjacent granulation tissue often shows considerable fibrosis.

Management

Any related dental cause is treated and swellings are incised and drained as necessary. A 3-week course of penicillin is used for acute infections and a 6-week course is

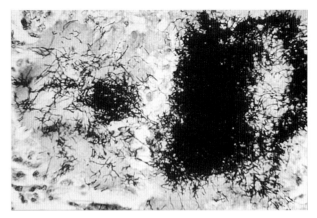
Fig. 55 Gram-stained actinomycosis.

used for chronic infections. Alternatively, erythromycin, tetracycline or clindamycin may be used.

Osteomyelitis

Osteomyelitis is inflammation of the medullary cavity of a bone caused by an infection. It is quite rare but is seen particularly in those patients whose defence against infection is compromised because of local or systemic factors. It is a serious condition requiring urgent specialist management. In contrast, localised bone infection following tooth extraction is referred to as **osteitis** or dry socket and can be managed in primary care (Ch. 6).

Acute osteomyelitis
Clinical features

Symptoms are of pain, tenderness and swelling in the affected area. As such, these symptoms are essentially those of an acute dental infection. The mandible is affected more frequently than the maxilla. An important symptom is a developing numbness over the chin as a result of mental nerve involvement.

Radiology

The typical feature is a rarefying osteitis (see acute periapical periodontitis, above). This may extend through a large area of bone, involving the inferior dental canal and lower cortex of the mandible (Fig. 56).

Pathology

True acute osteomyelitis is rare because spread of infection into bone is usually a chronic process or develops on a background of chronic inflammation. Acute osteomyelitis is considered to involve rapid spread of infection within the marrow spaces. By the time that the bone matrix is affected, the condition is classified as chronic osteomyelitis.

Management

Benzylpenicillin or clindamycin and metronidazole are normally started and altered as necessary according to the results of pus sensitivity testing. The patient may require hospital admission for incision and drainage, but it is preferable to limit any dentoalveolar surgery to the extraction of grossly mobile and non-vital teeth. Antibiotics should be continued for at least 2 weeks after control of the acute infection.

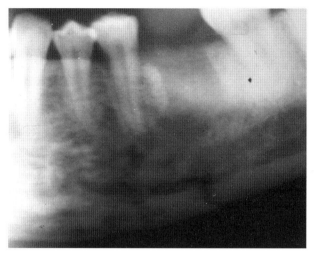

Fig. 56 Radiograph of acute osteomyelitis. This occurred after extraction of the first molar.

Chronic osteomyelitis

The natural course of acute osteomyelitis is that it develops into a chronic disease with pus accumulation and the formation of islands of necrotic bone (sequestra). Predisposing factors are depressed immune or inflammatory response, for example diabetes or long-term corticosteroid use and bone abnormalities such as Paget's disease or cemento-osseous dysplasia.

Clinical features

Pain and swelling are always present, although this is likely to be less severe than in the acute form. Paraesthesia tends to persist in mandibular lesions. One or more soft-tissue sinuses are typically present, draining pus. The affected bone may become enlarged owing to periosteal reaction.

Radiology

In addition to the rarefying osteitis seen in acute lesions, irregular radio-opaque areas (sequestra) surrounded by radiolucencies are visible. A late sign of chronic osteomyelitis is radiological evidence of periosteal new bone, visible as one or more thin shells of radio-opacity at the lower border of the mandible or above the buccal/lingual cortices (Fig. 57).

Pathology

Fragments of dead bone (sequestra) are characterised by the presence of empty osteocyte lacunae and degenerative changes to the matrix. Often the surfaces are scalloped as a result of previous osteoclastic activity. If a sequestrum communicates with the exterior, then bacterial plaque may form on some surfaces. Sequestra may be surrounded by necrotic debris and acute inflammatory cells. Pus may fill the adjacent marrow spaces while granulation tissue infiltrated by chronic inflammatory cells is present at the junction between vital and non-vital bone. Osteoblasts rim the surface of the surrounding vital bone and both endosteal and subperiosteal bone deposition may be seen.

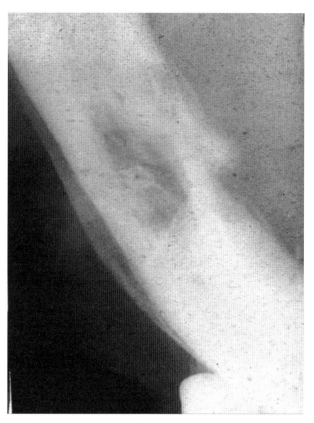

Fig. 57 Occlusal radiograph of the lower right molar region in chronic osteomyelitis. Note the bone destruction within the jaw and sequestration lingually. Buccally there is periosteal new bone formation.

Management

Antibiotics are given as for acute infection. Any sequestra that have not spontaneously separated should be surgically removed. Quite extensive sequestrectomy may be necessary, which may necessitate subsequent reconstruction. Hyperbaric oxygen therapy may be helpful in difficult cases. The patient breathes 100% oxygen in a special chamber for a prescribed number of sessions.

Garré's osteomyelitis

Garré's osteomyelitis is a chronic sclerosing osteomyelitis with a proliferative periostitis. This rare condition is usually associated with either a chronic periapical periodontitis or, sometimes, a chronic pericoronitis.

Clinical features

This condition is usually seen in children and younger adults in the body and ramus of the mandible. Swelling is the principal feature. Symptoms and signs of an overlying periapical periodontitis will usually be present.

Radiology

There is an area of sclerosing osteitis in the mandible. Periosteal new bone will be evident at the periphery of the jaw.

Pathology

Garré's osteomyelitis is characterised by the formation of periosteal new bone. The latter is trabecular in nature;

cortical bone is lacking and there may be 'onion skin layering' of the reactive bone.

Management

Removal of the diseased tooth will result in resolution, with gradual remodelling of the bone cortex eventually resulting in restoration of the normal contour.

Osteoradionecrosis

Clinical features

A reduction in vascularity, secondary to endarteritis obliterans, and damage to osteocytes as a consequence of ionising radiotherapy can result in radiation-associated osteomyelitis or osteoradionecrosis. The mandible is much more commonly affected than the maxilla, because it is less vascular. Pain may be severe and there may be pyrexia. The overlying oral mucosa often appears pale because of radiation damage. Osteoradionecrosis in the jaws arises most often following radiotherapy for squamous cell carcinoma. Scar tissue will also be present at the tumour site, often in close relation to the necrotic bone.

Radiology

Osteoradionecrosis appears as rarefying osteitis within which islands of opacity (sequestra) are seen. Pathological fracture may be visible in the mandible.

Pathology

The affected bone shows features similar to those of chronic osteomyelitis. Grossly, the bone may be cavitated and discoloured, with formation of sequestra. Acute inflammatory infiltrate may be present on a background of chronic inflammation, characterised by formation of granulation tissue around the non-vital trabeculae. Blood vessels show areas of endothelial denudation and obliteration of their lumina by fibrosis. Small telangiectatic vessels lacking precapillary sphincters may be present. Fibroblasts in the irradiated tissues lose the capacity to divide and often become binucleated and enlarged.

Management

Prevention of osteoradionecrosis is essential. Patients who require radiotherapy for the management of head and neck malignancy should ideally have teeth of doubtful prognosis extracted at least 6 weeks prior to treatment. However, a delay to starting the radiotherapy is unacceptable and if teeth are extracted only within a couple of weeks of treatment, osteoradionecrosis may still result. This risk may have to be taken. There are also other factors that increase the risk of developing osteoradionecrosis, such as the dose of radiation, the area of the mandible irradiated and the surgical trauma involved in the dental extractions. Patient factors, such as age and nutrition, and others that have a bearing on wound healing will also influence the risk. A more conservative approach to pre-radiation extractions can be adopted in the maxilla. When extraction of teeth is required in patients who have had radiotherapy to the jaws, a specialist opinion should be sought.

Surgical management of osteoradionecrosis is similar to osteomyelitis. Sometimes, the changes can be extensive, necessitating partial jaw resection to remove all necrotic bone.

Bisphosphonate-associated necrosis of bone

Bisphosphonates are a class of drug used for treatment of a variety of bone conditions, including osteoporosis, Paget's disease of bone, osteogenesis imperfecta and as part of management of bony metastatic disease. Their mode of action is upon osteoclasts, slowing bone remodelling and turnover, but they also have a prominent antiangiogenic effect. In the past few years, there have been increasing numbers of reports of necrosis of bone in the jaws of patients being treated with these drugs, principally where the more potent nitrogenous drugs have been administered intravenously. The evidence suggests that the disease can be a late effect of bisphosphonate use, even occurring after cessation of therapy. The aetiology of the necrosis of bone in the jaws is not clearly understood, but seems to be related to inhibition of bone remodelling, killing of osteoclasts and decreased intra-osseous blood flow.

Clinical features

Patients may present with poor wound healing, soft-tissue breakdown and exposure of bone. There may be superadded symptoms and signs of osteomyelitis (see above). The disease affects the mandible more frequently than the maxilla. The apparent trigger for development of the condition may be an extraction, implant placement or other minor surgical procedure. The criteria for diagnosis are: history of current or prior treatment using bisphosphonate drugs, exposed bone in the jaws that has been present for more than 8 weeks and no previous history of radiotherapy.

Radiology

Plain radiographic appearances are identical to those of osteoradionecrosis (see above). CT may offer improved sensitivity over plain radiographs, while MR scans may be useful in delineating sequestra and showing soft-tissue involvement. Radioisotope bone scans are highly sensitive but have limited specificity.

Pathology

The bone often becomes black or dark green in colour due to the products of bacterial colonies forming in the marrow spaces once the necrotic bone becomes exposed to the oral cavity. Microscopically the surfaces of the non-vital bone are scalloped due to osteoclastic action. The osteocyte lacunae are empty and in the later stages the bone matrix collagen breaks down. Granulation tissue may form at the interface with vital bone and a dense chronic active inflammatory reaction is seen. Sequestration and trans-mucosal elimination are often found.

Management

As is the case for patients who have had radiotherapy to the head and neck, prevention of the condition is paramount so as to reduce the chance of surgery being necessary. Special care should be taken with any patient attending the dentist who is, or has, undergone bisphosphonate treatment. Where an extraction or other surgical treatment is required, the wisest course is to refer the patient to a specialist. Patients receiving intravenous bisphosphonates for metastatic bone disease are more at risk than those receiving oral bisphosphonates for osteoporosis. Modification or cessation of oral bisphosphonates may be considered in consultation with the treating physician and the patient. Any surgery should be undertaken as atraumatically as possible and patients should be reviewed regularly after surgery.

Management of bisphosphonate-associated necrosis of bone is essentially the same as that for osteoradionecrosis, being a combination of antibiotics and careful surgery, along with cessation of bisphosphonate use. Hyperbaric oxygen therapy may also have value. Immediate reconstruction of any resection using non-vascularised or vascularised bone may be problematic as necrotic bone may develop at the recipient site.

Periostitis

Proliferative periostitis sometimes causes jaw swelling and ulceration. The condition arises as a result of chronic irritation to the periosteum, often from foreign material, which enters through an ulcer. Vegetable pulse material is the best-known example. Leguminous grains from cooked food accumulate under an ill-fitting denture and are forced into the periosteum. The resulting chronic inflammatory processes, including a foreign body reaction to the starch, cause cortical erosion and periosteal swelling. The lesion, which may be mistaken for a malignant process clinically, is referred to as a **vegetable pulse granuloma**.

Augmentation materials that have been implanted into the jaws sometimes become infected and cause periostitis and osteitis. A rare cause of periosteal expansion is metastatic deposition of carcinoma.

Five

Self-assessment: questions

Multiple choice questions

1. A dense bone island (DBI; idiopathic osteosclerosis):
   a. Is a mixed radiolucent/radio-opaque lesion
   b. Causes external bony swelling
   c. Is found only in relation to teeth unresponsive to sensitivity tests
   d. Requires no treatment
   e. Is also known as an 'enostosis'

2. Periosteal new bone formation is seen in:
   a. Chronic osteomyelitis
   b. Cherubism
   c. Langerhans cell histiocytosis
   d. Metastatic bronchial carcinoma
   e. Paget's disease of bone

3. Orofacial infections are:
   a. Common following contaminated facial laceration
   b. A common source of lost working days
   c. Usually of fungal or viral aetiology when affecting the oral mucosa
   d. Best managed by prescribing an antibiotic empirically rather than waiting for the results of a culture and sensitivity investigation
   e. Commonly the result of endogenous commensal organisms

4. Penicillins:
   a. Are the most commonly used antimicrobial drugs in dentistry
   b. Are described as being non-toxic
   c. Such as amoxicillin are more readily absorbed from the gastrointestinal tract than phenoxymethylpenicillin (penicillin V)
   d. Are more useful than metronidazole when anaerobic activity is required
   e. Such as benzylpenicillin produce rapid high plasma levels when given by the intravenous route

5. Apical surgery:
   a. May be carried out using a semilunar incision when the tooth is restored with a crown
   b. Is indicated when surgical repair of a root perforation is required
   c. May be undertaken on posterior teeth
   d. Need not involve the removal of all the gutta-percha from the walls of the cavity in the root end
   e. May be described as successful even when there is no regeneration of periapical bone

Extended matching items

Options:

A Chronic periapical periodontitis
B Cellulitis
C Acute periapical periodontitis
D Garré's osteomyelitis
E Pericoronitis
F Acute pulpitis
G Chronic osteomyelitis
H Acute alveolar abscess
I Chronic pulpitis
J Bisphosphonate-associated necrosis of bone

Lead in: Match the clinical and radiological signs and symptoms from the list below with the likeliest diagnosis above.

1. *Clinically:* painful, diffuse, reddened swelling affecting the right side of the face, centred on the cheek, causing partial closure of the eye. This developed overnight. The previous 3 days there had been, according to the patient, 'an abscess' present on UR3. The patient feels unwell and there is lymphadenopathy present. UR3 is grossly carious. *Radiologically:* UR3 has a periapical rarefying osteitis.

2. *Clinically:* a 20-year-old male presents with pain and swelling at the 'back of his mouth' on the right side. It has been present for a couple of days. On examination, he has a tender, palpable, upper right cervical lymph node. There is some trismus. Intra-orally, there is swelling of the gingivae distal to LR7. UR8 is erupted and traumatising this swelling when in occlusion. *Radiologically:* LR8 is present but mesioangularly impacted against LR7.

3. *Clinically:* a dull, throbbing pain associated with LL6, made worse on touching and when trying to eat. This tooth is heavily restored. It does not respond to sensitivity testing. *Radiologically:* LL6 has periapical rarefying osteitis associated with both roots.

4. *Clinically:* severe, sharp pain on right side of the face. Difficult to localise, but is precipitated particularly by hot drinks and comes in waves lasting several minutes. *Radiologically:* there is nothing unusual to see extra-orally. In the mouth, there are many heavily restored teeth, but no obvious carious lesions. On closer examination, using a pledget of cotton wool soaked in ethyl chloride, UR5 is hypersensitive, but it is not tender to percussion.

5. *Clinically:* pain of left side of the face that is hard to localise, although LL5 is tender on touching and eating. This has been present for a few days, but this morning the patient reports that the pain was a bit easier, although some swelling has arisen next to the LL5. On examination, there is tenderness when palpating the left side of the face over the premolar region of the left mandible. Intra-orally, LL5 is grossly carious and tender to pressure. There is fluctuant swelling in the buccal sulcus next to LL5. The tooth does not respond to sensitivity tests. *Radiologically:* LL5 has a periapical rarefying osteitis.

6. *Clinically:* occasional dull ache from UL1. The tooth is restored with a crown. No tenderness to pressure. No soft tissue abnormality. *Radiologically:* round, 0.5 cm

diameter periapical radiolucency, with loss of lamina dura, associated with UL1.

7. *Clinically:* an 8-year-old child presents with a firm swelling associated with the left body of mandible. He complains of occasional 'toothache' on that side. On examination, a hard but mild swelling can be palpated, principally on the buccal aspect of the alveolus, deep in the buccal sulcus, extending forwards to the canine region. He has gross caries of his first permanent molars. LL6 is sore when you press on it. *Radiologically:* LL6 shows a periapical condensing (sclerosing) osteitis. An occlusal radiograph, taken to assess the buccal swelling, shows a thin layer of periosteal new bone adjacent to the original buccal cortical margin of the mandible.

8. *Clinically:* a 75-year-old woman attends complaining of 'an infection' in her left lower jaw that has been present for a few weeks, since she had her LL5 extracted, and which now is causing her a lot of distress. She cannot wear her lower partial denture. She suffers from severe osteoporosis, having sustained several vertebral fractures over the last 5 years. On examination, there is swelling extra-orally over the left jaw and some cervical lymphadenopathy. Intra-orally, she has a partially dentate mouth, with missing molars on the lower left. Her alveolar ridge distal to LL5 is swollen and a draining sinus is visible buccally. LL5 socket is still partly open. *Radiologically:* there is a 2 × 3 cm area of radiolucency with a central area of radio-opacity located in LL5 and LL6 region.

9. *Clinically:* a 45-year-old male presents with a long-standing pain and swelling related to the left lower jaw. He also says that in the last week he is getting a tingling sensation in his left lower lip that aggravates him. He 'generally doesn't believe in dentists' and he has been self-treating for 2 months using various herbal remedies, to no avail. On examination, there is swelling of the lower part of the left face overlying the body of mandible. The swelling is tender and, upon this, there is a localised reddened area that has crusted over. Intra-orally, there are many carious teeth and poor oral hygiene. The LL6 and LL7 are little more than retained roots. There is buccal swelling next to LL6 and, adjacent to it, an obvious sinus in the buccal sulcus. *Radiologically:* LL6 and LL7 roots all show periapical radiolucency. Below these, there is a more extensive area of rarefying osteitis, within which can be seen some islands of radio-opacity.

10. *Clinically:* a dull, throbbing pain that arises spontaneously from the upper left molar region and which usually lasts for a few hours. Occasionally the pain is stimulated by hot drinks. The symptoms have been occurring irregularly for some months. On examination, there are no extra-oral abnormalities and no soft tissue abnormalities intra-orally. There are some large restorations in the upper left teeth, but only UL7 gives an abnormal response to pulp testing. It is not tender to percussion. *Radiologically:* apart from confirming a very deep amalgam restoration in UL7, there are no abnormal radiological findings.

Case history questions

Case history 1

Mary is a 40-year-old dental phobic. She attended 4 weeks ago as a casual patient for extraction of a grossly decayed lower left first molar. She has reluctantly returned now complaining of awful pain on the lower left, swelling in that region and in the submandibular region, a numb lip on the lower left and a bad taste. Radiographs are taken (Fig. 58).

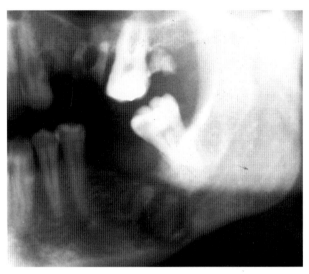

Fig. 58 Radiograph taken of the patient in Case history 1.

Describe your assessment, likely diagnosis and management.

Case history 2

Chris is 25 years of age. He attends your surgery complaining that he has pain and swelling at the back of his mouth on the lower right side, a bad taste, bad breath and that he cannot open his mouth properly. He has lymphadenopathy of the right submandibular and cervical nodes. You know from a previous visit that he has a partially erupted lower third molar.

Describe your assessment, likely diagnosis and management.

Case history 3

Susan is a 55-year-old regular patient at your surgery. You have spent many months restoring her dentition with crowns, bridges and endodontic treatments. She says that while she was away on her annual holiday she suffered an 'abscess' on a lower front tooth that was treated by antibiotics. While she is pain free now, she has noticed a small 'spot' on her chin that weeps fluid occasionally.

Describe your assessment, likely diagnosis and management.

Case history 4

Figure 59 shows radiographs of a patient who attends your surgery with toothache. She complained of a dull aching pain on the upper right, with some tenderness in the upper buccal sulcus. The pain is unaffected by thermal stimuli.

Describe your assessment and likely diagnosis.

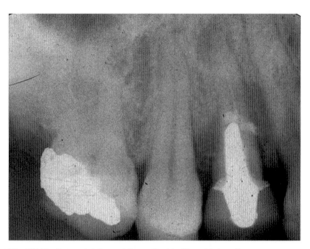

Fig. 59 Radiograph taken of the patient in Case history 4.

Viva questions

1. What is the significance of the radiological sign of loss of lamina dura?
2. When would you use antibiotics to treat an infection of dental origin?
3. What is an abscess?
4. Can you distinguish between a periapical granuloma and a radicular (periodontal) cyst on a radiograph?
5. What is pyrexia?
6. What is endarteritis obliterans?
7. How may infection spread from pericoronitis of a lower third molar tooth?
8. What are the clinical differences between acute pulpitis and acute periapical periodontitis?

Self-assessment: answers

Multiple choice answers

1. a. **False.** DBI has a uniform radio-opacity, very much the same in density as the cortical bone at the lower border of the mandible.
   b. **False.** DBI is entirely within the normal boundaries of the jaw.
   c. **False.** DBI typically forms close to the roots of teeth and is frequently joined to the lamina dura. However, the vitality of the teeth is irrelevant.
   d. **True.**
   e. **True.**

DBI is usually seen in the premolar/molar region of the mandible. Most authorities consider them to be a developmental, self-limiting entity. A typical size is around 1 cm, but occasionally much larger ones occur. The margins are well defined but the shape is irregular, with no radiolucent margin. Despite their innocuous nature, they are sometimes seen in association with external root resorption. If multiple DBIs are seen in the jaws, you should consider familial adenomatous polyposis (Gardner's syndrome) in the diagnosis.

2. a. **True.** One or more 'layers' of very thin bone form parallel to the periphery of the jaw as a late radiological feature. The thin bone is usually best identified on fine-detail intra-oral radiographic film.
   b. **False.** Cherubism leads to jaw enlargement, but not by proliferative periostitis.
   c. **True.** Langerhans cell histiocytosis has similar appearances to osteomyelitis.
   d. **False.** Metastatic lesions of prostate carcinoma will produce a proliferative periostitis, but bronchial carcinoma will not. Metastatic breast carcinoma sometimes stimulates new bone formation. In such cases, the appearance contrasts markedly with the new bone formed in osteomyelitis, being in spicules at right angles to the bone surface. This 'sunray' appearance is also classically seen in osteogenic sarcoma.
   e. **False.** The bone changes in Paget's disease frequently produce a parallel trabecular pattern and bony enlargement, but there is no periosteal new bone.

3. a. **False.** The orofacial region is well vascularised and few facial lacerations become infected. Similarly, few compound fractures of the mandible become infected. Impairment of this vascularity by radiotherapy or conditions such as diabetes mellitus significantly increase the risk of infection.
   b. **True.** Orofacial infections represent a significant proportion of attendances for dental care provided by general dentists and for hospital specialist services. Infections cause pain and disability and result in lost working days. Occasionally, the infections can be life threatening; untreated, many acute infections persist as chronic infections with associated morbidity.
   c. **True.** The major oral mucosal infections are of fungal, usually candidal, or viral origin. Other superficial mucosal surfaces of the body such as the vagina show similar infections.
   d. **False.** Orofacial infections require the appropriate management dependent on the nature of the infection. An antimicrobial drug may only be required for the management of a dentoalveolar infection if there are signs of spreading infection, pyrexia or should the patient be immunocompromised. Frequently, a surgical intervention such as tooth extraction is more appropriate than chemotherapy. The choice of antimicrobial agent should depend on the results of laboratory investigation unless there is a clinical urgency to prescribe empirically until the results are known. In dentistry, empirical prescribing is, in fact, common because the likely pathogen may be known, as may the usual sensitivity of that pathogen.
   e. **True.** Infection with a mixture of non-specific microorganisms that normally reside in the oral cavity is common. Dentoalveolar and salivary gland infections are examples of these.

4. a. **True.** The penicillins are the most widely used of all antimicrobial drugs in dentistry.
   b. **True.** The commonly used penicillins are non-toxic. The big problem with the penicillins is allergic reaction. A patient who is allergic to one penicillin is likely to be allergic to all penicillins, and 10% also show cross-reactivity to cephalosporins.
   c. **True.** Amoxicillin is well absorbed when given by mouth irrespective of the presence of food in the stomach and produces high plasma and tissue concentrations.
   d. **False.** Metronidazole is very effective against strict anaerobes and some protozoa. It is bactericidal and the drug of choice for acute ulcerative gingivitis; may be used alone or in combination with a penicillin for dentoalveolar infections.
   e. **True.** Benzylpenicillin produces particularly high plasma levels of antibiotic following intravenous injection and is, therefore, of use in severe infections where this is important.

5. a. **True.** A semilunar incision is positioned away from the gingival margin and this may, therefore, offer an advantage when apicecting crowned teeth as contraction of the wound margin may, on occasion, permit exposure of the crown/tooth margin when a full flap design is used. However, it is difficult to predict the size of the underlying periradicular lesion and a semilunar flap design may not be able to ensure that its margins are closed over sound bone. Closure should be with a long-lasting resorbable suture, or non-resorbable suture to prevent wound dehiscence.

b. **True.** Apical surgery is indicated:
   - where non-surgical root canal treatment has failed and re-treatment cannot be undertaken
   - in the presence of periradicular pathology when conventional root canal treatment cannot be undertaken because of a developmental or iatrogenic condition
   - where histopathological examination of periradicular tissue is required
   - where repair of a root perforation is required.

c. **True.** Apical surgery may be undertaken on posterior teeth but access is more difficult and the surgery technically more difficult as a result. It is not unusual to apicect one or two buccal roots of a maxillary molar tooth if these are the only roots with associated pathology and not treat the palatal root. Anatomical structures such as the maxillary antrum and inferior alveolar nerve are relevant to surgery on posterior teeth.

d. **False.** It is important to remove all traces of gutta-percha from the walls of the root-end cavity to ensure a good peripheral seal with the filling material.

e. **False.** Surgical endodontic treatment is described as successful when clinically there are no symptoms or signs of disease and radiologically there is no reduction in periradicular rarefaction and there is a normal lamina dura and osseous pattern. Clinical outcomes associated with failure are swelling, presence of a sinus tract, pain, pain on percussion, altered soft-tissue sensation as a consequence of nerve damage and damage to an adjacent tooth. The most significant radiological outcome associated with failure is lack of bony regeneration.

Extended matching items answers

EMI 1

1. **B.** The sudden appearance of a diffuse swelling is the key finding. The lax tissues around the eye can swell in a striking way due to oedema during a cellulitis. It is often surprising to the inexperienced to find a relatively minor lesion on a tooth as a cause of so major a clinical problem.

2. **E.** This is straightforward once all the symptoms and signs are revealed. On extra-oral examination alone, however, all we have are signs of infection. The intra-oral appearance, with the upper third molar occluding on the gingivae distal to the lower second molar, is an everyday sign of pericoronitis. The radiography merely confirms what is already a very likely diagnosis.

3. **C.** A non-vital tooth that is tender to touch leads to the diagnosis of acute periapical periodontitis. Of course, it is possible to think of other causes, such as a fractured root in a root-filled tooth, but the radiography provides the final confirmation of the straightforward diagnosis.

4. **F.** These symptoms and signs should be familiar to every dentist and student. The absence of tenderness to percussion or any radiological signs excludes an acute periapical periodontitis from the differential diagnosis. The thermal sensitivity is a classic sign.

5. **H.** The initial symptoms fit with acute periapical periodontitis, a finding that is consistent with the radiological signs. The appearance of a fluctuant swelling, however, indicates a collection of pus (abscess).

6. **A.** This needs no real explanation; the radiological appearance is diagnostic.

7. **D.** A firm swelling in a child's jaw could, of course, be due to several different conditions. The symptom of toothache and a grossly carious molar make for a straightforward cause-and-effect relationship, but could be coincidental to the bony swelling. Similarly, the periapical condensing osteitis could make for a simple diagnosis of chronic periapical periodontitis. The key feature here is the radiological finding of periosteal new bone. This sign makes the diagnosis almost certain.

8. **J.** The clinical features indicate chronic infection, but the radiological sign of a radiolucent area with a central radio-opacity are consistent with a sequestrum lying within an area of bone destruction. The history of a recent extraction provides a precipitating event. While chronic osteomyelitis is a suitable diagnosis, the history of severe osteoporosis raises the possibility of bisphosphonate-associated bone necrosis. Someone of this age with severe osteoporosis would certainly be offered treatment and bisphosphonates would be the obvious choice. Bone necrosis is more commonly associated with high-dose bisphosphonates used in management of metastatic malignancy, but there are numerous cases appearing in the literature of patients using oral bisphosphonates developing the condition.

9. **G.** The tingling lower lip should set the alarm bell ringing, as this sign is a feature of a significant problem (i.e. involvement of the ID canal by some pathosis). The draining extra-oral and intra-oral sinuses indicate an infection, while the radiological picture fits with sequestration of bone. Together with the history of a problem over several weeks, these features fit with chronic osteomyelitis. No periosteal new bone was noted in the history, but that is a feature usually only picked up on true occlusal and, sometimes, panoramic radiographs and may be quite a subtle change.

10. **I.** These symptoms and signs are all typical of chronic pulpitis. The pain is not so severe as with acute pulpitis, although occasional acute flare-ups may occur. An important finding is that the tooth was not tender to percussion, as that sign would have suggested periapical inflammation.

Case history answers

Case history 1

While most patients returning with postextraction pain will have alveolar osteitis ('dry socket'), there are a number of features here that indicate that the diagnosis is not so straightforward.

Assessment should begin with a thorough clinical examination. Extra-oral examination should include careful palpation of lymph nodes and assessment of the numbness affecting her lip (see Ch. 2 for details on both of these). Intra-oral examination should not only involve examination of the socket but also of other teeth on the lower left as it is always possible that the recent extraction is not the cause of the current problem. Examine the socket; after 4 weeks, a socket should be filled with maturing granulation tissue and early bone deposition will be occurring. Clinically, therefore, the socket should be largely closed over (although a defect is often still evident with larger molar teeth) and the mucosa should not be inflamed.

The pain, swelling and numbness affecting the mental nerve all suggest a pathological process involving the bone of the mandible distal to the mental foramen. Starting from first principles, differential diagnosis might include infection (osteomyelitis), fracture of the mandible and malignancy in the jaw. Suitable radiology will now help to narrow down the differential diagnosis. The radiographs show a 'mixed lesion' (i.e. radiolucent and radio-opaque) in the mandibular body. This is compatible with osteomyelitis rather than the other possible diagnoses, although it is possible that a fracture may have occurred secondary to the infection.

Management would be principally by antibiotic therapy and surgical removal of the sequestered bone. Such management would be carried out under the care of a hospital specialist.

Case history 2

Follow the standard assessment procedures described in Chapter 3 of extra-oral examination, intra-oral examination (to the degree possible where there is trismus) and appropriate special tests. The last would probably be limited to extra-oral radiography in this case, using either a lateral oblique film or a panoramic examination (preferably by a field size collimation to exclude other regions of the mouth).

All the symptoms suggest infection as a cause. Your knowledge about the impacted lower third molar make acute pericoronitis a likely diagnosis. If we assume that this is the case, then your management should include:

1. Irrigate beneath the operculum using saline or chlorhexidine solution.
2. If access will allow, relieve any traumatic occlusion on the operculum by grinding the cusps of the opposing tooth. Often the opposing tooth is a non-functional third molar; if you expect that the lower third molar will never erupt into function, then the opposing tooth may be best extracted to relieve the pericoronitis.

3. Prescribe antibiotics (the swelling and lymphadenopathy suggest that this is appropriate).
4. Advise frequent hot salt mouthwashes.
5. Arrange a review appointment. In a case as severe as this an early (24–48 hours) appointment would be appropriate, but you should arrange another visit once the infection has resolved to allow a considered assessment of the third molar (see Ch. 6).

Case history 3

Follow the standard assessment procedures described in Chapter 2 of extra-oral examination, intra-oral examination and appropriate special tests. Examine the 'spot' on her chin carefully. The description of it as 'weeping' fluid, along with the history, suggests that it may be a draining sinus from a chronic dental abscess.

The lower anterior teeth should be examined particularly carefully. Look in the labial sulcus and palpate it to identify any swelling, tender areas or other (intra-oral) sinuses. Examine the teeth and assess for mobility and tenderness to pressure that might indicate periapical or periodontal pathology. Periapical radiographs of suspect teeth should be taken and you should carefully compare these with any previous radiographs to identify deterioration in any pre-existing periapical lesions. Occasionally it might be possible to pass a gutta-percha point through an open sinus and take a radiograph. The rationale for this is that the radio-opaque gutta-percha will 'point' towards the origin of the infection. Practically this can be uncomfortable and only worthwhile where there is real uncertainty over the origin of the infection.

Management will commence with identification of the tooth causing the problem. Once a diagnosis of chronic abscess is made, appropriate treatment would be endodontic therapy (orthograde or, if not possible, retrograde with apicectomy). Alternatively, if this fits with the overall treatment plan, extraction may be preferred.

Case history 4

Clinical features

Obtain a complete history first. How long has the pain been present? Have there been previous episodes or is this the first? Carry out a complete examination. Test each tooth for sensitivity with a cotton wool pledget soaked in ethyl chloride. Use gentle finger pressure on each tooth, followed up by percussion if there is no abnormal response. Record the responses and note if you manage to reproduce the pain the patient is complaining of.

Radiology

The radiograph shows a large restoration in the molar and a post crown on the first premolar. In the premolar the root filling looks insubstantial and there is a periapical granuloma present. At the level of the end of the post there is radio-opaque material overlying the tooth and bone. Also at this level and further coronally lamina dura is lost along the root surface.

Likely diagnosis

The lack of any aggravation of the pain by thermal stimuli suggests that this is not pulpitis. The dull aching pain, along with the tenderness in the buccal sulcus, suggests chronic periapical periodontitis is a likelier diagnosis. On radiological grounds, there is only one likely tooth with problems: the first premolar. The apical granuloma suggests chronic inflammation, but you should bear in mind that the radiograph is a snapshot in time and that the lesion could be healing (although the poor root filling suggests otherwise). The interesting finding is the collection of signs around the end of the post. The radio-opaque material overlying the root here is probably extruded cement from when the post was cemented. This at least suggests a perforation and may indicate a fracture of the root at this level. Clinical examination might reveal mobility of the crown if a fracture were present.

Viva answers

1. Loss of lamina dura may be localised to a single tooth or generalised in the dentition. Localised lamina dura loss, usually around a tooth apex, is a sign of acute inflammation (or recent acute inflammation) of dental origin. In chronic inflammation, the 'lamina dura' persists as the margin of a granuloma or cyst. Lamina dura loss laterally on the root may occur in relation to a lateral canal or, more commonly, through loss of periodontal attachment in periodontal disease. Generalised loss of lamina dura occurs in hyperparathyroidism and Paget's disease of bone, while thinning occurs in osteoporosis and Cushing's syndrome.

2. The primary aim in treating dental infections is to achieve drainage of pus. The second aim is to remove the cause of the infection. In many cases, the two are achieved simultaneously by extraction of a tooth or a pulpectomy. Antibiotics would be used in dental infections if drainage of pus could not be achieved. They may also be used in addition to the usual surgical procedures if there is a local or generalised predisposition to infections (e.g. Paget's disease, immunocompromised patients).

3. An abscess is a pathological cavity filled with pus and lined by a pyogenic membrane. It is a common condition in dentistry as it may result from periapical periodontitis, periodontal disease, pericoronitis or infection of a cyst. Management involves drainage of the pus; this is usually undertaken by extracting the associated tooth or via the root canal.

4. No; at least it is no better than an informed guess. A periapical granuloma is usually no larger than 1 cm in diameter. Radiolucencies greater than this are more

likely to be cysts, but there is overlap in size around this threshold.

5. Pyrexia or abnormally high body temperature is an important physical sign. Most pyrexias result from self-limiting viral infections, characterised by influenza-like symptoms, although in dentistry the majority will result from oral infections that require active treatment. In general, a pyrexia may result from infections, neoplasms, connective tissue diseases or other causes such as drug reactions. Pyrexia is a sign of systemic toxicity; when it is associated with a dental infection it is an indication for the prescription of an antimicrobial drug and perhaps even hospital admission depending on the seriousness. Temperature has been traditionally measured by placing a mercury thermometer under the tongue, into the rectum or under the axilla. Electronic temperature sensors are now used against the tympanic membrane as they provide more rapid measurement and avoid the use of mercury. Normal temperature is in the range 35.8–37.1 °C.

6. The term endarteritis obliterans is used to describe a process of internal (intimal) proliferation within a blood vessel. It causes obliteration of the lumen, resulting in cessation of blood flow. Endarteritis obliterans may arise as a result of several inflammatory processes but is an important feature of radiation damage. Following irradiation, endothelial cell loss results in exposure of the subendothelial collagen. This prompts platelet adherence, thrombosis and organisation of the lumen by fibrosis. The reduced vascular supply to tissues may result in impaired wound healing or necrosis.

7. A pericoronal infection may spread via the lymphatic system and along tissue planes with serious consequences. Infection may present buccally in the vestibular sulcus or may spread lingually to the sublingual and submandibular spaces. The pharyngeal tissue spaces may also be involved. Unchecked, such spread may compromise the airway and on occasion necessitate advanced surgical airway management by way of tracheostomy.

8. These differ in symptoms and signs. Acute pulpitis involves severe, sharp pain of several minutes duration that is precipitated mainly by hot and cold stimuli. It is often poorly localised. Acute periapical periodontitis gives symptoms of a dull, throbbing ache, usually well-localised to a tooth. In acute pulpitis, a tooth is not tender to pressure but is hypersensitive to thermal stimuli, while in acute periapical periodontitis the tooth is tender to pressure and (usually) unresponsive to thermal stimuli.

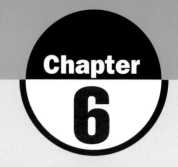

Removal of teeth and surgical implantology

Overview

In this chapter, the surgical treatment of teeth is described. The indications for dental extraction are listed together with the information that must be elicited before a tooth is extracted. Forceps and surgical techniques of extraction are outlined and the complications that can follow extraction are outlined with the treatment response. The clinical and radiological assessment and treatment are described for impacted and ectopic teeth, lower and upper third molars, mandibular second premolars and maxillary canines.

The final section of the chapter deals with surgery to assist retention of conventional dentures and the surgical placement of implants.

6.1 Dental extractions

Learning objectives

You should:
- understand the indications for removal of a tooth
- know how to complete the preoperative assessment
- know the techniques available for extraction
- be aware of the potential complications following extraction and their treatment.

Assessment for extraction

Indications for dental extraction

Teeth may require removal for many reasons including the following:

- gross caries
- pulpitis
- periapical periodontitis
- pericoronitis
- abscess resulting from periapical periodontitis, periodontal disease or pericoronitis
- fractured teeth

- when associated with other pathology such as a cyst, fracture of the jaw or tumour
- when misplaced, impacted or supernumerary
- as part of orthodontic treatment
- when retained (primary teeth).

History and clinical examination

The assessment of the patient has already been described in Chapter 2. A thorough medical history prior to any surgical procedure is obviously essential. This will identify patients who may require special preparation prior to even the simplest dental extraction. Such patients may include those taking anticoagulant medication or those that have undergone irradiation, amongst many others. The information obtained will also determine the advisability of carrying out the treatment in a primary care setting (general dental practice and community clinics) as opposed to in a hospital. The home circumstances and availability of an escort may also be important if considering conscious sedation or general anaesthesia.

The clinical examination includes the subjective assessment of the patient's anxiety and likely cooperation by observation of the patient's behaviour. These may also be gauged from answers to questions about the previous dental experience. The sex, general build of the patient or other factors may give an indication as to the expected ease or difficulty of the extraction. For example, an extraction is likely to be more difficult in heavily built men; elderly patients may have more brittle teeth and Afro-Caribbeans more dense alveolar bone, while child patients may have reduced access and less cooperation.

The intra-oral examination should include a note of the access to and position of the tooth. The crown of a heavily restored tooth is more likely to fracture during extraction, while endodontically treated teeth may be more brittle.

Radiological examination

Preoperative radiographs need not be taken prior to all extractions, but there are situations when radiographic assessment is essential to demonstrate root morphology, anatomical relationships or associated pathology (Box 5). Mandibular and maxillary third molar teeth are known to show a wide variability in root morphology, and so pre-extraction radiographs should be taken. It is also essential to know the relationship of the inferior alveolar canal in the case of the lower third molar. In general, where any difficulty is anticipated, it would be wise to take a radiograph before rather than during the extraction, so that the procedure may be planned appropriately. Where a radiograph is judged to be necessary a periapical view should be the first

> **Box 5** Checklist of situations where a pre-extraction radiograph is reasonable
>
> - Third molars
> - Isolated (lone-standing) upper molars
> - Previous history of difficult extractions
> - Heavily restored (e.g. crowned, root-filled) teeth

choice, although other films may be substituted or used in addition when indicated (e.g. panoramic or lateral oblique for lower third molar).

Treatment planning

The information from the history and examination is used to formulate the best plan for the patient. This will include measures for adequate preparation for the procedure and also the selection of anaesthesia: whether local anaesthesia, conscious sedation with local anaesthesia or general anaesthesia. Anticipated difficulties are better discussed with the patient before treatment rather than during treatment, when they may be perceived as excuses for inadequate planning or experience.

Surgical techniques

Instrumental extraction

To extract a tooth from the alveolus, the periodontal attachment must be disrupted and the bony dental socket enlarged to allow withdrawal of the tooth. To achieve this, various instruments have been developed:

- *elevators:* curved chisel-shaped instruments that fit the curvature of tooth roots; an elevator has a single blade
- *luxators:* similar to elevators but finer blade
- *forceps:* have paired blades that are hinged to permit the root to be grasped
- *peritome:* has a finer blade with which to sever the periodontal attachment and is preferred where it is important not to damage the bony support of the tooth, for example when immediately replacing a tooth with a dental implant.

There are several different forceps extraction techniques described and so some basic principles and guidance are required when learning. Forceps are used to disrupt the periodontal attachment and dilate the bony socket either directly, by forcing the blades between tooth and bone, or by moving the tooth root within the socket, or both. Once this has been done, the tooth may be lifted from its socket. The movements that are required to complete the extraction may be described as a *preliminary movement* to sever the periodontal membrane and generally dilate the socket, followed by a *second movement* to complete the dilation and withdraw the tooth. The first movement requires that force is directed along the long axis of the tooth, pushing the blades of the forceps towards the root apex. This force is then maintained during the second movement, which is dependent on the tooth root and bone morphology. If a tooth has a single round root, then it may be rotated. Where the buccal bone plate is relatively thin, it may be possible

to distort it significantly by moving the forceps applied to the tooth root in a buccal direction. The second movement depends on the tooth and may be described as:

- upper incisors and canines: rotational
- upper premolars: limited buccal and palatal
- upper molars: buccal
- lower incisors and canines: buccal
- lower premolars: rotational
- lower molars: buccal.

Alternative techniques for forceps movement are advocated by some, including a 'figure of eight' movement to expand the socket for molar teeth. Elevators may be used to carry out the first movement prior to completion of the extraction with forceps. Sometimes teeth and roots may be removed with elevators alone. There are many different designs of elevator (Fig. 60). The most commonly used are:

- *Coupland's elevators:* a straight blade in line with the handle; available in three sizes referred to as 1, 2 and 3
- *Cryer's elevators:* a triangular blade at right angles to the handle; available as a right and left pair
- *Warwick James elevators:* a small blade that is rounded at its tip rather than pointed; this is set at right angles to the tip in a right and left pair, but a straight Warwick James is also available.

It is important that elevators are used appropriately, with their blades between root and bone rather than between adjacent teeth, or else both teeth will be loosened.

There are many designs of forceps. The blades vary in size and shape according to the root morphology of the tooth/teeth for which they are designed. For example, lower molar forceps incorporate a right angle between blades and handles, while the blades each have a central projection to accommodate the bifurcation. Upper 'root' forceps have narrower blades than the equivalent upper premolar forceps.

It may be difficult to apply forceps to teeth that are outside of a crowded dental arch and elevators may be more

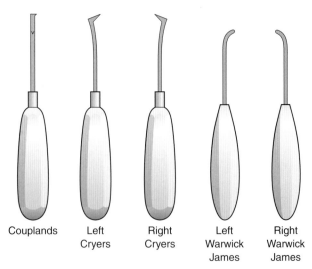

| Couplands | Left Cryers | Right Cryers | Left Warwick James | Right Warwick James |

Fig. 60 Elevators commonly used in oral surgery.

appropriate for initiating the extraction or for the whole procedure. The applied force should be controlled and limited when using both elevators and forceps so that the soft tissues are not accidentally injured or the jaws fractured. Only with experience is it possible to know that the usual force is not producing the expected result, when further investigation is required with a radiograph (if not already available) or a transalveolar approach required.

The non-dominant hand is used to support the mandible against the force of the first movement when extracting lower teeth. It is also used to retract the intra-oral soft tissues and, by supporting the adjacent alveolus, provide feedback of movement as a measure of control.

The patient should have eye protection; if the treatment is carried out under local anaesthesia, then the patient may be placed in a position between sitting up and supine or treated supine. Treatment under conscious sedation or general anaesthesia will dictate the supine position. Lower right quadrant extractions are best performed with the operator standing behind the patient; for all other extractions, the operator should stand in front of the patient.

Surgical removal of teeth

Teeth resistant to forceps extraction and those that fracture during extraction need to be removed surgically. However, it may be acceptable to leave a very small root apex if there is no associated periapical pathology and the anticipated surgical morbidity is significant. The patient must be told if any fragments are to be retained.

Teeth are surgically removed by a transalveolar approach. The procedure is described in Box 6.

Box 6 Technique for surgical tooth removal by transalveolar approach

1. A mucoperiosteal flap is raised, with a broad base to ensure good blood supply. Incisions should be full thickness and the flap should be retracted to ensure good access and visibility of the area without causing undue trauma to the soft tissues. Papilla should be included in the design of a flap and not divided or they are unlikely to maintain their viability.

2. Bone is removed with an irrigated bur to permit adequate access for application of elevators and for removal of the tooth. A chisel and mallet may be used to remove bone if the operation is being undertaken under general anaesthesia.

3. The tooth is divided with a bur as necessary.

4. Elevators are used to sever the periodontal membrane and dilate the socket; the tooth is then removed.

5. The wound is cleaned with irrigation and bone is filed, as appropriate.

6. Haemostasis.

7. The wound is closed with sutures. The flap should be designed so that its margins will rest on sound bone at closure.

Postoperative care

Control of postoperative pain is important (Chapter 4). Some clinicians prescribe antibiotics if bone removal is necessary.

Patients should be given a written set of postoperative instructions (Fig. 61) and these should be also given verbally before the patient leaves.

Complications of dental extractions

Postoperative pain

Discomfort after the surgical trauma of dental extractions is to be expected and may be alleviated with an analgesic such as paracetamol or a non-steroidal anti-inflammatory drug (NSAID) such as ibuprofen.

Severe pain after a dental extraction is unusual and may indicate that another complication has occurred.

Postoperative swelling

Mild inflammatory swelling may follow dental extractions but is unusual unless the procedure was difficult and significant surgical trauma occurred.

More significant swelling usually indicates postoperative infection or presence of a haematoma. Management of infection may require systemic antibiotics or drainage. A large haematoma may need to be drained. Less likely is surgical emphysema (see below).

Trismus

Trismus or limited mouth opening after a dental extraction is unusual and is likely to be infective in origin.

Fracture of teeth

Teeth may fracture during forceps extraction for a variety of reasons and this is not an unusual event.

ON THE DAY OF TREATMENT

- Do not rinse your mouth for at least 24 hours.
- Avoid hot fluids, alcohol, hard or chewy foods. Choose cool drinks and soft foods.
- Avoid vigorous exercise.
- Smokers should avoid smoking.
- Should the wound start to bleed, apply a small compress. This can be made from some cotton wool in a clean handkerchief. Place this on the bleeding point and bite firmly on it for 5–10 minutes or longer if necessary.
- If you cannot stop the bleeding yourself, please seek professional advice.
- Any pain or soreness can be relieved by taking the prescribed medication. If none was prescribed, take tablets such as paracetamol (Panadol) 2 tablets every 4 hours as required. Do not take more than the recommended number per day.

STARTING 24 HOURS LATER

- Gently rinse the wound with hot saltwater mouth rinses (or other rinse as recommended) for a few days. This should be carried out three times a day after each meal.

Fig. 61 A typical instruction leaflet given to patients after an extraction.

The crown may fracture because of the presence of a large restoration, but this may not prevent the extraction from continuing as the forceps are applied to the root. However, if the fracture occurs subgingivally, then a transalveolar approach will be necessary to visualise the root.

If a small (3mm) root apex is retained after extraction, this may be left in situ, providing it is not associated with apical infection. The patient must be informed of the decision to leave the apex to avoid the morbidity associated with its surgical retrieval and the decision recorded. Antibiotics should be prescribed.

Excessive bleeding

It may be difficult to gauge the seriousness of the blood loss from the patient's history, because they are usually anxious. However, it is important to establish whether or not the patient is shocked by measuring the blood pressure and pulse. This can be done while the patient bites firmly on a gauze swab to encourage haemostasis. Typically, if the systolic pressure is below 100 mmHg and the heart rate in excess of 100 beats/min, then the patient is shocked and there is an urgent need to replace lost volume. This may be done by infusion of a plasma expander such as Gelofusine or Haemaccel or a crystalloid such as sodium chloride via a large peripheral vein. For this purpose, the patient should be transferred to hospital. More commonly, the patient is not shocked and can be managed in the primary care setting.

The next step in management is to investigate the cause of the haemorrhage by taking a history and carrying out an examination.

History

- Local causes
  - mouthrinsing
  - exercise
  - alcohol
- General causes
  - previous postextraction or surgical haemorrhage
  - medications
  - liver disease
  - family history of disorders of haemostasis.

Examination

Determine the source of the haemorrhage by sitting the patient upright (unless feeling faint) and using suction and a good light. This is commonly from capillaries of the bony socket or the gingival margin of the socket, or more unusually from a large blood vessel or soft-tissue tear.

Achieve haemostasis

If the history has suggested a general cause, then local methods will not adequately result in haemostasis and the patient should be transferred to hospital where specialist haematological management is available. Otherwise the following techniques are used:

- socket capillaries: pack the socket with resorbable cellulose, such as Surgicell

- gingival capillaries: suture the socket with a material that will permit adequate tension, such as vicryl or black silk
- large blood vessel: ligate vessel, usually by passing a suture about the vessel and soft tissues.

Dry socket (alveolar osteitis)

In some cases, a blood clot may inadequately form or be broken down. Predisposing factors of osteitis include smoking, surgical trauma, the vasoconstrictor added to a local anaesthetic solution, oral contraceptives and a history of radiotherapy. The exposed bone is extremely painful and sensitive to touch.

Dry socket is managed by:

- reassuring the patient that the correct tooth has been extracted
- irrigation of socket with warm saline or chlorhexidine mouthrinse to remove any debris
- dressing the socket to protect it from painful stimuli: bismuth–iodoform–paraffin paste (BIPP) and lidocaine (lignocaine) gel on ribbon gauze are useful.

Postoperative infection

In some cases, sockets may become truly infected, with pus, local swelling and perhaps lymphadenopathy. This is usually localised to the socket and can be managed in the same way as a dry socket, although antibiotics may be necessary in some instances. A radiograph should be taken to exclude the presence of a retained root or sequestered bone (Fig. 62). Positive evidence of such material in the socket indicates a need for curettage of the socket.

Osteomyelitis

Osteomyelitis (Ch. 5) is rare but may be identified by radiological evidence of loss of the socket lamina dura and a rarefying osteitis in the surrounding bone, often with scattered radio-opacities representing sequestra (see Figs 56 and 57).

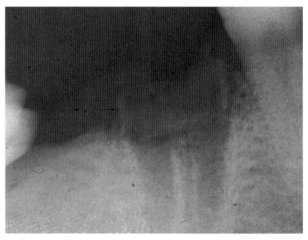

Fig. 62 Intra-oral film of a patient with persistent post-extraction infection. The bone of the crest of the socket is detached, acting as a sequestrum.

Damage to soft tissues

Crush injuries can occur to soft tissues when a local or general anaesthetic has been used and the patient does not respond to the stimulus and, therefore, inform the operator. This may happen to a lower anaesthetised lip when extracting an upper tooth; the lip can be crushed between forceps and teeth if it is not rotated out of the way.

Damage to nerves

Paraesthesia or anaesthesia can result from damage to the nerves in the intradermal canal during extraction of lower third molars.

Opening of the maxillary sinus

Creation of a communication between the oral cavity and maxillary sinus, an oroantral fistula (OAF), may result during extraction of upper molar teeth. This is described in Chapter 7.

Loss of tooth

A whole tooth may occasionally be displaced into the maxillary sinus, when it is managed as for displacement of a root fragment, as described in Chapter 7.

A tooth may also be lost into the infratemporal fossa or the tissue spaces about the jaws, but this usually only occurs when mucoperiosteal flaps are raised.

Loss of tooth fragment

Typically, a fractured palatal root of an upper molar tooth is inadvertently pushed into the maxillary sinus by the misuse of elevators. Rarely, a fragment may be lost elsewhere, such as into the inferior alveolar canal.

Fracture of the maxillary tuberosity

Fracture of the maxillary tuberosity can result from the extraction of upper posterior molar teeth; it is described in Chapter 7.

Fracture of jaw

A fracture of the jaw is a rare event and is most likely to be the result of application of excessive force in an uncontrolled way. More commonly, small fragments of alveolar bone are fractured, which may be attached to the tooth root. Any loose fragments should also be removed.

Dislocation of the mandible

Dislocation may occur when extracting lower teeth if the mandible is not adequately supported. It is more likely to occur under general anaesthesia and should be reduced immediately.

Displacement of tooth into the airway

The airway is at risk when extracting teeth on a patient in the supine position. It can be protected when the patient is being treated under general anaesthesia but not when the patient is conscious or being treated under conscious sedation. It is, therefore, essential that an assistant is present and high-velocity suction and an appropriate instrument for retrieval of any foreign body are immediately available.

A chest radiograph is essential if a lost tooth cannot be found, to exclude inhalation.

Surgical emphysema

Air may enter soft tissues, producing a characteristic crackling sensation on palpation. However, this is unlikely if a mucoperiosteal flap has not been raised. Air-rotor dental drills should not be used during surgery because they may force air under soft-tissue flaps.

The patient should be reassured and antibiotics prescribed.

6.2 Impacted and ectopic teeth

Learning objectives

You should:

- understand the terms impacted and ectopic and know which teeth are likely to be affected
- be able to examine and assess patients with impacted/ectopic teeth
- understand the treatment options
- know the surgical techniques, their application and complications.

Assessment

In the context of teeth, the term **ectopic** is applicable to a tooth that is malpositioned through congenital factors or displaced by the presence of pathology. It includes **impacted** teeth. Impaction may occur because there is no path of eruption because the tooth develops in an abnormal position or is obstructed by a physical barrier such as another tooth, odontogenic cyst or tumour.

Most commonly affected

- mandibular third molars
- maxillary third molars
- maxillary canines.

Less commonly affected

- mandibular second premolars
- supernumerary teeth.

An impacted tooth may be *completely impacted*, when entirely covered by soft tissue and partially or completely covered by bone within the bony alveolus, or *partially erupted*, when it has failed to erupt into a normal functional position. The terms unerupted and partially erupted are commonly used for normally developing as well as impacted teeth. It is important, therefore, to distinguish between impaction and normal development.

Third molars. These usually erupt between 18 and 24 years but, frequently, eruption occurs outside these limits. One or more third molars fail to develop in approximately one in four adults. Impaction of third molars predisposes to pathological changes such as pericoronitis, caries, resorption and periodontal problems.

Impacted maxillary canines. These may be associated with resorption of adjacent lateral incisor roots, dentigerous cyst formation and infection.

Impacted lower second premolars. These are often lingually positioned and may have an unfavourable root morphology.

History and clinical examination

The patient may have noticed that a tooth is missing or this may not be apparent until observed at a routine dental examination. It is unusual for unerupted teeth to cause pain unless there is associated infection. The signs and symptoms of pericoronal inflammation are described in Chapter 5. Pericoronitis can be associated with any impacted tooth but is of particular concern when it involves the mandibular third molar because of the greater potential to spread via the tissue spaces and compromise the airway.

On examination, missing teeth should be noted and also any caries or mobility of adjacent teeth. Signs of infection will include swelling, discharge, trismus and tender enlarged cervical lymph nodes.

Radiological examination

Radiological examination should be based upon clinical history and examination. Routine radiographic examination of unerupted third molars is not recommended. Radiological assessment is essential prior to surgery but does not need to be carried out at the initial examination if infection or some other local problem is present.

The views used are:

- periapical, dental panoramic tomography (DPT) (or lateral oblique) and, rarely, computed tomography (CT) for lower third molars
- DPT (or lateral oblique, or adequate periapical) for upper third molars
- parallax films (two periapicals or one periapical and an occlusal film) for maxillary canines
- periapical and true occlusal radiograph for mandibular second premolar; a DPT (or lateral oblique) should be used if the periapical does not image the whole of the unerupted tooth.

Radiological assessment of impacted teeth should cover:

- type and orientation of impaction and the access to the tooth
- crown size and condition
- root number and morphology
- alveolar bone level, including depth and density
- follicular width
- periodontal status, adjacent teeth
- relationship or proximity of upper teeth to the nasal cavity or maxillary antrum
- relationship or proximity of lower teeth to the interdental canal, mental foramen, lower border of mandible.

Diagnosis

When documenting the diagnosis, it is important to state 'impacted tooth' and the problem associated with this tooth. The mere presence of an impacted tooth may not in itself justify the treatment planned for the patient. It is better therefore to state 'impacted lower third molar and recurrent pericoronitis', for example.

Treatment options

The initial management of pericoronal infection may include irrigation beneath the operculum, grinding the cusps (or extraction) of any opposing tooth in the case of a lower third molar, and antibiotic therapy, as described in Chapter 5.

Review of the patient is necessary to assess the long-term management of the impacted tooth or teeth. Treatment options are:

- observation
- surgical removal
- operculectomy
- surgical exposure
- surgical reimplantation/transplantation.

In the case of impacted third molars, the decision is usually between observation or removal, as the outcomes for the alternative treatments offer limited therapeutic success. The decision to recommend removal takes into account the likely surgical morbidity and the risk of continuing and recurring pathology. In the case of maxillary canines, surgical exposure is a good option if there is sufficient space in the arch to accommodate the tooth or if space can be created orthodontically. Lower second premolars may also be exposed, but this is less commonly undertaken than for maxillary canines. The medical history, social history and age of the patient may all have an influence on the decision making.

Indications for removal of third molars

There has been disagreement about the appropriateness of removing third molars without associated pathology in order to prevent potential development of pathology (prophylactic removal) but there is no controversy about the value of removing teeth that are associated with pathology. In the UK several bodies have published guidelines to help clinicians with decision making about wisdom teeth but the research evidence on which these are founded has been of poor quality. They have generally encouraged a more conservative approach (retention of wisdom teeth) than found in other parts of the world, particularly the USA. The following indications have been suggested for the removal of wisdom teeth in the national health service of the UK:

- pericoronitis
- unrestorable caries
- non-treatable pupal/periapical pathology
- cellulitis/abscess/osteomyelitis
- internal/external resorption of the tooth or adjacent teeth
- fracture of the tooth
- disease of the follicle, including cyst/tumour
- tooth impeding surgery or reconstructive jaw surgery
- tooth involved in tumour or in field of tumour resection.

The decision to remove wisdom teeth or not will be based on the relative benefits and harms, in the context of the best research evidence, clinical experience and the patient values, as described in Chapter 1. Impacted third molar teeth that are not to be removed should be kept under review to ensure that no pathological process develops. Caries involving the second molar adjacent to partly erupted impacted retained wisdom teeth may develop. The decision will therefore take many factors into account including the caries risk in addition to general health and local factors.

Most commonly the benefits include alleviation of the symptoms and signs of pericoronitis and its potential consequences. The symptoms of pericoronitis are pain, bad taste, swelling of the pericoronal tissues and face, and restricted mouth opening (trismus). The local infection may spread, resulting in a regional lymphadenopathy, pyrexia and malaise. Rarely the swelling may threaten the patency of the airway and breathing. The potential harms are described below under 'complications'.

Surgical techniques

Lower third molar surgery

The operation is described in Box 7. The area of bone that is removed and the path of withdrawal of the tooth depends upon the type of impaction (Fig. 63).

Upper third molar surgery

The procedure follows the same principles as for lower third molars, although obviously no lingual nerve protection is required and, frequently, bone removal is not necessary. It is important to maintain good vision of the

---

Box 7 Surgical technique for removal of lower third molar

1. A buccal mucoperiosteal flap is raised to provide adequate access.

2. A lingual flap is raised and the lingual nerve is protected with an appropriate instrument. This aspect is controversial and some would avoid raising a lingual flap and restrict their approach to the buccal only. This latter approach requires tooth division more frequently and is carried out in an attempt to reduce the incidence of lingual nerve damage and resulting sensory disturbance. The avoidance of a lingual flap has been the popular technique in the USA, while raising a lingual flap and protecting the nerve, with a retractor such as a Howarth, has been common in the UK.

3. Bone removal may be required and this may be undertaken with an irrigated bur in a handpiece or a chisel. The lingual split technique involves the removal of a segment of lingual bone plate with a chisel after the nerve has been protected. The advocates of this technique suggest that while temporary nerve damage may occur, permanent damage is reduced when compared with the use of burs for bone removal.

4. The tooth may then need to be divided before elevation and removal. (Fig. 63 shows areas of bone removal and paths of withdrawal.)

5. The wound is irrigated and inspected before the soft tissues are closed with an appropriate suture material.

---

surgical site and to position an instrument carefully to keep the soft-tissue flap open and direct the elevated tooth into the mouth, to prevent its entry into the infra-temporal fossa. The usual path of withdrawal is shown in Figure 64.

Maxillary canines

A buccal or palatal approach is made, appropriate to the position of the tooth. The palatal approach must take into account the greater palatine artery, which is incorporated into a large flap design with the sacrifice of the nasopalatine neurovascular bundle (Fig. 65). Bone is then removed and the tooth elevated and removed. If the tooth is to be exposed, the bone is removed without damaging the tooth and a defect created when repositioning the flap, which is maintained by interrupting healing by the placement of a pack, sutured in place.

If it is apparent that the tooth cannot be moved by orthodontic means, then it is possible carefully to remove it with as little damage as possible to the periodontal ligament and splint it into position in a surgically created socket. This transplantation technique has become less popular over the years as it has become apparent that the long-term success is not good and resorption frequently occurs, albeit after some years.

Mandibular second premolars

It is important that the mental nerve is identified and protected while raising a buccal mucoperiosteal flap. It is frequently necessary to divide the tooth and remove the crown before the root can be delivered by elevation.

Supernumerary teeth

Commonly, supernumerary teeth occur in the anterior maxilla and are exposed via a buccal or palatal flap and bone removal. It is important to identify the supernumerary teeth clearly before removal and this can be difficult when there are also developing permanent teeth present.

Complications of treatment of impacted and ectopic teeth

The potential complications of the surgical removal of impacted teeth are postoperative pain, swelling, infection and trismus. When surgery involves the removal of lower third molars a less common but more debilitating outcome for the patient is lingual or inferior alveolar nerve damage, resulting in altered sensation of the tongue or skin of the lower lip and chin. Taste sensation may also be impaired. Sensory disturbance may be temporary, described as recovery of normal sensation within 4–6 months, or may persist, described as permanent. The degree and description of altered sensation is variable and includes reduced sensation (hypoaesthesia), abnormal sensation (paraesthesia) and unpleasant sensation (dysaesthesia). The incidence of temporary and permanent lingual nerve damage following the surgical removal of third molar teeth varies considerably between reports and may be related to a number of factors including the surgical technique and the skill

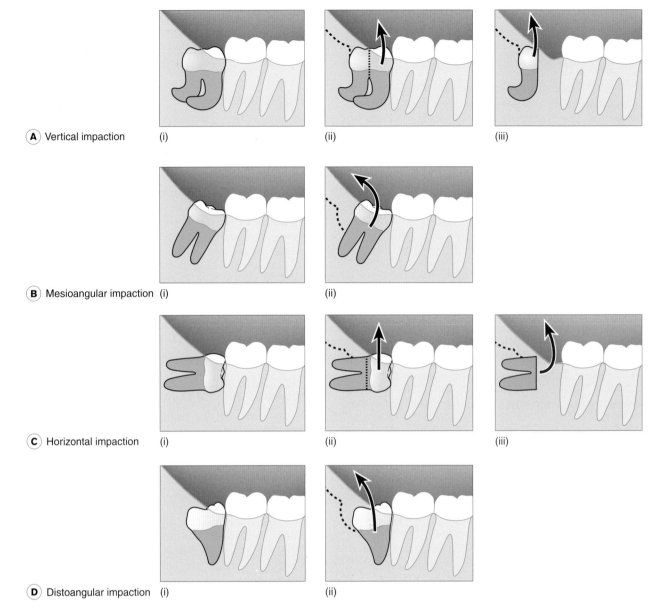

(A) Vertical impaction   (i)   (ii)   (iii)

(B) Mesioangular impaction (i)   (ii)

(C) Horizontal impaction   (i)   (ii)   (iii)

(D) Distoangular impaction (i)   (ii)

Fig. 63 Examples of various types of third molar impactions. **A,** Vertical impaction with unfavourable root morphology requiring bone removal and vertical sectioning. **B,** Mesioangular impaction requiring bone removal and a mesial application point to elevate and upright to remove. **C,** Horizontal impaction requiring bone removal, sectioning of the crown to permit removal of crown and then roots in stages. **D,** Distoangular impaction requiring significant bone removal to permit elevation distally for removal without reimpaction.

of the surgeon. The incidence of temporary lingual nerve disturbance has been reported to be 0% to 23% and that of permanent disturbance to be 0% to 2%. Inferior alveolar nerve damage is less common than lingual nerve damage.

Fig. 64 Path of withdrawal of maxillary third molar.

6.3 Preprosthetic surgery

Learning objective

You should:
- know the surgical procedures that can be used to prepare for retentive conventional dentures.

Preprosthetic surgery refers to the surgical procedures that can be used to modify the oral anatomy to facilitate the construction of retentive conventional dentures. Some of these traditional techniques have been less commonly needed since the introduction of osseointegrated implants into clinical practice. However, implant treatment sometimes

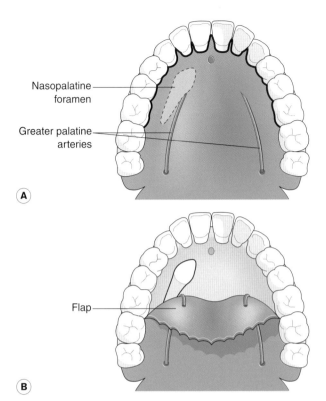

Nasopalatine foramen

Greater palatine arteries

A

Flap

B

Fig. 65 Surgical approach for the removal of an impacted palatal canine. **A,** An incision is made about the palatal gingival margins. Greater palatine arteries and nasopalatine foramen are shown. **B,** A palatal mucoperiosteal flap is raised to provide access to the palatal canine tooth.

requires additional surgical intervention and this may also be referred to as preprosthetic surgery.

Retained teeth/roots removal

Retained dental roots can become superficial as the alveolar ridge resorbs. This may lead to ulceration of the overlying mucosa or the area can become infected. Such roots should be surgically removed with minimal bone loss. The importance of preserving alveolar bone whenever oral surgery procedures are undertaken cannot be overstated.

Denture irritation hyperplasia

Long-term use of ill-fitting dentures can lead to hyperplasia of the mucosa. This may then prevent the construction of new well-fitting dentures. The initial treatment is to persuade the patient to stop wearing the denture and this will permit some reduction in the volume of hyperplastic tissue. Small amounts of hyperplastic tissue may be excised under local anaesthesia. Larger amounts should be excised with a laser or cutting diathermy or the defect grafted with palatal mucosa to facilitate haemostasis and reduce scar contracture.

Tori

Bony prominences can be surgically reduced using a bur or chisel if it is not possible to adjust the denture to accommodate them.

Muscle attachments

Prominent muscle attachments from the facial muscles or tongue can displace a denture when they contract. Surgical procedures allow these muscles to be stripped from their bony insertions. In some cases, it may be important to re-attach a muscle in a more favourable position. The word **fraenoplasty** is used for the removal of muscle attachments for preprosthetic purposes (Figs 66 and 67) and **fraenectomy** when removal is carried out for orthodontic purposes, as the techniques differ in these different situations. When carrying out a fraenectomy for orthodontic reasons such as to permit closure of a median diastema, it is important to excise the frenum thoroughly and to ensure that no muscle remnants remain in the alveolar bone between the central incisor teeth (Fig. 68).

Alveolar ridge augmentation

Resorbed and defective alveolar ridges may be built up with bone grafts and bone substitutes to facilitate the construction of dentures. However, these procedures are rarely performed now because they do not provide good results in the long term. Bone grafts resorb and bone substitutes such as hydroxyapatite granules become displaced. The advent of osseointegrated implants has superseded the need for much of this surgery, although alternative

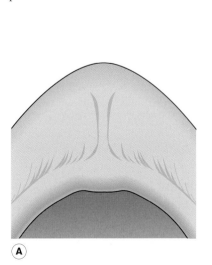

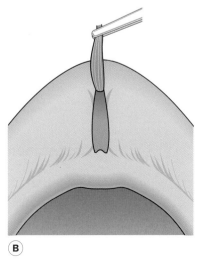

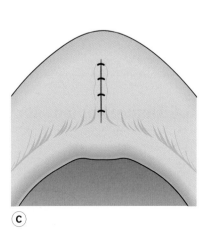

A　　　　**B**　　　　**C**

Fig. 66 Fraenoplasty technique for prominent labial fraenum of the edentulous maxilla.

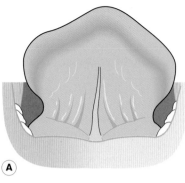
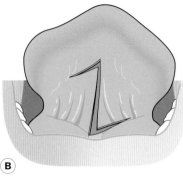
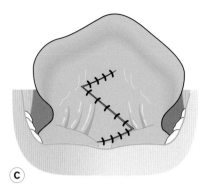

(A) (B) (C)

Fig. 67 Fraenoplasty for prominent lingual fraenum using a Z-plasty technique.

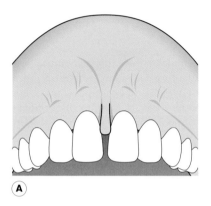
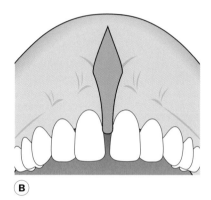
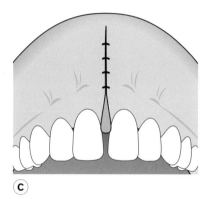

(A) (B) (C)

Fig. 68 Fraenectomy technique for orthodontic purposes where there is a prominent maxillary fraenum and midline diastoma.

techniques of bone augmentation prior to implant placement have developed, as described below.

Sulcus deepening

Inadequate alveolar ridge height can be treated by deepening the sulcus by a vestibuloplasty procedure rather than augmenting the ridge. Such procedures may leave a raw area of soft tissue, which can be covered by a skin or mucosal graft. The major problem with these techniques is the significant wound contracture, which reduces the sulcus height again. Many variants of the surgical procedure have been developed in an attempt to improve the long-term outcome from these operations.

Nerve repositioning

With atrophy of the mandible, the mental nerve can come to lie on the ridge and denture trauma can cause significant pain. The mental foramen can be surgically moved into an inferior position to alleviate this problem.

6.4 Dental implant surgery
• • • • • • • • • • • • • • • •

Cobalt chrome subperiosteal implants developed in the 1940s and titanium blade implants developed in the 1960s are now little used. Reference to implants today generally means **osseointegrated implants**, which have superseded other types because of their high success rate. Osseointegration is the word used to describe the healing of bone around implants so there is direct anchorage of the implant that is then maintained during functional loading without the growth of fibrous tissue at the bone–implant interface. P.-I. Branemark discovered osseointegration, developed its application over a number of years and first presented his work and results in 1977. Development of many dental implant designs based on the root-form model has followed, as has development of implants for maxillofacial reconstruction and for use in orthopaedic surgery.

The aims of placing osseointgrated dental implants are:

1. Replacement of dentition and supporting tissues to restore function and appearance
2. Alveolar bone preservation.

Assessment
• •

Indications for implant treatment

There are a number of indications for implant treatment:

- severe denture intolerance for the following reasons:
  - severe gagging
  - severe ridge resorption with unacceptable stability or pain

- – psychological
- prevention of severe alveolar bone loss
  - – moderate ridge resorption in young individuals, under 45 years of age
  - – moderate ridge resorption in one jaw opposing natural teeth with a good prognosis
- developmental anomalies
  - – oligodontia
  - – cleft palate
- trauma resulting in loss of teeth and supporting tissues
- complete unilateral loss of teeth in one jaw where dentures are not tolerated or an edentulous span is considered too difficult to manage by other means
- maxillofacial and cranial defects
  - – intra-oral implants may be required for reconstruction in situations of extensive ridge deformities, patent clefts or after major jaw resection
  - – extra-oral implants may be required for the reconstruction of ears, eyes or nose in situations of congenital absence, trauma or surgical ablation.

Figure 69 shows a dentate maxilla and edentulous mandible in a 44-year-old female. The mandible has already shown significant atrophy, and placement of four anterior mandibular implants will enable a stable retentive prosthesis to be provided and preserve the mandibular bone in this area.

Assessment for oral implant surgery

The appropriateness of implant treatment for a patient is the joint decision of the restorative dentist and the surgeon in discussion with the patient. The history should elicit the patient's precise current complaint. The reason for tooth loss or absent teeth should be noted together with details of any prosthesis and current problems. An indication of patient motivation should be obtained before embarking on implant treatment that may be lengthy and complex.

The medical history may reveal relevant information. Any systemic condition or drug that impairs wound healing will compromise the healing of the implant fixtures, that is, the osseointegration process. This does not mean

that patients with such conditions are absolutely excluded from being offered implant treatment, but rather that they may have an increased risk of treatment failure and therefore the patient should be fully informed of the likely outcome. The decision to provide or not provide treatment will take into account the severity of need.

Dental implant treatment is less successful in patients who smoke. Smoking is not an absolute contraindication to dental implant treatment but patients who smoke should be made aware that they have a significantly increased risk of implant failure and are therefore advised to seek smoking cessation therapy prior to the commencement of dental implant treatment. Neither is dental implant treatment contraindicated in patients who have lost teeth because of periodontitis as the evidence suggests that the difference in survival of superstructure and implants is not significantly different at 10 years from that in patients who did not have periodontitis. However, there may be slightly increased peri-implant marginal bone loss in patients with a history of periodontitis so patients should be warned of possible increased failure rate.

Patients receiving bisphosphonates need careful consideration (see also Ch. 5). Procedures that involve direct osseous injury should be avoided in those receiving intravenous bisphosphonates and placement of dental implants could lead to bisphosphonate-related osteonecrosis. However, elective dentoalveolar surgery including dental implant placement does not seem to be contraindicated in patients receiving oral bisphosphonates. Strong research evidence for the production of clinical guidelines has been lacking and so patients should be counselled regarding possible implant failure and osteonecrosis of the jaws as part of the consent process. Patients are best managed by a specialist and should be placed on a regular review schedule.

Clinical examination

A full clinical oral examination is carried out. It is important to assess the bone volume available at sites of potential implant fixture placement. Classification systems are available for bone resorption and bone density. The amount of attached gingiva should also be noted as this may be atrophied if there has been tooth loss for a long time. Some clinicians gauge the alveolar bone volume present beneath soft tissue by penetrating the mucosa with graduated sharp probe or other instrument under local anaesthesia. This procedure is described as ridge mapping.

Presurgical investigations

Study models and imaging are used to give information on *quantity* and *quality* of bone. Quantification of bone requires radiological techniques that are accurate and precise.

Imaging

Radiography and CT can be used.

Periapical view. A periapical view of the implant site(s) is advised because of the better image resolution than is possible on panoramic radiographs. The sites should be examined for root fragments or other abnormalities. However, in edentulous patients, particularly in the mandible, good quality images may be difficult.

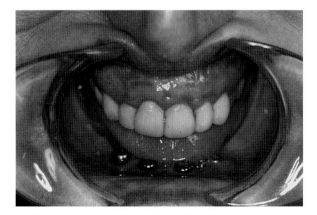

Fig. 69 Four anterior mandible implants with gingival formers after surgical exposure and prior to restoration.

Panoramic view. This may not be appropriate for a single anterior maxillary implant but is usually appropriate for implants in other sites because the full depth of the jaws is imaged. Usefulness of panoramics is greatly enhanced by using individually made baseplates/templates, which are worn during radiography. These incorporate metallic markers so that the radiograph can be related to the mouth; ball bearings of known size allow calculation of magnification.

Lateral cephalometric radiograph. This view gives a crude cross-sectional image of the midline regions of both jaws for anterior implants.

Cross-sectional tomography. Specialised tomographic equipment is available to provide cross-sectional spiral tomograms of the jaws. The sites for tomography are planned from an initial panoramic film. Each spiral tomogram is produced independently (cf. CT, below), so this is suitable for single or multiple implant placement.

Computed tomography. Many hospital-based CT scanners have 'dental' software that permits life-size cross-sectional reconstructed images of the jaws to be produced (Fig. 70). As all of a jaw must be scanned, even to produce just one or two cross-sections, this technique is best reserved for multiple implant placements. Radiation doses are much higher than with radiography. Artefacts may be produced by dental restorations and errors introduced by movement. Cone beam CT produces high-definition digital images with reduced patient radiation exposure and much reduced imaging time. This 3-D imaging equipment has less space requirement than for a conventional scanner and is available for use in primary care. Image analysis software may be used for planning to allow the surgeon to 'virtually' place implants with due regard for avoidance of vital structures and then surgical guides can be constructed to accurately transfer the plan to the patient.

Surgical techniques

Bone augmentation

It may be necessary to augment the alveolus of the maxilla or mandible if there is inadequate bone volume to place an implant. Various materials may be used for this augmentation.

Autogenous bone. Grafts harvested from intra- or extra-oral sites of the same patient are considered the material of choice but require a donor site operation, with associated morbidity (Fig. 71). Each donor site has its own advantages and disadvantages. The anterior iliac crest of the hip is a popular site as it affords large bone volumes, whereas the calvarium is used less commonly because of the clinical significance of possible complications, such as dural tear and epidural haematoma. The posterior iliac crest offers greater volume than the anterior but the patient must be positioned prone during surgery so is less commonly used. Patients should be warned of postoperative pain and reduced mobility, scar and possible altered sensation of the lateral thigh skin when undergoing anterior iliac crest surgery.

Split rib has also been used but the bone resorbs quickly. Intra-oral sites avoid extra-oral scars but offer more limited availability of volume. The mandibular symphisis (chin), retromolar or ramus and maxillary tuberosity sites are all used. Autogenous grafts have the advantage of being both osteoconductive and osteoinductive, that is they act as a scaffold into which bone can grow from the adjacent recipient bed and also contain undifferentiated cells that convert into osteoblasts and allow osteogenesis at sites away from the recipient bed. When large defects require reconstruction a vascularised graft such as that harvested pedicled on the deep circumflex iliac arterial system may be required (DCIA flap).

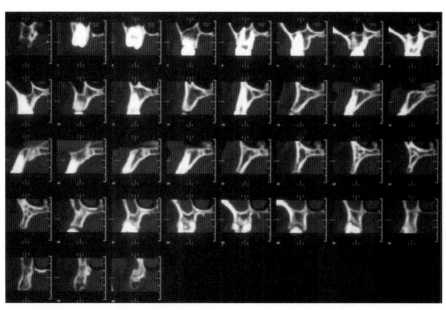

Fig. 70 Cross-sectional reconstructed images of the jaws produced from a computed tomographic scan using 'dental' software.

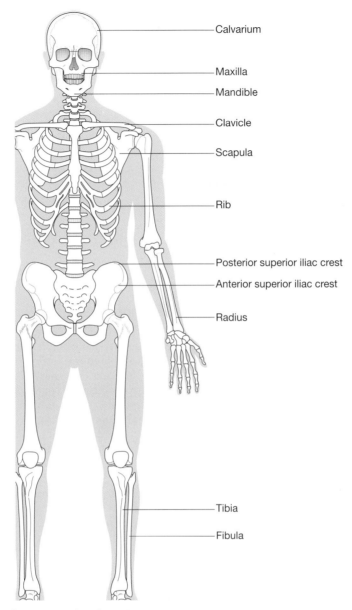

Calvarium

Maxilla

Mandible

Clavicle

Scapula

Rib

Posterior superior iliac crest

Anterior superior iliac crest

Radius

Tibia

Fibula

Fig. 71 Intra- and extra-oral sites for autogenous bone harvesting.

Alloplastic materials. Synthetic materials include hydroxyapatite, tricalcium phosphate and bioactive glasses. These are osteoconductive.

Ceramics. Calcium phosphate ceramics and glass ceramics are used, of which tricalcium phosphate and hydroxyapatite are the most useful clinically. These are biologically active, that is they release calcium and phosphate ions into tissue and encourage bone formation. However, they are mechanically weak.

Metals. Pure titanium or titanium alloys are the most useful. They are mechanically strong, although not biologically active. This has led to the development of a hydroxyapatite surface on titanium.

Allografts. Human bone grafts can be harvested from cadavers and are available in forms such as demineralised freeze-dried bone. The processing activates bone morphogenic proteins, which means that they are osteoinductive but may not be free from the risk of infectivity.

Xenografts. Animal bone grafts harvested from species such as cow (Bio-Oss) or coral (Algipore) can be used. The organic component is removed during processing so that they should be free from the risk of infectivity. They are osteoconductive.

Bone grafting techniques

Onlay grafting. Donor bone blocks may be attached on to the recipient site as an onlay and fixed with screws or plates.

Interpositional grafting. The alveolus may be sectioned from the basal bone and donor bone blocks inserted between the two.

Sinus elevation or lift. A Caldwell–Luc (see Ch. 7) window is infractured into the sinus to create a new floor of the sinus. The space between the alveolus and this new floor is then packed with graft material, which indirectly increases the vertical height of the alveolar ridge (Fig. 72). This sinus lift plus grafting technique was first described by Hilt Tatum.

All bone screws and plates are removed at implant placement if not before. The graft requires sufficient time to revascularise before implants are placed so that osseo-integration can occur but not such a prolonged time that resorption occurs because is has no physiological stress. Opinions vary with surgeons placing implants between 3 months and 9 months. Sometimes implants are placed at the bone grafting surgery. In this case implants are retained by friction of fit with osseointegration occurring later as the bone becomes revascularised.

Stimulation of bone regeneration

Bone morphogenic proteins have been identified and are now produced commercially in an attempt to accelerate bone regeneration.

Implant placement

The technique for implant placement is outlined in Box 8.

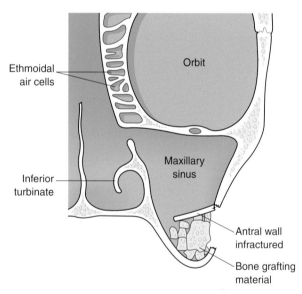

Fig. 72 Coronal section to show sinus lift procedure.

Ethmoidal air cells

Orbit

Inferior turbinate

Maxillary sinus

Antral wall infractured

Bone grafting material

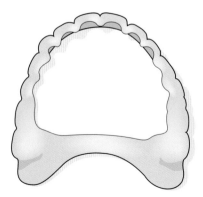

Fig. 73 A surgical guide or stent.

Box 8 Technique for implant placement

1. A mucoperiosteal flap is raised and the alveolar ridge may need to be smoothed or reduced.

2. A surgical guide or stent is usually used (Fig. 73) to indicate the correct position for implant placement and mark the positions before proceeding to use various drills appropriate to the system being used. Holes are prepared, of the exact dimensions to accept an implant, by incremental drilling at slow speed to avoid overheating of bone (Fig. 74A). It is critical that bone does not heat to 42 °C or the injury to bone will impair osteointegration. Copious irrigation with sterile saline is therefore necessary.

3. The implant is then pressed (Fig. 74B) or screwed (Fig. 74C) into position. The position is crucial and a high degree of parallelism is necessary when placing multiple implants.

4. The soft-tissue flaps are then closed with sutures (Fig. 74D).

Implant exposure

The submerged implants are usually uncovered or exposed at about 4–6 months following placement, although it is also possible to carry out a one-stage implant procedure when implants are exposed at the placement surgery. The overlying soft tissue is punched out or a crestal flap is raised and repositioned. The implant cover screw is removed and a 'gingival former' or healing abutment attached so that this projects through the gingival tissue, which can then heal and mature about the implant (Fig. 75).

Immediate loading of implants

It is crucial that implants are immobile during healing. This is why they are frequently buried so that forces are not transmitted. However, in situations where there is excellent primary stability because of the bone density at a site such as the anterior mandible, then the implant will remain immobile and heal normally even when loaded early or even immediately.

Postoperative care

This consists of prescribing analgesia and a chlorhexidine mouthrinse and advising the patient not to smoke. Suture removal is arranged for 7–14 days postoperatively if non-resorbable sutures have been used.

Soft-tissue surgery

Surgery may be necessary to ensure that there is kera-tinised tissue about the implant and that the soft-tissue contour permits adequate oral hygiene maintenance.

Timing of implant placement

Immediate implant placement

Following tooth extraction, an implant may be placed immediately into the socket after preparation. This pre-vents the bone resorption that normally follows tooth loss and reduces the number of surgical procedures. While connective tissue may grow into gaps between the implant and socket, the procedure has a high success rate.

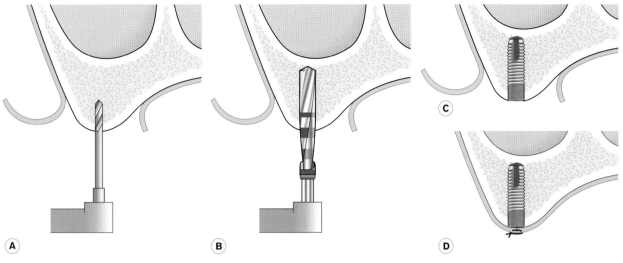

A   B   C   D

Fig. 74 Implant placement technique.

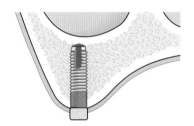

Fig. 75 Implant exposure with attachment of healing abutment.

Delayed immediate implants

Implants may be placed at 6–8 weeks after tooth extraction into the surgically prepared socket. Little bone resorption will have occurred and, because the soft tissues will have healed, it will be easier to obtain closure of the flaps over the implant.

Implant success

Biological failure occurs when osseointegration is not established or is not maintained. When not established in the first place, implant failure is described as 'early failure' and will be observed before or at abutment connection. When osseointegration does occur but then is lost, the implant is described as a 'late failure' as this is observed at any time after abutment connection. When an implant is not osseointegrated, a peri-implant radiolucency is observed radiographically and the implant is clinically mobile. The site in the mouth of a patient is a significant contributory factor to failure. A general trend towards maxillas having almost three times more implant losses than mandibles has also been reported in the edentulous situation. Failure may occur as failure to heal after placement, a later failure involving gradual bone loss and leading to loosening of the implant. Frequently the failing implant causes no discomfort.

Six

Self-assessment: questions

Multiple choice questions

1. When extracting primary teeth:
   a. The same principles are applied as for permanent teeth
   b. General anaesthesia may be required
   c. It is essential to protect the airway during the removal of teeth under general anaesthesia to prevent blood, tooth fragments or teeth entering the airway
   d. It is essential not to retain any roots as these may impede the eruption of the permanent successor
   e. A surgical procedure may be required if the tooth has become submerged.

2. When removing a lower third molar tooth:
   a. The patient need not be warned about possible lingual nerve damage if the removal is to be by extraction with forceps
   b. Any bone removal should be undertaken with an irrigated bur rather than a chisel and mallet when using local anaesthesia alone
   c. Horizontally impacted teeth present the greatest surgical challenge
   d. The relationship to the inferior alveolar canal can be determined by radiographic assessment
   e. General anaesthesia is usually indicated.

3. The following radiological signs are associated with an increased risk of nerve injury during third molar surgery:
   a. Presence of an enlarged pericoronal space (follicle)
   b. Interruption of the lamina dura ('white lines') of the interdental canal overlying the tooth
   c. Darkening of the root where it is crossed by the interdental canal
   d. Periradicular bone sclerosis
   e. Diversion of the interdental canal.

4. The surgical removal of a tooth:
   a. Rather than forceps removal is likely to make subsequent replacement with a dental implant less feasible
   b. Will cause pain, the intensity of which will be determined by the amount of bone removal and overall surgical difficulty
   c. Requires that the patient be prescribed antibiotics to reduce the likelihood of postoperative infection
   d. Always requires a radiograph as part of the surgical planning
   e. Should always proceed immediately in the event of a failed forceps extraction.

5. Preprosthetic surgery:
   a. Is less frequently required now that dental implants can provide effective tooth replacement rather than dentures
   b. To ensure an adequate margin of keratinised mucosa is present about dental implants is important for success of the implant
   c. Can be carried out to increase the space between the maxillary tuberosity and mandibular retromolar pad
   d. Should be used to reduce a torus mandibularis that is discovered on clinical examination
   e. For sulcus deepening may require the construction of an acrylic stent to be worn postoperatively.

Extended matching items

EMI 1. theme: Complications associated with the removal of teeth

Options:

A Prescribe analgesia
B Cold compress
C Warm compress
D Prescribe antibiotics
E Check body temperature
F Check blood pressure
G Suture socket
H Place haemostatic pack in socket
I Place dressing with lidocaine (lignocaine) in socket
J Undertake radiographic examination

Lead in: Select the most appropriate management from the list above for each of the following cases. Each option can be used once, more than once or not at all.

1. A patient complains of severe pain 2 days following the surgical removal of a lower impacted third molar.
2. A patient complains of severe pain 1 week after an uneventful removal of a mobile lower first molar tooth with forceps. On examination there is exposed bone present in the socket that is very sensitive to touch.
3. A patient returns, still bleeding from an extraction socket several days after the removal of a tooth. The patient is anxious, sweaty and pale.
4. A patient complains of a bad taste 2 months following the removal of a lower third molar tooth. On examination there is a discharging sinus buccal to the site where the tooth was removed.
5. A patient has post-extraction bleeding from gingival tissue around the socket and returns 2 hours after the surgery.

EMI 2. theme: Dental implant surgery

Options:
A Immediate dental implant placement
B Dental implant placement
C Immediately loaded implant
D Chin block bone harvesting for grafting
E Iliac crest bone harvesting for grafting
F Maxillary overdenture supported by implants
G Maxillary fixed bridgework supported by implants

H Mandibular overdenture supported by implants
I   Mandibular fixed bridgework supported by implants
J   No treatment

Lead in: Select the most appropriate first stage of treatment from the list above for each of the following cases. Each option can be used once, more than once or not at all.

1. A 20-year-old male has lost all four upper incisor teeth following an alleged assault. He lost three of the teeth at the time of the injury and one other a little later. On clinical examination he has significant buccal bone loss to the alveolus in the edentulous area and also significant loss of alveolar height.

2. An upper right lateral incisor tooth has undergone conventional and surgical endodontic treatment previously and the tooth now requires removal because of recurrent periapical infection and gingival recession leading to a poor appearance. The patient would much prefer an implant option for tooth replacement.

3. A 60-year-old male patient is to lose all of his remaining maxillary teeth due to periodontal disease. He has a severe gag reflex and has been unable to tolerate a partial denture at all. He is very anxious to have tooth replacement following the extractions.

4. An adult patient who had a cleft palate surgically closed as a child still has a small patent cleft (oronasal fistula) to the anterior of the palate. She does not want further surgery for this cleft and is now to lose her remaining maxillary teeth.

5. A 45-year-old female patient has fractured the tooth root about a post crown that was restoring an upper right central incisor tooth. A periapical radiograph shows that there is no evidence of periapical pathology.

Case history questions

Case history 1

Mrs Jones is a frail 75-year-old lady who complains of pain beneath her lower denture. On examination, you discover a partly erupted lower left third molar tooth. She requests that you extract it. A digital panoramic tomograph (DPT) is shown in Figure 76.

Discuss the management of this patient.

Case history 2

Matthew is 17 years old and presents to your practice asking if he can have dental implants to replace his missing teeth (Fig. 77). Matthew has several permanent teeth missing and has worn partial dentures for many years.

Discuss your management.

Viva questions

1. What is combination syndrome?
2. What are the principles of flap design?
3. The root of which tooth is most often displaced into the maxillary antrum during forceps extraction?
4. When removing a lower molar tooth surgically, should you section the roots completely with a bur?
5. In which anatomical areas are vertical releasing incisions contraindicated in flap design?
6. Why is it contraindicated to curette a local osteitis (dry socket) to stimulate haemorrhage?
7. What are dental implants?
8. Which oral site has the highest implant failure rate?
9. Do implants require regular maintenance after placement?
10. What are the two most common features of a failed implant?

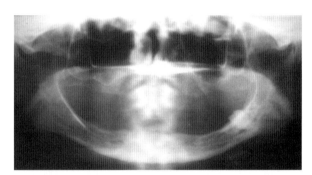

Fig. 76 Radiograph showing patient in Case history 1.

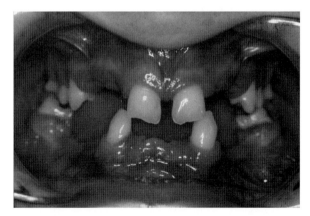

Fig. 77 Intra-oral photograph showing patient in Case history 2.

Self-assessment: answers

Multiple choice answers

1. a. **True.** Primary teeth are extracted following the same principles as for permanent teeth; however, it is important to recognise that the molar roots are closely associated with the developing tooth germs, which must be carefully avoided. Smaller forceps help to facilitate this.

   b. **True.** The use of general anaesthesia in dentistry is reducing in the UK but may be indicated for the removal of primary teeth, especially when multiple teeth need to be removed or the child is young or uncooperative.

   c. **True.** Airway protection during dental extraction under general anaesthesia is afforded by placing a gauze throat pack. This is necessary because the usual airway protective reflexes, principally the vocal folds, do not function in unconsciousness. Even when the endotracheal intubation is used during anaesthesia, it is still good practice to place a throat pack.

   d. **False.** In some cases it is better to leave small fragments of root in situ rather than damage the permanent successor by excessive use of elevators. The retention of a root fragment will not impede the eruption of the permanent successor. However, thought will have to be given to its removal at a later stage as frequently it will come to lie in a partly erupted position adjacent to the crown of the tooth, and this may lead to caries.

   e. **True.** A tooth is described as submerged if the occlusal surface is at a lower level than the neighbouring teeth. The second primary molar is the most common tooth to become submerged and the condition is more likely in the mandible than maxilla and is often associated with a missing permanent successor. These submerged primary teeth may become ankylosed and are very difficult to remove.

2. a. **False.** The planned extraction with forceps may become a surgical procedure involving the raising of soft-tissue flaps and bone removal. Also, it is possible to cause lingual nerve damage with forceps alone in the region of the lower third molar, although this is rare.

   b. **True.** Most patients would find it unacceptable to have a chisel and mallet used on them when conscious. This is an effective technique when general anaesthesia is used and particularly useful for the removal of distolingual bone from about distoangularly impacted third molars.

   c. **False.** Distoangular teeth are usually more difficult to remove because on elevation they move distally and a significant amount of bone removal must be anticipated.

   d. **True.** The inferior alveolar canal may lie below the roots of the third molar or may be intimately related to it. If the canal is seen to converge as it crosses the root then this suggests that the root is notched by the nerve or, if almost interrupted, then the nerve may perforate the root.

   e. **False.** The choice of anaesthesia is determined by the anticipated difficulty of the surgery, the patient, previous experience of dentistry, their level of anxiety and degree of cooperation, the medical history and the social history. Taking all these factors into account, the removal of a single third molar may require general anaesthesia but does not usually do so. Conscious sedation is a more likely option.

3. a. **False.** It is irrelevant.

   b. **True.** Suggests that the bony wall of the canal is disrupted in some way by the roots.

   c. **True.** May indicate a groove in the root.

   d. **False.** Is irrelevant, although it is possible that sclerotic bone might lead to a more difficult removal of the tooth.

   e. **True.** Particularly where there is a marked 'dog leg' course to the canal over the root, suggests a close relationship.

4. a. **True.** Generally this is true if bone removal is required as part of the surgical removal procedure. It is important that teeth are removed as untraumatically as possible and with as little bone removal as possible as this may compromise implant placement, which requires sufficient bone to support the implant adequately.

   b. **False.** Bone removal will usually cause more pain than no bone removal, but the amount of bone removal and the overall surgical difficulty are not good predictors of postoperative pain. More important factors are the cultural experiences, personality and anxiety of the patient.

   c. **False.** If bone is not removed then antibiotics are unnecessary. If bone removal is undertaken, then many clinicians do prescribe antibiotics. However, the use of a chlorhexidine gluconate mouthrinse just before the surgery is likely to be of more use in the prevention of postoperative infections.

   d. **True.** A radiograph is not always necessary for extractions to be undertaken with forceps. However, if it is anticipated that a surgical approach will be necessary or a forceps extraction fails and a surgical approach must be adopted, then a radiograph is essential.

   e. **False.** While it is usually preferable to limit the number of surgical episodes for the patient, it may be necessary to investigate the cause of the failed extraction with forceps further before proceeding. A radiograph will be required if one is not already available. The dentist may need to refer the patient to a specialist if further surgery beyond the skill of the dentist is required or adequate facilities are not available.

5. a. **True.** While preprosthetic surgery referred in the past to a means of improving the retention of conventional dentures, it now also refers to that required to facilitate soft-tissue health about osseointegrated implants. However, since the introduction of implants, significantly less preprosthetic surgery is required because implants have overcome many of the problems that surgery and dentures were trying to address.
   b. **True.** Sufficient keratinised mucosa about implants is essential to maintain health of the surrounding soft tissues. Non-keratinised mucosa about implants usually leads to pocketing and peri-implantitis, which ultimately leads to failure of the implant.
   c. **True.** A hyperplastic maxillary tuberosity can be reduced in size by excising a wedge of soft tissue.
   d. **False.** Mandibular tori are found as painless bony enlargements of the lingual plate in the premolar region. They are bilateral in 80% of cases. They only need surgical reduction if they are interfering with the lingual flange of a denture and preventing adequate retention.
   e. **True.** An acrylic stent lined with adapted gutta-percha may be useful especially to stabilise and protect a soft-tissue graft; however, their efficacy is now doubted and patients usually find them uncomfortable.

Extended matching items answers

EMI 1

1. **A.** The surgical removal of third molar teeth may cause postoperative pain that is severe in intensity. It is not unusual for some patients to remain in pain for several days after surgery. Reassuring the patient and encouraging regular use of appropriate analgesia should be adequate. Clinical examination should of course be carried out and further investigation by way of radiographic examination may be appropriate should there be any reason to suspect root retention or fracture.
2. **I.** Pain at 1 week after surgery is unlikely to be related to surgical trauma, especially if the surgery was very simple. It is more likely that the patient is experiencing pain because of dry socket (alveolar osteitis) or infection. As there is exposed bone then alveolar osteitis is more likely and a dressing with lidocaine would be helpful.
3. **F.** A patient who looks unwell as described may be surgically shocked and this should be investigated by checking the blood pressure and pulse.
4. **J.** A radiograph should be taken to investigate the possibility of a retained root or sequestered bone as these are the most common cause of such infection.
5. **G.** Suturing the dental socket will put the surrounding tissues under tension and stop the bleeding. During the extraction the local anaesthetic may have contained epinephrine (adrenalaine) which reduced local bleeding.

EMI 2

1. **E.** If there is a significant three-dimensional defect to the alveolus then bone augmentation will be required to facilitate later placement of dental implants. Harvesting bone from the iliac crest of the hip provides large quantities of bone very suitable for this augmentation. Some surgeons may prefer to use intra-oral harvesting only and there are regional variations around the world sometimes dependent on training and access to facilities.
2. **D.** There will be significant buccal bone loss because of the previous endodontic surgery and the horizontal bone loss associated with this tooth. Any implant placement is likely to require prior bone augmentation surgery. Bone harvested from an intra-oral site will usually provide the appropriate bone volume.
3. **G.** If the patient has a gag reflex that cannot be reduced by restorative or behavioural means then it may be appropriate to consider implant treatment to retain fixed bridgework. An overdenture retained by implants will be much less bulky than a conventional denture and may prove adequate.
4. **F.** An overdenture retained by implants will serve the purpose of tooth replacement and bone preservation but also permit closure of the oronasal fistula.
5. **A.** The fractured tooth root may be removed and a dental implant placed at the same time. This will reduce the number of surgical episodes.

Case history answers

Case history 1

A thorough history should be taken to establish the nature of the pain experienced by the patient. Is this mild discomfort as a result of denture-induced trauma to the soft tissues about the partly erupted tooth or is this severe pain as a result of pericoronitis or pulpitis or even an acute abscess? A medical history is more likely to yield positive findings in this age group that may be relevant to her dental management. For example, non-steroidal anti-inflammatory analgesics are contraindicated for her pain control and paracetamol or codeine would be more appropriate. The medical history may contraindicate general anaesthesia and the age is a relevant risk factor in any such decision. Does Mrs Jones live alone, is she far from the practice and how does she travel? These may be relevant to the extent of treatment that you may wish to undertake in your practice. The radiograph shows a deeply impacted lower third molar tooth in an otherwise edentulous mandible. The bone will be less flexible and more brittle than in a young person and this is going to be a difficult surgical procedure. The patient needs to be referred to an oral surgeon. Tooth removal would involve significant bone removal to facilitate elevation with as little effort as possible.

Case history 2

A history would confirm that several permanent teeth never erupted rather than these teeth required extraction because of caries or trauma. A family history of this problem may be present. Such oligodontia may or may not be associated with other features comprising a syndrome. The medical and social history may be important in determining the choice of anaesthesia and extent of any treatment that may be required. Smoking will reduce the success rate of implant treatment. A clinical examination would note the teeth present and their health and also the dimension of the edentulous alveolar ridges. A DPT radiograph would confirm that there are no unerupted teeth. There are too few teeth to support fixed bridges. Implants would be preferable to partial dentures, especially in a young person. However, it appears that the edentulous alveolar ridges are very narrow and undercut and it would not be feasible to place implants without significant bone grafting. Figure 78 shows a corticocancellous block of iliac crest graft bone fixed in place as a buccal onlay in one of the edentulous spaces to widen the ridge for later implant placements. The patient will obviously require referral to an implant team that is familiar with the management of such problems.

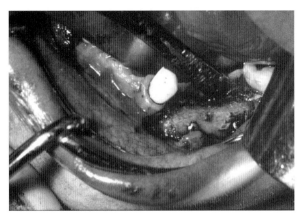

Fig. 78 Photograph showing a corticocancellous block of iliac crest graft bone fixed in place as a buccal onlay at surgery for the patient in Case history 2.

Viva answers

1. Combination syndrome is when there is excessive resorption of the edentulous maxilla in the anterior region as a consequence of the forces generated by the opposition of natural mandibular teeth.

2. The base of the flap should be broader than the apex to ensure an adequate blood supply. The flap should be wide enough to provide good access to the underlying operative field. The design should permit tension-free closure with margins over sound bone.

3. The palatal root of the maxillary first molar tooth is most frequently dislodged into the maxillary antrum during forceps extraction.

4. The lingual plate is thin and undercut and so it is important not to section mandibular molar roots completely through to the lingual side because of the risk of sectioning the lingual nerve with the bur.

5. Vertical relieving incisions are contraindicated in the palate, lingual aspect of the mandible, buccal aspect of mandible in the area of mental nerve, and over the maxillary canine eminence.

6. Curetting a dry socket delays healing rather than accelerating it. Any early attempts at healing will be destroyed.

7. Dental implants are tooth root analogues, usually made of titanium, that are placed into alveolar bone to act as abutments for prostheses. The healing process of implants is described as osseointegration and results in a relationship between implant and bone that mimics ankylosis of a tooth to bone.

8. Implants placed in the anterior maxilla are the most likely to fail because only relatively short implants can be placed at this anatomical site.

9. Implants like natural teeth require regular maintenance. Plastic-tipped instruments are available for professional cleaning as metal instruments would scratch the titanium surface. Meticulous home care is required to be undertaken by the patient.

10. Bone loss, as demonstrated by a standardised radiograph, and mobility of the implant are the most consistent features of a failed implant.

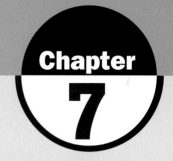
Diseases of bone and the maxillary sinus

Overview

This chapter covers the basic anatomy and diseases of the bones of the face and the maxillary sinus. Most diseases of the jaw are odontogenic in origin but the jaws can also be affected by systemic disease and by local non-odontogenic conditions. The clinical and radiological features, pathology and management of non-inflammatory/infective lesions are described. Chapter 4 deals with inflammations and infections of bone.

The maxillary sinus is affected by inflammation, cysts and tumours as well as the consequences of dental pathology and procedures. Pathology of the sinus often presents with toothache.

7.1 Diseases of bone

Learning objectives

You should:
- know the normal structure of the jaw
- understand how bone is formed
- know the clinical and radiographic features of the diseases that can affect the bones of the face
- understand the management of these diseases.

Normal jaw skeleton

The mandible and maxillary bones form in membrane and are unusual in that they contain odontogenic epithelium and neurovascular bundles within their substance. Most diseases arising in the jaws are of odontogenic origin, but both non-odontogenic local and systemic disorders may affect the jaws.

The mandible is formed of a cortex and rather coarse trabecular medulla. A depression into the cortex may form around the submandibular salivary gland during development. It can give rise to a radiolucent area at the angle of the mandible, referred to as **Stafne's cavity** (Fig. 79). It is important to be aware of this normal structure, which appears below the inferior alveolar nerve canal on radiographs, to avoid confusion with bone cysts. Another important normal structure is the **torus mandibularis**. Tori are

smooth bone prominences found on the lingual aspect of the mandible below the canine/premolar teeth (Fig. 80). They are often bilateral and may consist of single, double or triple prominences. The maxilla is often extensively pneumatised to form the **maxillary sinus**, described later in this chapter. The hard palate forms by elevation and fusion of embryonic shelves. A bony prominence may form in the midline, which is referred to as **torus palatinus**. Both the torus palatinus and **pterygoid hamulus** can be discovered by anxious patients and reassurance may be required.

At a histological level, bone is composed of mineralised collagenous matrix containing osteocytes. It is organised into an outer cortex and an inner cancellous (trabecular) structure, which is adaptive to stresses (Fig. 81). Endosteal surfaces are lined by bone lining cells; remodelling is achieved by the coordinated activity of **osteoclasts** (bone-resorbing cells) and **osteoblasts** (bone-forming cells) in bone metabolic units. Bone is surrounded by periosteum, which is continuous with oral mucosa in certain places in the jaws. The vascular supply to bone is via periosteal vessels and marrow spaces. Fatty and haemopoetic marrow may be present in the jaws.

Bone fractures and tooth extraction sockets heal by similar processes, which involve demolition of blood clot, formation of initial woven bone in a fibrous scaffold and subsequent remodelling to restore normal architecture. In tooth sockets, there is simultaneous epithelial healing. Alveolar remodelling occurs over a prolonged period, resulting eventually in a rounded ridge form. The lamina dura can be detected radiographically for up to 2 years after extraction.

Benign fibro-osseous lesions

Benign fibro-osseous lesions are characterised by the replacement of normal bone by fibrous tissue in which there is formation of mineralised cemento-osseous matrix.

Fibrous dysplasia

Fibrous dysplasia is caused by mutation of the GNAS1 gene. Normal bone is replaced with fibrous tissue, which, in turn, undergoes gradual calcification. Monostotic (single bone) and polyostotic (more than one bone) types are seen. Around 30% of those affected have the polyostotic form of the disease.

Clinical features. An affected bone or area within a bone undergoes painless expansion. Other symptoms are few, but when the skull base is involved neurological signs may occur, presumably owing to pressure on foramina. In the jaws, teeth are often affected, with effects

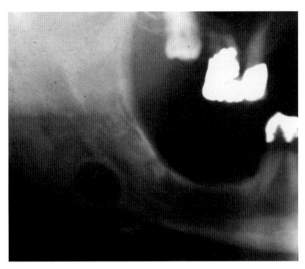

Fig. 79 Stafne bone cavity. This radiograph shows the typical appearance of a rounded well-defined radiolucency with corticated margins, below the inferior dental canal.

upon eruption and developing malocclusion. The maxilla is affected twice as commonly as the mandible. The disease is most commonly unilateral but may involve multiple craniofacial bones and typically produces a visible facial asymmetry (Fig. 82). Fibrous dysplasia develops during childhood, usually before 10 years of age, with no sex predilection (except Albright's syndrome: see below). The disease becomes quiescent in early adult life, but the deformity persists.

The polyostotic form of fibrous dysplasia shares these general characteristics but has additional signs. There are two types: Jaffe's type and Albright's syndrome. In the first, multiple bones are affected and there are patches of skin pigmentation (café-au-lait spots). In Albright's syndrome, which is unusual in that it is almost always a disease of females, there are also various endocrine abnormalities such as precocious puberty, hyperthyroidism and hyperparathyroidism.

Pathology. The histopathological appearance is dependent on the stage of disease development. Initially, normal bone is replaced by cellular fibrous tissue within which, as the disease progresses, irregular islands and fine trabeculae of metaplastic woven bone develop. As the lesion matures so too does the connective tissue, becoming more collagenous, while the bone is remodelled to a lamellar pattern. The lesional tissue merges with the adjacent normal tissue.

Radiology. Radiology shows:

• enlargement of a bone
• altered trabecular pattern
• generally poorly defined margins.

Initially an affected area appears radiolucent, reflecting the fibrous tissue content. As bone forms, the lesion becomes more radio-opaque. The alteration in trabecular pattern is particularly notable: the trabeculae are very small and fine, resulting in a picture that has been described as like 'ground glass', although coarser forms are often described as resembling a 'fingerprint' or 'orange peel' (Fig. 83). Where teeth are present, another commonly noted sign is loss of lamina dura. With age, there is a tendency for lesions to increase their radio-opacity. While lesions classically merge into surrounding normal bone, mandibular lesions sometimes have better defined margins.

Management. There is no ideal treatment for fibrous dysplasia. Observation may be appropriate if the lesion is minor but development of any neurological signs or disfigurement would indicate a need for surgical or medical management. Surgery involves recontouring of

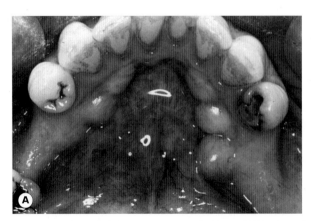

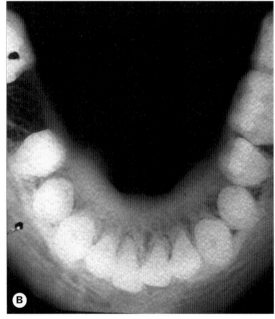

Fig. 80 Torus mandibularis. **A,** Clinical appearance. **B,** True occlusal radiograph of the mandible showing bilateral protruberances of the lingual cortical bone.

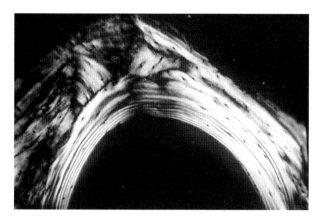

Fig. 81 Bone structure as seen at low magnification in a histological section.

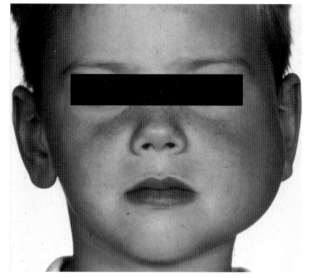

Fig. 82 Clinical picture of a fibrous dysplasia.

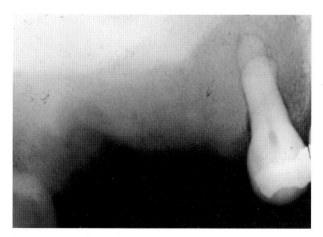

Fig. 83 Periapical radiograph of a patient with fibrous dysplasia of the right maxilla. The premolar has lost its lamina dura and the bone has a striking appearance, with an homogeneous finely stippled trabecular pattern.

the bony areas involved or resection and reconstruction. Medical management may involve the use of drugs that inactivate osteoclasts (bisphosphonates) and, therefore, limit invasion of lesions into normal bone. Medical management is undertaken by a physician, and consideration must be given to the unwanted effects of the drugs, particularly in children.

Cemento-ossifying fibroma

The cemento-ossifying fibroma shares much with fibrous dysplasia in its histopathology, but clinically and radiologically it is different. Its general behaviour is typical of a benign neoplasm in bone.

Clinical features. This fibroma typically affects young adult females, usually in the mandible. Its clinical presentation is that of any benign lesion, being that of a slowly growing swelling and developing asymmetry. The slow growth means cortices stay intact, so the swelling is firm to touch and painless.

Pathology. The histopathological features of the ossifying fibroma are similar to those observed in fibrous dysplasia; however, in contrast to fibrous dysplasia, the lesional tissue of the ossifying fibroma is well demarcated from the surrounding normal bone.

Radiology. In the early stages, the predominantly fibrous component means that it appears as a 'cyst-like' well-defined, corticated radiolucency. With time, radio-opaque foci appear and these increase in number and size until the lesion becomes predominantly radio-opaque. A thin radiolucent line often remains around the radio-opaque centre. Teeth in the path of the lesion may be displaced or resorbed (as is the case with any benign lesion).

Management. Surgical enucleation of the lesion is usually adequate.

Paget's disease of bone

In Paget's disease there is abnormal formation and resorption of bone. It is usually polyostotic, but invariably some bones in the skeleton will remain normal while others will be at different stages of the disease. Its aetiology may be viral.

Clinical features

Paget's disease affects individuals in middle and old age. Males are more commonly afflicted than females. The clinical symptoms reflect the enlargement and weakening of bone that results from Paget's disease. Slowly growing swelling of bones may lead to shape changes and enlargement of the skull and jaws (Fig. 84). Deformity of bones, typically of those bearing weight, may lead to bowing of legs and spinal curvature. Bone pain may occur and, if the skull base is affected, various neurological effects may develop.

In the jaws, the maxilla is affected more commonly than the mandible. In contrast to fibrous dysplasia, the disease is bilateral in the jaws. Spacing of teeth may develop and dentures may cease to fit. Extraction of teeth may be difficult, as a result of hypercementosis and ankylosis, and can be complicated by excessive bleeding, infection and slow healing. Other complications of Paget's disease include high-output cardiac failure and an increased risk of sarcoma, in particular osteosarcoma.

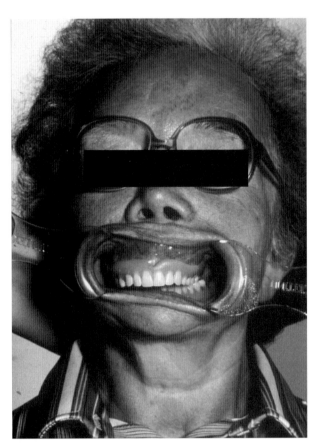

Fig. 84 Clinical picture showing lengthened maxilla due to bone expansion in a patient with Paget's disease.

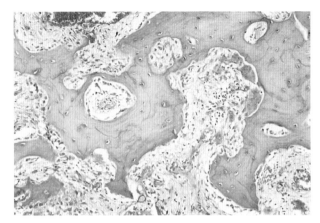

Fig. 85 Mosaic histopathology in Paget's disease.

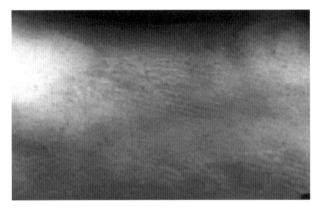

Fig. 86 Intra-oral radiograph of the mandible of an edentulous patient with Paget's disease of bone. There are two main features of note. There is an altered trabecular pattern with an impression of linearity/parallel lines. Mesially and distally there are densely radio-opaque areas ('cotton wool' radio-opacities).

Pathology

Paget's disease can be roughly divided into three overlapping phases. During the first of these osteoclastic activity predominates, normal bone is resorbed and is replaced by well-vascularised cellular fibrous tissue. The surface of the bone is rimmed by giant osteoclasts resting in Howship's lacunae. As the disease progresses, this osteolysis is accompanied by osteogenesis as new bone forms within the cellular fibrous tissue in the second phase of the disease. This combination of bone resorption and deposition gives rise to the classic mosaic appearance of bone in Paget's disease (Fig. 85). The basophilic reversal lines that outline 'the pieces of the mosaic' mark switches in activity from bone resorption to bone deposition. Ultimately, in the third phase, osteoblastic activity predominates and the trabeculae of bone fuse together to give rise to masses of dense, sclerotic bone that is relatively avascular. Cementum is affected by Paget's disease in a similar manner to bone, resulting in hypercementosis and, when bone and cementum fuse, ankylosis.

Radiology

There are three stages:

- *radiolucent (osteolytic):* bone resorption results in radiolucency and cortical thinning; the lamina dura of teeth may disappear

- *mixed:* the bony trabecular pattern is altered and often appears like 'ground glass' or may show a striking appearance of lines with few connections (Fig. 86); a few radio-opaque patches may appear in the bone
- *radio-opaque (osteoblastic):* with time, the radio-opaque patches increase in number, grow and coalesce; tooth roots often have hypercementosis.

The affected bone will always enlarge. In maxillary lesions, the enlargement encroaches on the maxillary sinuses, often obliterating them entirely (Fig. 87).

Management

If Paget's disease is suspected, the serum alkaline phosphatase level should be measured. This is elevated while serum calcium and phosphate levels are normal. Observation only may be appropriate in an elderly patient with no symptoms. However, medical treatment is indicated in those with pain or neurological signs. This consists of calcitonin and bisphosphonates, which inhibit osteoclast activity and slow rather than stop the disease process. Oral surgery should be avoided if possible, and patients given antibiotic cover when it is necessary.

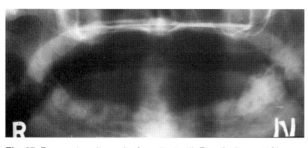

Fig. 87 Panoramic radiograph of a patient with Paget's disease of bone. There are several dense radio-opacities within the mandible. The largest, in the lower left third molar region, subsequently underwent infection and sequestration.

Giant-cell granuloma (central giant-cell granuloma)

Giant-cell granuloma (GCG) is a non-neoplastic lesion of bone.

Clinical features

GCG occurs most commonly in younger age groups (first to third decades) and has a greater incidence in females. The mandible is more likely to be affected and the anterior parts of the jaws are favoured. Presentation is usually that of a painless swelling, which may be accompanied by displacement of teeth.

Pathology

This lesion is identical histologically to the giant-cell epulis (peripheral giant-cell granuloma) and the brown tumours of hyperparathyroidism (see below) and must be distinguished on clinical grounds. GCGs are characterised by the presence of multi-nucleate osteoclast-like giant cells lying in an extremely vascular stroma. The giant cells vary in size, shape, intensity of staining and the number of nuclei that they contain. The fibroblastic stroma is densely cellular and rich in capillaries, with which the giant cells are often intimately related. Extravasated red blood cells and deposits of haemosiderin may be present. Evidence of dys-

trophic calcification and metaplastic bone formation may also be seen. In some lesions, fibrous septa delineate foci of giant cells.

Radiology

A round or ovoid radiolucency can be seen with a well-defined, non-corticated margin. Expansion is a common feature, with cortical thinning and sometimes perforation, producing a soft-tissue mass. Occasionally there is wispy internal calcification. Displacement of teeth often occurs but resorption is less common (Fig. 88).

Management

It is important to distinguish the GCG from hyperparathyroidism. This is normally done by estimating serum calcium, which is raised in hyperparathyroidism. Patients with hyperparathyroidism are referred to a physician for further investigations and treatment (see below). Surgical curettage of a GCG is usually adequate. This treatment may need to be repeated if there is recurrence; sometimes a wider resection may be indicated. Radiotherapy is contraindicated, as with any benign bone lesion.

Osteoporosis

Osteoporosis is a disease characterised by a microarchitectural deterioration of bone structure and a low bone mineral content, leading to increased bone fragility and an increase in fracture risk. It is a generalised disease, the effects of which are of greatest clinical importance in the hip, spine and forearm, but which will also occur in the jaws.

Clinical features

Osteoporosis may be primary, or may occur secondarily in association with other diseases or with drug therapy (e.g. corticosteroid use). There is a normal distribution of bone mineral density (BMD) in the population and osteoporosis in a particular bone is defined as a BMD lower than 2.5 standard deviations below the mean value for a young adult of the same sex. Women are more likely to suffer from the disease. Bone mineral loss is accelerated at the

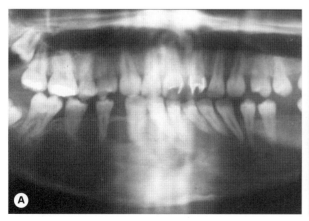
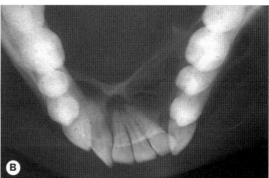

Fig. 88 Granuloma. **A**, A panoramic radiograph of a 20-year-old female who presented with a painless swelling of the anterior mandible with displacement of teeth. **B**, True occlusal radiograph of the same patient, showing the marked buccal and lingual expansion. The expanded cortices are very thin, suggesting rapid growth.

menopause or following hysterectomy. Patients may suffer from loss of height, a developing kyphosis and greater susceptibility to fractures. In the jaws, there may be a lower success rate with implant treatment and there seem to be associations with periodontal bone loss and resorption of the residual alveolar ridge.

Pathology

The trabeculae of cancellous bone are affected by a combination of thinning, reduction in number and discontinuities. Cortical bone undergoes endosteal and subperiosteal resorption and may ultimately resemble cancellous bone histologically.

Radiology

There is greater radiolucency of bone and cortical thinning. The vertebrae undergo compression fractures. In the jaws, the cortex at the lower border of mandible becomes thinner (Fig. 89) and the trabecular pattern becomes sparse.

Management

Management comprises medical treatment, exercise and lifestyle advice. Medical therapies include hormone replacement therapy (in women), bisphosphonate drugs, vitamin D, fluoride and other drugs.

Hyperparathyroidism

Hyperparathyroidism is an endocrine abnormality in which there is an excessive amount of parathyroid hormone (PTH). This causes bone resorption and hypercalcaemia. The disease may be primary, caused by excessive PTH formation by a parathyroid tumour (usually a functioning adenoma), or secondary to hypocalcaemia resulting from poor diet, vitamin D malabsorption, liver or kidney disease.

Clinical features

This disease usually affects the middle aged and is more often seen in women. Hypercalcaemia leads to clinical symptoms through renal calculi, peptic ulceration, bone pain and psychiatric problems. In the jaws, teeth may become loose or even be exfoliated.

Pathology

Cortical bone is more severely affected than cancellous bone. The increase in osteoclastic activity results in thinning of the cortices with loss of lamina dura. Marrow is replaced by fibrovascular tissue; brown tumours of hyperparathyroidism may develop (Fig. 90).

Radiology

There is increased radiolucency of bone, either generalised or localised. The earliest sign is subperiosteal resorption of the terminal phalanges. In the jaws, lamina dura of teeth is classically lost, along with the cortex of the inferior dental canal. There may be demineralisation of the cortex of the lower border of the mandible. Localised fairly well-defined radiolucencies (brown tumours) may be seen throughout the skeleton but are more common in facial bones than elsewhere (Fig. 91).

Management

If hyperparathyroidism is suspected, assays of serum calcium, phosphate and alkaline phosphatase should be carried out by a physician. Both serum and urinary calcium levels and serum PTH levels are usually raised and serum phosphate levels decreased. Alkaline phosphatase levels are raised in severe disease. The most frequent cause of primary disease is an underlying parathyroid adenoma.

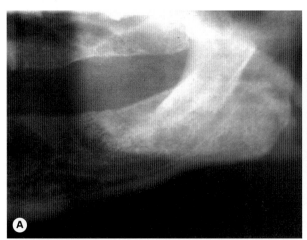 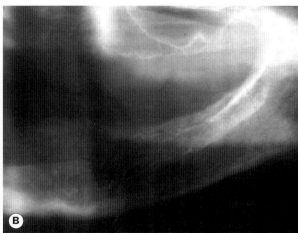

Fig. 89 Parts of two edentulous mandibles as seen on panoramic radiographs. **A**, A thick cortex can be seen at the lower border of the jaw. **B**, The thinned cortex here is typical of a patient with osteopenia or osteoporosis.

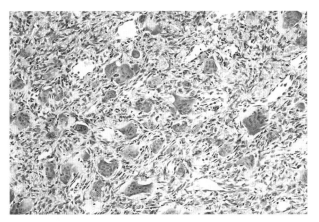

Fig. 90 Histopathology of the brown tumour of hyperparathyroidism, showing numerous multinucleate giant cells.

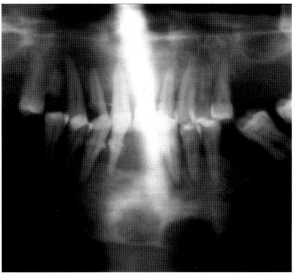

Fig. 91 Brown tumours of hyperparathyroidism. There are two fairly well-defined radiolucencies in the symphysis and parasymphysial region of the mandible; these were brown tumours. Lamina dura is also difficult to identify on the teeth. The radiolucency in 12 region may be inflammatory rather than related to the systemic disease.

Genetic disorders

Numerous genetic disorders affect the jaws, and a good reference source for evaluation of individual cases is the On-line Mendelian Disorders in Man (OMIM) database (*http://www.ncbi.nlm.nih.gov/Omim*). A number of disorders have effects in the jaw bones:

- familial adenomatous polyposis (Gardner's syndrome): multiple osteomas and odontomes, hazy sclerosis and hypodontia may be found in the jaws; numerous polyps develop in the large bowel and there is a very high risk of malignant change (adenocarcinoma of the bowel)
- osteogenesis imperfecta: multiple bone fractures occur after minor trauma and soft tissues are typically lax, with hernia formation; the sclera may look blue and some patients develop dentinogenesis imperfecta; short stature is typical
- osteopetrosis: also known as marble bone disease, the medullary cavity infills with dense bone; the maxillary sinus may fail to pneumatise and bone appears dense and structureless on radiographs; there may be partial failure of tooth eruption
- vitamin-D-resistant rickets (hypophosphataemia)

- cleido-cranial dysplasia
- cemento-osseous dysplasia
- McCune–Albright syndrome.

Bone tumours

A simple classification of bone swellings is given in Box 9. Osteomas occur most frequently in the paranasal sinuses and are dealt with in the section on maxillary sinus. Primary malignant bone tumours are rare and include osteosarcoma, chondrosarcoma and multiple myeloma. Direct invasion of bone by squamous-cell carcinoma arising in the oral mucosa is common in advanced oral cancers. Metastatic deposition of carcinoma from colon, lung, breast, kidney and other primary sites is more likely to be the cause of a destructive malignant lesion in bone than primary sarcoma.

Box 9 Simple classification of bone swellings in the jaws

Benign
Torus mandibularis and torus palatinus
Reactive exostosis
Osteochondroma
Haemangioma
Osteoma
Osteoblastoma
Chondroma
Central giant-cell granuloma
Fibrous dysplasia
Cemento-ossifying fibroma
Cemento-osseous dysplasias

Malignant
Osteosarcoma
Chondrosarcoma
Myeloma
Metastatic deposits in bone

7.2 Diseases of the maxillary sinus

The maxillary sinus (antrum) has a close anatomical and pathological relationship with the oral cavity. It is relevant in dentistry because:

- patients with maxillary sinusitis or other pathoses may present to the dentist believing they have toothache
- patients with dental pathology in the maxilla may develop secondary signs and symptoms in the sinus
- dentists may intrude into the maxillary sinus during surgery or other dental procedures.

Anatomy

The normal sinus in adults is pyramidal in shape. At birth, it is very small, growing laterally from its point of origin above the inferior turbinate bone until, by about the ninth year, it extends to the zygoma. Lateral growth ceases by 15 years of age. Radiologically, the sinus appears as a triangular-shaped radiolucency on occipitomental radiographs (Fig. 92). On intra-oral radiographs, the antrum

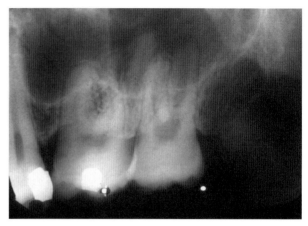

Fig. 93 Periapical radiograph of the left upper molar region. The normal sinus floor is seen overlying the roots of the molars, with a vertical septum directly above the first standing molar. A curving radiolucent band runs across the sinus: this represents the groove in the bony wall containing the postero-superior alveolar nerve and vessels.

is demarcated by the prominent lamina dura of its walls. A variable feature is the presence of one (or more) septum within the antral space. On intra-oral radiographs, neurovascular channels, which groove the bony walls, may be seen as sinuous radiolucent lines overlying the sinus (Fig. 93).

Histology

The antral lining is composed of pseudostratified ciliated columnar epithelium rich in mucus-secreting goblet cells. Deep to this epithelium, within a lamina propria composed of loose connective tissue, lie mucous, seromucous and serous glands.

Anomalies

Hypoplasia and hyperplasia of the maxillary sinuses are frequently seen. These anomalies may be unilateral or bilateral and are identified by chance on radiography. Hypoplasia can be misinterpreted on radiography as sinus opacity due to disease, while hyperplasia that extends the anterior alveolus may be interpreted as a cystic lesion.

Inflammation ('sinusitis')

Chronic maxillary sinusitis

Chronic inflammation of the mucosa lining the sinus is common, particularly amongst those living in polluted environments and in smokers. It is also associated with allergies. Symptoms and signs may be few or none, only occurring during acute exacerbations of inflammation. There may be nasal stuffiness and discomfort on pressure to the infra-orbital area.

The main radiological finding is thickening of the mucosa lining the antrum. This reduces the size of the air space on sinus radiographs (usually the occipitomental radiograph, although mucosal thickening may be seen on periapical and panoramic radiographs; Fig. 94). While the thickening is often even in width, 'lumpy' (polypoid) mucosal thickening is also seen. Occasionally the mucosal thickening may be severe enough to exclude virtually

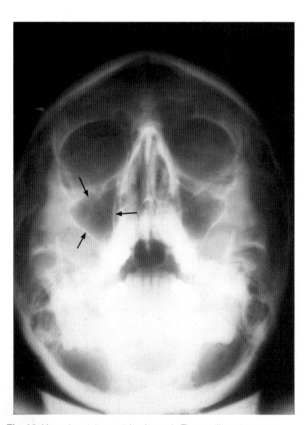

Fig. 92 Normal occipitomental radiograph. The maxillary sinuses are uniformly radiolucent (arrowed on patient's right).

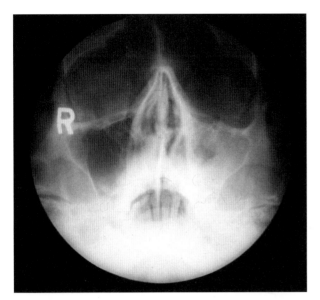

Fig. 94 Chronic maxillary sinusitis affecting the left sinus. The peripheral radio-opacity in the left sinus is mucosal thickening and contrasts well with the normal right sinus.

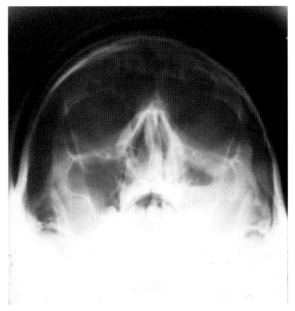

Fig. 95 Acute maxillary sinusitis affecting the left sinus. There is an obvious fluid level in the left sinus, along with mucosal thickening visible along the orbital floor. The right sinus is normal.

all air from the sinus, producing a radiologically opaque antrum. Long-standing chronic sinusitis may stimulate sclerosis of the bony wall of the antrum. Destruction of bone in the walls of the sinus is very unusual and should be interpreted as a sinister sign (see malignancy, below).

In chronic sinusitis, the antral mucosa is oedematous and contains a dense infiltrate of lymphocytes, plasma cells and macrophages. Eosinophils are often present, especially in allergic disorders.

Mild chronic sinusitis may be associated with few symptoms and is very common. No treatment may be necessary in such cases. Where treatment is appropriate, promoting drainage is the usual goal of treatment because obstruction of the ostium is often a feature. Endoscopic surgery is the usual mode of treatment. Polyps may need to be surgically excised.

Acute maxillary sinusitis

Acute sinusitis often occurs in association with a cold or influenza. Chronic sinusitis is a predisposing factor. Occasionally, patients may interpret symptoms as 'toothache' and present to their dentist.

Pain, stuffiness, nasal discharge, tenderness over the cheek and tenderness of posterior teeth on the affected side are all symptoms. There may be general malaise and lymphadenopathy. Acute sinusitis is associated with accumulation of inflammatory exudate and neutrophils/eosinophils in the sinus. This may appear as an air/fluid level on radiography (Fig. 95), or, if all air is displaced, as a totally opaque antrum. Antibiotic therapy, decongestants and inhalations are used in combination. Treatment of an underlying chronic problem may be necessary after resolution of the acute sinusitis.

Mucosal cysts of the antrum

A common phenomenon is the appearance of mucosal cysts in the lining mucosa of the maxillary antrum. Such cysts may be of retention or extravasation type. These cysts can be found in all age groups but are more common in males. They are usually not associated with symptoms, but some patients report symptoms of sinusitis, presumably when the normal flow of secretions is obstructed by the cyst.

The mucosal cysts are similar to salivary mucocoeles. The retention cyst is characterised by the presence of a lining of pseudostratified ciliated columnar epithelium while the extravasation type lacks an epithelial lining. The wall of both types consists of connective tissue infiltrated by chronic inflammatory cells.

These cysts appear as clearly defined dome-shaped radio-opacities overlying the antrum. While small cysts may be seen on periapical radiographs, they are more often noticed as a chance finding on panoramic radiographs (Fig. 96). It is important to exclude odontogenic cysts in differential diagnosis. Odontogenic cysts may expand up from the maxillary alveolus into the antral space and be seen as a dome-shaped radio-opacity. However, the radio-opaque cortex of the antral floor will be raised up around

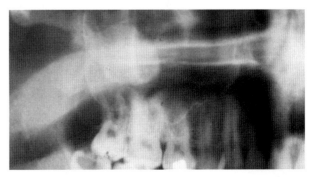

Fig. 96 Mucus retention cyst of the right antrum.

the periphery of an odontogenic cyst, while the antral floor will be in its normal position below a mucosal retention cyst.

No treatment is normally indicated. Cysts may spontaneously rupture or persist for months or even longer periods. If symptoms of sinusitis are present, then referral to the patient's medical practitioner is advisable.

Benign tumours

Osteoma

Osteoma is a benign tumour that is relatively common in the paranasal sinuses. However, it is most common in frontal and ethmoid sinuses. It is common in males.

The tumour is usually asymptomatic and, therefore, may be discovered by chance on dental radiography. Symptoms of sinusitis may occur if the osteoma obstructs normal flow of secretions into the nose. Very large lesions may cause expansion of the palate or a swelling of the face.

Osteomas may be of cancellous or compact types. In the former, the tumour is composed of slender trabeculae of cancellous bone with fibrofatty marrow. The latter consists of dense lamellar bone with inconspicuous marrow spaces.

A well-defined, usually round/ovoid radio-opacity overlies the sinus. As osteomas may be predominantly compact bone (compact or 'ivory' osteoma) or mainly trabecular bone (cancellous osteoma), the degree of radio-opacity may vary.

Surgical excision of the tumour via a Caldwell–Luc approach is the treatment of choice.

Odontogenic cysts and benign tumours

Any odontogenic cyst or tumour involving the maxilla may secondarily involve the maxillary antrum.

Frequently symptoms/signs are few or are those usually associated with cyst/benign tumour growth (Ch. 10). If the lesion is large and has involved a great part of the antrum, sinusitis-like symptoms may develop if the normal flow of secretions into the nose is obstructed.

Periapical radiographs may be misleading unless examined carefully. A radiolucent cyst or tumour may be misinterpreted as the antrum. However, lamina dura will be lost from involved teeth. There may be displacement and resorption of roots. On occipitomental radiographs a dome-shaped radio-opacity may be evident arising from the antral floor. (It is an important principle to understand that a lesion which is radiolucent in bone, such as a cyst, will appear radio-opaque in the antrum when surrounded by relatively less dense air.)

Malignancy

Symptoms of sinusitis may be early features of the disease. Paraesthesia or anaesthesia of the infra-orbital nerve can occur. As the disease progresses, it may destroy the bone of the antral wall and lead to various signs such as oral swelling, nasal obstruction or eye symptoms or signs. However, importantly for the dentist, alveolar bone involvement may cause loosening of teeth. Occasionally, malignancy may present with a soft-tissue mass growing out of a maxillary extraction socket (Fig. 97).

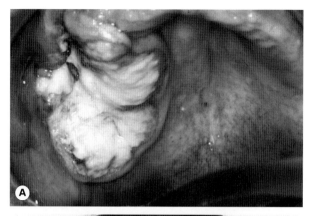

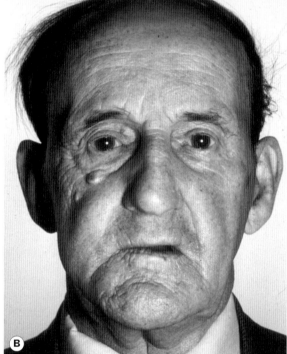

Fig. 97 Antral carcinoma. Intra-oral (**A**) and extra-oral (**B**) views. Note loss of nasolabial fold on the right side.

Squamous-cell carcinomas, displaying typical histological features, form the bulk of maxillary sinus malignancies (approximately 80%). Adenocarcinomas and undifferentiated carcinomas constitute much of the remainder. Less-common malignant neoplasms arising in this site are malignant melanoma, lymphoma and sarcoma.

On dental radiographs, antral radio-opacity may be difficult to discern without a normal antral air shadow available with which it can be compared. On a panoramic radiograph, recognition may be easier because of the comparison with the contralateral side. Where bone has become involved, the radio-opaque lamina dura of the sinus floor may become indistinct or disappear altogether. At a later stage, teeth may lose all supporting bone ('floating teeth', Fig. 98) and, if the malignancy extends into the mouth, a soft tissue mass may be observed (Fig. 98) (although this will be self-evident clinically).

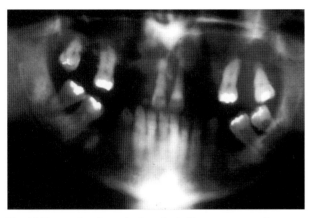

Fig. 98 Panoramic radiograph of a patient with a squamous-cell carcinoma of the left maxillary sinus. There is complete absence of bone supporting the upper left third molar tooth and the sinus floor is not visible.

Management of antral cancer is difficult, in part because the tumour may be advanced at initial presentation having increased in size unimpeded within the sinus. Surgical removal of the tumour is necessary by partial or total maxillectomy together with radiotherapy. However, recurrence is common. Chemotherapy is used in combination with surgery for some tumours. The defect may be lined with a skin graft and an obturator constructed, possibly retained by osseointegrated implants. Alternatively, very large defects may require a microvascular free flap for reconstruction.

Antral response to inflammation of dental origin

Where the lamina dura of a posterior maxillary tooth is also the cortical bone of the antral floor, periapical inflammation of dental origin may provoke a localised inflammation of the antral lining.

Clinical features

Symptoms and signs are of periapical periodontitis.

Pathology

There are features of chronic sinusitis.

Radiology

There is a rounded radio-opacity immediately above the affected tooth ('antral halo').

Management

Treatment of the diseased tooth is required.

Displacement of roots into the sinus

Root displacement into the sinus usually arises when an upper posterior tooth fractures during extraction and where the antrum is anatomically closely involved with the roots. Pre-existing periapical inflammation causing bone destruction is a predisposing factor. Incorrect application of an elevator during attempted removal results in the root slipping upwards into the antrum, usually beneath the mucosal lining but sometimes into the antral air space. Diagnosis is usually immediate, although occasionally

a root may be displaced laterally/medially beneath the mucoperiosteum of the alveolar bone and misinterpreted as being in the antrum. Alternatively, a whole tooth may occasionally be displaced into the antrum.

The first step is to take a periapical radiograph of the socket. The root may be visible immediately above the socket. If it is not visible, larger radiographs (oblique occlusals, panoramic) may be appropriate to discover the root. Parallax films (e.g. a periapical and an oblique occlusal) can help to interpret position. In a hospital situation, occipitomental radiographs are usually taken: these may show various degrees of antral opacity from a sinusitis arising in response to the root.

If the root is beneath the antral lining, it may be retrieved by raising a buccal mucoperiosteal flap and carefully removing buccal bone to expose it. If the root is within the antral air space then it is retrieved by a Caldwell–Luc approach, which provided better access to the antrum. The Caldwell–Luc antrostomy is performed by raising a buccal mucoperiosteal flap in the canine fossa region to expose the anterior wall of the antrum (Fig. 99). The infra-orbital nerve is identified and protected behind a retractor before bone is removed to open a 15-mm-diameter window into the anterior antrum. With a good light and suction, the contents of the maxillary sinus are searched for the tooth or root, which is retrieved with an appropriate instrument such as a Ficklings. The intra-oral wound is closed. This surgical procedure is best carried out under general anaesthesia and with antibiotic cover. The bony defect in the anterior sinus wall undergoes fibrous healing.

Oroantral communication

Oroantral communication may occur following displacement of a root into the antrum or simply after extraction of an upper posterior tooth. A prerequisite for its occurrence is a close relationship between tooth/root and antrum, while previous destruction of periapical bone by an inflammatory lesion is a predisposing factor.

The presence of a communication is often missed. Careful examination of the socket may clearly show a

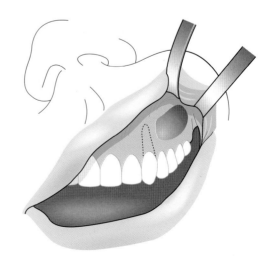

Fig. 99 The Caldwell–Luc surgical procedure showing the site of the window into the anterior antrum.

'hole' into the antrum. Sometimes air bubbles may be evident in the socket. Classic features include liquids passing from the mouth into the nose via the antrum and air passing in the opposite direction if a patient attempts to blow the nose. If a communication is left it will eventually epithelialise, forming an oroantral fistula (OAF). Symptoms of sinusitis often occur.

An intra-oral film will probably reveal absence of lamina dura from the socket. Occipitomental radiography may reveal nothing immediately after creation of a communication, but signs of sinusitis (see above) often develop with time.

Presumably some undiagnosed OAF close spontaneously but more often they are difficult to manage. The surgical technique of choice depends on the time of diagnosis, with either a buccal or a palatal flap used.

A newly created OAF should be closed immediately. An OAF that is diagnosed later should be allowed a period of 6 weeks to close spontaneously. The reason for this is that an attempt to close the fistula earlier is likely to fail because the tissues are more friable during their initial healing phase and more difficult to manage. After 6 weeks, if the OAF persists, then it should be surgically closed with a buccal flap but the epithelial tract that has formed must be excised first.

Buccal advancement. A buccal flap should be used to close a newly created OAF and this should be carried out by the dentist immediately. The intention is to completely close the fistula to facilitate healing by primary intention (Fig. 100). The buccal flap, therefore, has to be advanced sufficiently to achieve this and this may require incising the periosteum of the mucoperiosteal flap. Mattress sutures facilitate good closure and are removed after 10 days. A broad-spectrum antibiotic such as amoxicillin and 0.5% ephedrine nasal drops are prescribed and the patient instructed not to blow the nose. This procedure may be undertaken under local anaesthesia. The advancement of the buccal flap may result in a decrease in height of the buccal sulcus. It may be difficult to achieve tension-free closure of a large extraction socket.

Palatal flap. Alternatively, an OAF may be closed with a palatal flap. This may be necessary because a buccal advancement flap has failed or is not feasible. A palatal pedicle flap is raised so as to include a greater palatine artery (Fig. 101). This is rotated to close the defect and is

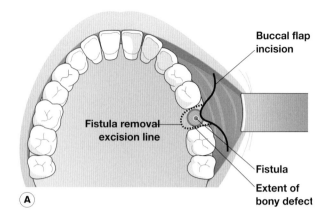

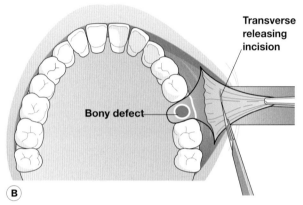

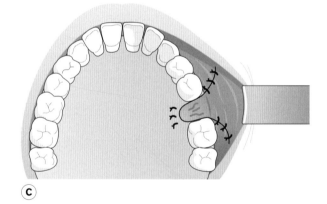

Fig. 100 Buccal advancement procedure to close an oroantral fistula.

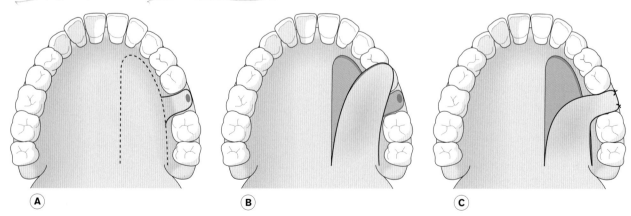

Fig. 101 The palatal flap procedure to close an oroantral fistula.

obviously more difficult the more posterior is the OAF. The denuded area of palatal bone is protected with resorbable cellulose such as Surgicell and heals by granulation. A palatal flap is very much more robust than a buccal flap but this technique is better undertaken under general anaesthesia.

Fracture of the maxillary tuberosity

Extraction of a posterior maxillary molar, usually lonestanding, is the scenario in which a fracture might occur. With the application of force to the forceps, an audible crack may occur and the alveolar bone of the tuberosity is felt, or seen, to move with the tooth.

A periapical or panoramic radiograph may show nothing unless the fracture is displaced. If the latter has occurred, discontinuity of the antral floor is the sign.

An OAF will inevitably be created and immediate closure with a buccal flap as described above is indicated. It is likely to be relatively straightforward to achieve primary closure if the fractured piece of bone is dissected free and removed. However, if the segment of bone is large, then one could consider management as per alveolar fracture (Ch. 8). This would involve splinting the bone by means of the tooth and then removing the tooth surgically with care 6 weeks later when the bony fracture can be assumed to have healed. However, if the tooth has been causing pain, this may not be an option.

Seven

Self-assessment: questions

Multiple choice questions

1. The following are features of osteopetrosis (marble bone disease):
   a. The maxillary sinus may be obliterated on occipitomental radiographs
   b. Osteomyelitis is a recognised complication
   c. Osteoclastic activity is normal
   d. Anaemia is uncommon because of extramedullary haemopoiesis
   e. Dense bone fills the medullary cavities, increasing bone strength

2. Fibrous dysplasia:
   a. Can affect a single bone, the craniofacial skeleton or multiple bones
   b. Does not require surgical removal but can be contoured when bone deformity occurs
   c. Radiographically evolves through radiolucency to ground glass and orange peel appearances
   d. Forms a sharp, discrete margin with adjacent normal bone
   e. May be a feature of Albright's syndrome

3. Giant-cell lesions in the jawbones:
   a. May occur in renal osteodystrophy
   b. May be treated by direct calcitonin injection
   c. Can be a feature of primary hyperparathyroidism
   d. Contain cells with histological and functional features of osteoclasts
   e. May perforate the alveolus

4. Chronic osteomyelitis:
   a. Is associated with sickle-cell disease
   b. Is an appropriate term to describe 'dry socket'
   c. The most common source of infection is blood-borne streptococci
   d. May produce bony sequestra, involucrum and chronic sinus tracts
   e. May lead to amyloidosis

5. In the maxillary sinus:
   a. If a posterior maxillary tooth or root is lost into the sinus during extraction, a flap may be raised immediately for retrieval
   b. Roots displaced between the bone floor and sinus lining should always be removed
   c. An established oroantral fistula should be treated by removal of any antral polyps, excision of the fistula and closure by advancing of a mucoperiosteal flap
   d. Spontaneous formation of an oroantral communication that is non-symptomatic can be managed appropriately by asking the patient to refrain from blowing the nose
   e. Maxillary sinusitis can result in a toothache-like pain that is poorly localised and made worse by tilting the head forwards

6. Of the bone tumours:
   a. Osteosarcoma is the most common malignancy found in bone
   b. Osteosarcoma tends to occur in two age peaks, juvenile and adult, except in the jaws where the peak age is around 25 years
   c. Osteomas may be solitary or multiple in the jaws
   d. Sun-ray spicules are a typical radiographic feature of cemento-ossifying fibroma
   e. Torus mandibularis should always be confirmed by undertaking trephine biopsy

Extended matching items

EMI 1

Options:
A Paget's disease of bone
B Osteonecrosis
C Marble bone disease
D Osteosarcoma
E Osteoma
F Condylar hyperplasia
G Cleido-cranial dysplasia
H Hyperparathyroidism
I Fibrous dysplasia
J Juvenile ossifying fibroma

Lead in: Match the case history from the list below that is most appropriate for each diagnosis above.

1. A 15-year-old girl presented with an expanding bone lesion around the roots of a lower first molar. A biopsy showed principally cartilage containing groups of pleomorphic chondrocytes. In one small area hyperchromatic and rapidly dividing osteoblasts were forming osteoid trabeculae.
2. A 14-year-old girl presented with an expanding bone lesion affecting the ascending ramus of the mandible. The radiographs showed a diffuse ground-glass appearance that merged with the surrounding bone. A biopsy showed interlacing fascicles of fibrous tissue containing fine trabeculae of woven bone.
3. A 63-year-old man was under the care of a haematologist for multiple myeloma. He was taking thalidomide and was also on intravenous bisphosphonates. He developed an area of exposed discoloured bone on the upper alveolar ridge.
4. A 15-year-old girl attended regarding 'missing' teeth. On the dental panoramic tomogram there were several unerupted teeth and the bone appeared unusually radio-opaque in quality. An occipito-mental radiograph showed that the maxillary sinuses were obscured.
5. A 22-year-old man attended for treatment. He had a history of Gardner's syndrome and noticed a bony hard lump on the ascending ramus of the mandible.

6. A 28-year-old woman presented for a check up. The dentist noticed that the occlusal plane was depressed on the left side. The molar teeth did not make contact with the maxillary teeth on that side, though wear facets were present.

7. A 9-year-old girl presented with failure of eruption of several permanent teeth. A dental panoramic tomogram showed that there were multiple supernumerary teeth in all quadrants of the jaws.

8. A 58-year-old man presented with a brown-red granular epulis. A periapical radiograph showed underlying bone destruction and a biopsy was reported as showing osteoclast-like giant cells in a spindle-cell background with numerous thin-walled vessels. Haemosiderin and extravasated red cells were abundant.

9. A 15-year-old girl presented with an expanding bone lesion in the ascending ramus of the mandible. It was well circumscribed and showed a ground-glass appearance. A biopsy showed interlacing fascicles of fibrous tissue containing fine trabeculae of woven bone.

10. A 63-year-old woman presented with exposed bone sequestrating from the maxillary alveolar ridge. Serum biochemistry showed that her alkaline phosphatase level was elevated twenty-fold over the top of the normal range.

EMI 2

Options:

A Acute sinusitis
B Osteoma of maxillary sinus
C Squamous-cell carcinoma of maxillary sinus
D Chronic sinusitis
E Oro-antral fistula
F Maxillary sinus hypoplasia
G Root within the sinus
H Odontogenic cyst in the sinus
I Mucosal cyst of the sinus

Lead in: Match the case history from the list below that is most appropriate for each diagnosis above.

1. A 12-year-old patient attending for orthodontic treatment has a panoramic radiograph take. There are no symptoms or signs related to the sinuses. The radiograph shows increased radio-opacity over the left maxilla and the line of cortical bone of the maxillary sinus floor is not obviously visible. An occipito-mental radiograph confirms the radio-opacity and seems to show that the left orbital floor is lower down than on the right.

2. A 45-year-old male attends for a routine dental check-up. He is a smoker. He says that he sometimes gets a dull ache from his upper teeth and also that he gets 'catarrh' a lot. He has periodontal disease and asks if his symptoms are due to his gum trouble.

3. A 27-year-old patient has a panoramic radiograph taken. This reveals a 2-cm-diameter round radio-opacity (of soft tissue density) overlying the right maxillary sinus, apparently arising from the sinus floor. The radio-opacity is uniform and has no line of cortical bone at its edge. The patient has no symptoms.

4. A 65-year-old man attends as a new patient. He would like something to fill the space where a tooth was removed on the upper left side, because food gets stuck in there. He says he has had 'sinus trouble' for a few years on the same side, and has to get antibiotics now and again when it gets painful. He last saw a dentist 3 years ago for some fillings and the extraction of the UL6. The UL6 extraction site shows a substantial defect, and the patient mentions that the extraction was difficult, 'needed stitches' and was very slow to heal.

5. A 35-year-old woman attends as an emergency complaining of toothache on the upper right side. It is a throbbing dull ache. She says her back teeth on the upper right are tender. She feels generally unwell and asks if she has an abscess developing. She says that she is still a bit 'blocked up' from a cold. On examination, she has tender, palpable right upper cervical lymph nodes. Intra-orally, she has a few carious teeth on the upper right, but all teeth test positively to sensitivity tests.

6. A 70-year-old woman complains of a painful upper left molar. On periapical radiography, apart from a periapical inflammatory lesion on the first molar, you notice a dense radio-opacity at the upper edge of the image, distant from the teeth. You refer the patient for a panoramic radiograph; this shows a 1 cm diameter, rounded, densely opaque radio-opacity overlying the middle of the left maxillary sinus. On enquiry, the patient gives no history of sinusitis.

7. A 65-year-old man complains of an upper left molar being very loose. He also says he has been suffering from what he thinks is sinusitis on the left side for a few weeks. His GP has given him antibiotics for this. On examination, he mentions that the left side of his upper lip has been tingling for a week or more. Intra-orally, you note that his UL7 is very loose and that the UL6 is also a little mobile. There is a little tenderness in his buccal sulcus next to these teeth. A periapical radiograph shows virtually no bone support on UL7 and the bone loss extends the full depth of the alveolus, including the apparent loss of the maxillary sinus floor.

8. A 24-year-old man complains of a swelling in his upper right buccal sulcus that has been slowly developing for some weeks or months. There are no other symptoms. On examination there is nothing to see extra-orally, but in his mouth there is a definite swelling adjacent to UR7 buccally. UR8 is not visible clinically, but the swelling extends distally to this region. On palpation the swelling is bony hard. Radiologically, panoramic radiography reveals a rounded radio-opacity at the posterior floor of the right maxillary sinus. At the edge of this soft tissue-density radio-opacity is a very thin margin with the density of bone. UR8 is visible, unerupted, in a high position overlying the

radio-opacity. UR7 roots are short and blunt-ended, suggesting external resorption.

9. A 30-year-old woman attends your practice as an emergency. She had an upper left second premolar extracted at another dental practice a week ago and 'had an awful time' when the tooth broke and the dentist was 'poking around' for ages. She doesn't want to see that dentist again. Now she is complaining of a throbbing ache and she feels 'blocked up' on the left cheek and sinus. In response to your questions, she says she has not been aware of drinks passing into her nose, but she has been using a straw when drinking to stop hot drinks going near the socket. On examination, there is a new socket, with a clot in place, but with evidence of substantial soft tissue trauma from the surgery. Periapical and panoramic radiographs reveal the outline of a normal socket. There is a 3 × 4mm radio-opacity of tooth or bone density immediately above the line of the maxillary sinus floor, just above the socket. The maxillary sinus has a band, of soft-tissue radio-opacity and about 10mm thick, running along its walls.

Case history questions

Case history 1

A 58-year-old woman noticed that her front teeth had become spaced and seeks advice from her dentist.
On entering the surgery, the dentist notices that she has difficulty in walking and does not respond to his questions. She has become increasingly deaf and her vision has also deteriorated. On examination, the maxilla and zygoma are enlarged and there is enlargement of the forehead.

1. What diagnosis would you suspect?
2. What information might be gained from oral radiographs and blood tests to support this diagnosis?
3. What are the principal histological features of this disorder?

Case history 2

A 60-year-old man has been treated for a T2N0M0 squamous-cell carcinoma by radical radiotherapy. He has a history of chronic alcoholism and was a heavy smoker. Six years after treatment, he develops a painful ulcer in the alveolar mucosa in the treated area following minor trauma. His pain worsens and the bone became progressively exposed. He is treated by a partial mandibular resection with graft.

1. What diagnosis is most likely?
2. How does radiotherapy damage tissues and what structural features might be seen in the bone?
3. What changes may arise in irradiated connective tissues 10 years after exposure?

Case history 3

A 6-year-old girl presents with dental pain. On examination, her teeth are discoloured and worn down. Her panoramic radiograph is shown (Fig. 102). She has a history of previous bone fractures and was of short stature for her age.

1. Which genetic bone disorder should be suspected?
2. What signs would be apparent on extra-oral examination of the face?
3. Which gene is likely to be mutated?
4. Which dental disorder is present?

Case history 4

A 35-year-old man presents with gross loosening of both his lower left premolar teeth. The gingivae around them looks swollen and is purple-brown in colour. A radiograph shows irregular bone destruction to the apices. Incisional biopsy shows multinucleated osteoclast-like giant cells in a haemorrhagic fibrous stroma.

1. Which investigations should now be performed?
2. If these prove negative, what treatment should be undertaken?
3. Which other lesions in the jaws contain multinucleate giant cells of this type?

Case history 5

A 63-year-old man presented complaining of an area of numbness in his left cheek. On objective sensory nerve testing, a patch of paraesthesia was found over the distribution of the left infra-orbital nerve. An occipitomental radiograph reveals opacity of the maxillary antrum and a biopsy is reported as showing squamous-cell carcinoma.

1. What other presenting signs of carcinoma of the maxillary sinus are known?
2. Which histological features may be expected in the biopsy?

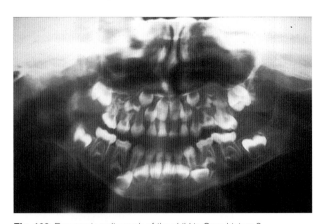

Fig. 102 Panoramic radiograph of the child in Case history 3.

3. Which imaging modalities can be used to provide information to aid treatment planning?

Viva questions

1. Which disorders are included in the spectrum of fibro-osseous lesions and how can they be distinguished?

2. What is dry socket and how is it treated?
3. How are the lesions of the cementoma group distinguished?
4. What are the clinical features of acromegaly?
5. Which local and systemic factors may delay healing and repair in bone?

Self-assessment: answers

Multiple choice answers

1. a. **True.** The medullary cavity tends to infill and the maxillary sinus cannot be seen. Unerupted teeth may be present.
    b. **True.** Infection tends to become chronic and this should be considered when extracting teeth. Specialist opinion is advised.
    c. **False.** Osteopetrosis is a rare genetic condition where there is defective osteoclast function.
    d. **False.** As the medullary cavity is obliterated, some compensation occurs by extramedullary haemopoiesis, but anaemia is common and bone marrow transplantation is sometimes needed.
    e. **False.** Despite obliteration of the medullary cavity, bones are fragile.
2. a. **True.** Monostotic, craniofacial and polyostotic forms are recognised.
    b. **False.** Surgical removal is not required, but bone recontouring may only be undertaken after skeletal maturity has been reached, to avoid recurrence.
    c. **True.** These reflect increasing formation and thickening of bone trabeculae in a fibrous matrix; the degree of radio-opacity also depends on lesional thickness.
    d. **False.** Fibrous dysplasia blends with adjacent normal bone and this feature distinguishes this fibro-osseous lesion from ossifying fibroma.
    e. **True.** Polyostotic fibrous dysplasia, skin pigmentation and sexual precocity are the principal features of Albright's syndrome.
3. a. **True.** Renal osteodystrophy is a complex disorder secondary to chronic renal failure and it may contain elements of hyperparathyroidism and osteomalcia. Osteolytic lesions containing giant-cell foci may occur in the jaws.
    b. **True.** An experimental study injecting calcitonin into giant-cell granuloma has been published. It is more usual to remove these lesions by curettage.
    c. **True.** Giant-cell lesions may form in primary hyperthyroidism as a result of parathyroid neoplasia or hyperplasia. Hyperparathyroidism can be excluded by estimating serum calcium when a giant-cell lesion in the jaw is diagnosed histologically.
    d. **True.** The osteoclasts in giant-cell granulomas contain tartrate-resistant acid phosphatase and can resorb mineralised matrix.
    e. **True.** Giant-cell lesions may perforate the alveolus and simulate a giant-cell epulis clinically.
4. a. **True.** Sickle-cell disease can lead to infarction and bone necrosis, followed by osteomyelitis and bone pain in the jaws.
    b. **False.** The term osteitis is preferred for local bone infection in dry socket. It may progress to osteomyelitis.
    c. **False.** Staphylococcal infection is the most common infective agent in osteomyelitis.
    d. **True.** Sequestra are separated fragments of necrotic bone; involucrum is a bone layer deposited upon the cortex following periosteal expansion. Chronic sinus tracts discharging pus from the necrotic bone in the medulla to the exterior are a feature of osteomyelitis.
    e. **True.** Amyloidosis may result from a variety of chronic inflammatory disorders where there is increased production of serum amyloid A precursor in the liver.
5. a. **True.** Depending on experience. If referral is decided upon, then the tooth or root is X-rayed before being removed surgically.
    b. **False.** If a small root produces no sinusitis and healing is demonstrated radiographically, surgical removal may not be essential.
    c. **True.** After closure, antibiotic therapy is often prescribed and the patient advised to refrain from blowing the nose.
    d. **False.** Appearance of a spontaneous oroantral fistula may be a result of dental infection, carcinoma of the maxillary sinus or other pathoses. Thorough investigation is essential.
    e. **True.** The teeth related to the affected sinus may be tender to percussion and there may be nasal stuffiness and discharge.
6. a. **False.** The most common malignant process in bone is metastatic deposition of carcinoma. Osteosarcoma is the most common primary bone malignancy.
    b. **True.** Some jaw osteosarcomas do occur in the juvenile age group, especially where there is a genetic predisposition to cancer.
    c. **True.** Multiple osteomas, odontomes and bone sclerosis may be features of Gardner's syndrome (familial adenomatous polyposis coli).
    d. **False.** Sun-ray spicules are a feature of osteogenic osteosarcoma.
    e. **False.** Normally a diagnosis of torus mandibularis can be made on purely clinical findings. Radiographic examination is used prior to biopsy when other bone lesions are suspected in other situations.

Extended matching items answers
EMI 1

1. **D.** Osteosarcoma is a malignant neoplasm of bone. A variety of histological patterns are known and a large amount of cartilage may be present. Formation

of osteoid by malignant osteoblasts is the defining histological feature. On radiographs the periodontal ligament may be widened, teeth may be displaced or resorbed and sometimes 'sun-ray spicules' may be seen.

2. **I.** The histological features are those of a 'fibro-osseous lesion'. Fibrous dysplasia merges radiographically with the surrounding bone whilst ossifying fibroma is well circumscribed. Fibrous dysplasia can affect one bone (monostotic) or several bones (polyostotic). The affected cells contain mutations of the GNAS gene.

3. **B.** Intravenous bisphosphonates such as pamidronate (Aredia) and zoledronic acid (Zometa) given to preserve bone mass in cancer have been linked to osteonecrosis in the jaw. Specialist advice should be sought when patients on these drugs need extractions.

4. **C.** Osteopetrosis is a complex genetic disorder characterised by reduced osteoclast action. Infantile (lethal) and late adult (benign) clinical patterns occur. This case fits with the 'intermediate' (childhood) pattern. Paranasal sinus malformations occur and the bone is sclerotic. The alveolus fractures easily when teeth are extracted.

5. **E.** Gardner's syndrome affects 1:8000 people and is characterised by polyps in the bowel that undergo malignant transformation. Dentists may identify the condition because multiple osteomas, odontomes and hazy sclerosis are often found in the jaws. The osteomas may be compact or cancellous and can occur on periosteal and endosteal surfaces.

6. **F.** The dental features suggest that the ascending ramus of the jaw on the left side continued growing after the right side ceased. This is typical of condylar hyperplasia. As the occlusal plane becomes depressed the corresponding maxillary teeth overerupt.

7. **G.** Cleido-cranial dysplasia is an autosomal dominant condition. The fontanelles fail to close and dental manifestations include multiple supernumerary teeth, peg teeth and retention of deciduous teeth.

8. **H.** These biopsy features may be seen in central or peripheral giant-cell granuloma, and also may occur in hyperparathyroidism. Serum calcium levels are typically elevated in hyperparathyroidism and the test may be used to exclude the hyperparathyroidism when giant-cell granuloma features are seen.

9. **J.** The high degree of radiographic circumscription is typical of ossifying fibroma when a fibro-osseous lesion is diagnosed histologically. Adult and juvenile types are seen and the new bone formed in the lesion may be trabecular or rounded (psammomatous) in form.

10. **A.** Highly elevated alkaline phosphatase is a good marker of Paget's disease of bone in the appropriate clinical setting. Bone sequestration is often secondary to chronic osteomyelitis in the jaws. Bisphosphonates are used to treat Paget's disease and also have been linked to jaw osteonecrosis.

EMI 2

1. **F.** Hypoplasia of the maxillary sinus is always discovered by chance during radiography. This patient is asymptomatic and has no clinical signs of disease. The absence of the line of the sinus floor on panoramic radiographs and increased radio-opacity is a key finding; in simple terms, the maxilla is filled with normal trabecular bone. It has been observed, however, that the orbital cavity may be larger in these patients, extending down into the maxilla. An 'opaque antrum' can, of course, be caused by a multitude of conditions and if you have any doubt about your diagnosis you should seek a second opinion.

2. **D.** Chronic sinusitis usually gives mild symptoms, but a dull ache in the cheeks is not unusual, along with nasal stuffiness and a post-nasal drip. It is common in smokers.

3. **I.** The round radio-opacity can be interpreted according to its characteristics of a uniform, round, soft tissue-density mass. Round radio-opacities can be produced by dental cysts and tumours, along with osteomas, but they have different radiological characteristics.

4. **E.** Of course, this patient may simply have been suffering from chronic sinusitis, but the history of a unilateral sinus problem, apparently arising over a similar time period since a difficult extraction of an ipsilateral upper molar, does raise the question of an oro-antral fistula. When a fistula has developed, the classic features of an oro-antral communication (drinks passing into the sinus and nose, air bubbles arising from the socket) may recede as mucosal thickening in the sinus may partly block off the hole.

5. **A.** The symptoms suggest an infective cause, and the principal differential diagnosis is dental abscess and acute maxillary sinusitis. The history of a recent cold is a strong hint. The sensitivity testing of the teeth is important. Radiography in a dental practice is only really useful in this context if, after clinical tests, you still think that the diagnosis is possibly a dental infection. Maxillary sinus infection is poorly shown by dental radiographs.

6. **B.** The dense radio-opacity is almost certainly an osteoma. In practice, rounded radio-opacities are much more likely to be mucosal cysts and these can look quite radio-opaque in contrast with the surrounding, low density, air. Osteomas should, however, be the density of bone. Osteomas are often chance findings on radiographs, although the maxillary sinus is a less common site than the frontal or ethmoidal sinuses.

7. **C.** The clues here are both clinical and radiological. The tingling of the upper lip indicates something affecting the maxillary division of the trigeminal nerve which, as its infra-orbital nerve component, passes along the roof of the maxillary sinus. A history of sinus-like symptoms is not unusual in malignancy of the sinus, while the loosening and exfoliation of teeth is also a frequent event. Radiologically, on dental radiographs, the destruction of the floor and walls of the maxillary sinus is a key sign; while a periodontal

abscess often leaves a tooth without any bony attachment, it would not destroy the sinus floor.

8. **H.** The painless, bony hard swelling suggests a non-infective lesion arising within the bone. The rounded radio-opacity can be differentiated from a mucosal cyst by its bony edge. Resorption and displacement of teeth is common with odontogenic cysts. In this case, the main differential diagnosis would include radicular cyst (from UR7 or UR6, if present), a dentigerous cyst involving UR8 and a keratocyst. The presence of UR8 overlying the lesion does not prove that this is a dentigerous cyst, as another type of lesion may simply have enveloped an unerupted third molar.

9. **G.** The recent traumatic extraction immediately raises suspicions about fractured roots and oro-antral communications, although the more common causes of post-extraction pain, such as dry socket, should also be considered. In this case, the latter is clearly not present as the clot is present in the socket. There were no clinical signs or symptoms of an oro-antral communication; indeed, the fact that she was using a straw to suck up drinks is a good clue that there is not an oro-antral communication (if there is a connection between nose and the mouth, you could only use a straw successfully by pinching closed your nostrils). The radiological features are most useful, as these show what is most likely to be a root. Its position is apparently just under a thickened sinus lining rather than free in the air space. Beware, however, of simple radiography; a root displaced into the buccal sulcus could appear superimposed over the maxillary sinus.

Case history answers

Case history 1

1. Paget's disease of bone results in enlargement of cranial bones and deformation of weight-bearing bones. The cranium is usually expanded in thickness and symptoms may arise from cranial nerve compression.
2. Radiographs of the jaws may show hypercementosis, cemental masses, abnormal trabeculation and a cotton-wool appearance in the jaws. The alkaline phosphatase level is markedly raised.
3. Disordered bone remodelling is seen; larger osteoclasts are present and the trabeculae show a scalloped outline. Numerous resting and reversal lines, resulting in a mosaic pattern, are seen and the vasculature may be increased. Globular cementum-like masses are seen in the jaws.

Case history 2

1. The features suggest osteoradionecrosis. Recurrent carcinoma is possible but less likely.
2. Radiotherapy damages tissues by producing free radicals. DNA damage may prevent cell division and repair. Endoarteritis obliterans results in reduced vascular supply to the tissues. Bone may become necrotic, showing osteocyte death, sequestration and

breakdown of the matrix. Infection may result in osteomyelitis.
3. Mutations and other genetic damage may lead to neoplasia in irradiated tissues. Osteosarcoma can arise in this way.

Case history 3

1. Osteogenesis imperfecta should be suspected. Increased joint mobility may also be present.
2. Blue sclera caused by thinness of the connective tissue may be seen. Some patients have characteristic 'Madonna facies'.
3. Collagen type I gene mutations have been described.
4. Dentinogenesis imperfecta is a feature of some forms of osteogenesis imperfecta, but either condition may arise as a separate disorder.

Case history 4

1. The serum calcium level should be measured and radiographs reviewed to exclude hyperparathyroidism.
2. The lesion should be treated by local removal with curettage.
3. Osteoclast-like giant cells are found in giant-cell granuloma, brown tumour of hyperparathyroidism, Paget's disease of bone, aneurysmal bone cyst and some fibro-osseous lesions, particularly cherubism.

Case history 5

1. Carcinoma of the maxillary antrum may be clinically occult and can present as maxillary swelling, loss of nasolabial skin crease, facial pain, cervical metastasis and symptoms similar to those of the temporomandibular disorder. Tumour fungating through premolar and molar maxillary extraction sockets is a classic sign.
2. Squamous-cell carcinoma is the most common malignancy arising in the maxillary sinus. Infiltrative pleomorphic and mitotically active squamous epithelium supported by fibrous stroma is seen. Keratin pearls may be present but some tumours are poorly differentiated.
3. Computed tomography, magnetic resonance and positron emission tomography are useful modalities for imaging maxillary sinus carcinoma.

Viva answers

1. Fibro-osseous lesions are grouped on the basis of their histology, consisting of cytologically bland fibroblastic fascicles in which bone trabeculae form. Radiographic examination is used to distinguish fibrous dysplasia from cemento-ossifying fibroma, as the former merges with surrounding bone while the latter has a sharply defined boundary. Cherubism and aneurysmal bone cyst have distinct clinical and radiographic features.
2. Dry socket is a local bone infection following tooth extraction. It is treated by irrigation with warm, mild antiseptic solution and placement of an obtudant dressing with antiseptic properties.

3. Cemento-ossifying fibroma is a solitary, slow-growing, circumscribed bone tumour; true cementoma is a sclerotic tumour of cementum most often associated with the roots of a lower first molar; cemento-osseous dysplasia is a genetic disorder most common in Negroids. Periapical, florid and focal forms are described as part of the spectrum.

4. Acromegaly results from excessive growth hormone secretion, most often from a pituitary adenoma. Condylar growth is reactivated and the mandible becomes enlarged and protrusive. The teeth become spaced and excessive growth of the lips, nose and facial tissues leads to coarse features. Hands and feet become spade like. Diabetes and visual disturbance may also develop.

5. Local features that delay healing in bone include mobility of a fracture, infection, foreign bodies and reduced local vascular supply. Systemic factors include diabetes mellitus, steroid therapy, osteoporosis and genetic disorders.

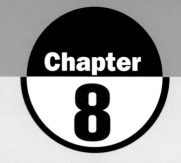

Oral and maxillofacial injuries

Chapter 8

Overview

This chapter concentrates on injuries to the face. It covers the primary survey procedure to identify and manage life-threatening injuries and the subsequent assessment and care of injuries that occur to teeth, soft tissues and bones of the face. The techniques available for fixing facial fractures are described.

8.1 Assessment of the injured patient

Learning objectives

You should:
- know how to carry out a primary survey to identify and manage life-threatening conditions
- know how to assess and document injuries
- be aware of the particular requirements for a child patient.

Primary survey

Guidelines for the management of the injury trauma patient initially developed by the American College of Surgeons have been widely adopted and disseminated through Advanced Trauma Life Support (ATLS) courses. These describe treatment priorities to achieve two aims: to save life and to restore function. A 'primary survey' is carried out simultaneously to identify and to manage life-threatening conditions and consists of the following:

- airway maintenance with cervical spine control
- breathing and ventilation
- circulation with control of haemorrhage
- disability owing to neurological deficit
- exposure and environmental control.

These are illustrated in Figure 103. Universal precautions of cross-infection control are adopted.

Airway

Airway management skills are necessary because the trauma patient will not be able to maintain his or her own airway if unconscious or if the airway is compromised by serious facial soft-tissue injury or facial fractures. However, airway skills are also important in other situations, such as when consciousness is altered by alcohol or other drugs, or when patients are treated with sedation and general anaesthesia. It is important to understand:

- how to recognise airway obstruction
- how to clear and maintain the airway with basic skills
- the role of advanced airway management including surgical management.

Airway obstruction may be recognised by the 'look, listen and feel' observations for breathing. Common causes of upper airway obstruction are the tongue and other soft tissues, blood, vomit, foreign body or oedema. Obstruction may be partial or complete:

- silence suggests complete obstruction
- gurgling suggests presence of liquid
- snoring arises when the pharynx is partially occluded by the tongue or soft palate
- crowing is the sound of laryngeal spasm.

Correction of airway obstruction is as described in Chapter 3 with the basic manoeuvre of chin lift or jaw thrust, use of oropharyngeal or nasopharyngeal airways and suction. The jaw thrust is the method of choice for the trauma victim as this avoids extension of a potentially injured neck, and the nasopharyngeal airway should be avoided if a fracture of the maxilla is suspected as it may pass into the cranial fossa. Airway compromise resulting from facial injury will require the early involvement of the oral and maxillofacial surgeon. Advanced airway management by way of endotracheal intubation is the 'gold standard' of airway maintenance and protection but is only carried out in the trauma situation after cervical spine radiograph has excluded bony injury.

Surgical airway intervention may be indicated, as a life-saving procedure, if it is not possible to intubate the trachea. This may consist of a needle cricothyroidotomy, in which a large-calibre plastic cannula is inserted into the trachea through the cricothyroid membrane

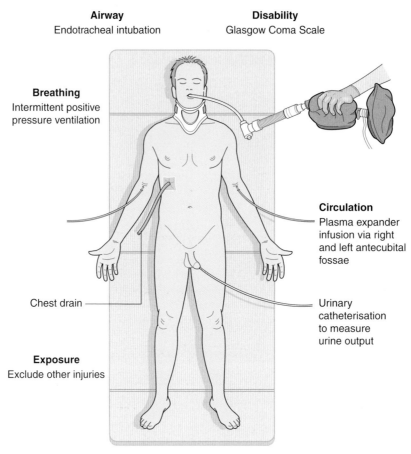

Airway
Endotracheal intubation

Disability
Glasgow Coma Scale

Breathing
Intermittent positive
pressure ventilation

Circulation
Plasma expander
infusion via right
and left antecubital
fossae

Chest drain

Urinary
catheterisation
to measure
urine output

Exposure
Exclude other injuries

Fig. 103 Trauma management primary survey.

(Fig. 104). Alternatively, a surgical cricothyroidotomy may be undertaken with a transverse incision through the membrane to permit placement of a small endotracheal tube. These measures can provide up to 45 minutes of extra time in which to arrange undertaking an emergency tracheostomy in a theatre environment. A transverse skin incision is made midway between the cricoid cartilage and the suprasternal notch followed by midline dissection of the infrahyoid muscles and division of the thyroid isthmus. Haemostasis is achieved and then the trachea is opened by cutting away part of the second and third rings to create a circular opening so that a tracheostomy tube may be placed and secured (Fig. 105).

Breathing

Once an airway has been established, then the adequacy of ventilation must be assessed. Artificial ventilation must be commenced immediately when spontaneous ventilation is inadequate or absent. Serious chest injuries such as tension pneumothorax and cardiac tamponade will compromise spontaneous ventilation. Early diagnosis of these potentially life-threatening conditions is essential so that they can be managed and permit adequate ventilation of the patient.

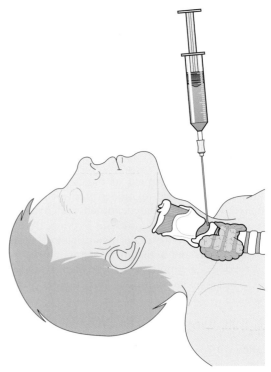

Fig. 104 Needle cricothyroidotomy.

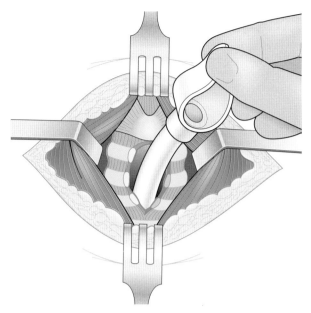

Fig. 105 Insertion of tracheostomy tube.

Circulation

Haemorrhage should be controlled by pressure to bleeding wounds or by applying an artery forcep or ligature to a severed artery as appropriate. Bleeding from a fractured maxilla will not be controlled unless it is manually repositioned, although this emergency is rare. If all local measures fail to control haemorrhage from the maxillofacial region then it may be necessary to consider ligation of the external carotid artery.

Intravenous fluids should be infused via a large peripheral vein such as in the antecubital fossa. When there is a need to maintain blood pressure, plasma expanders such as Gelofusine or Haemaccel are better than crystalloids such as sodium chloride as they remain in the vascular compartment for longer. Urinary catheterisation is required and adequate fluid replacement is monitored by documenting urine output, peripheral perfusion and temperature. The prognosis is better when the patient is warm with full veins and a good urine output.

Disability

A rapid initial assessment of conscious state can be made using the AVPU method: **A**lert, responds to **V**ocal stimuli, responds to **P**ainful stimuli or **U**nresponsive to all stimuli. Alternatively the Glasgow Coma Scale, which records the patient's motor, verbal and eye movements in response to stimulation, may be used.

Exposure and environmental control

All of the victim's clothing is removed to permit full assessment and exclude other injuries, taking into account the environmental conditions and respecting the patient's dignity.

Radiographic examination

Once immediate life-saving measures have been organised, essential radiography is undertaken. This is limited to cervical spine, chest and pelvis radiographs. The cervical spine is immobilised with a collar until any injury has been excluded.

Secondary survey

A secondary survey is carried out once the patient's general condition has been stabilised. This consists of a top-to-toe detailed patient examination of all body systems and a more thorough neurological examination, including testing of the cranial nerves. The particular role of the oral and maxillofacial surgeon in the secondary survey is to carry out a detailed examination of the head, neck and orofacial region. Appropriate radiographs or other investigations such as computed tomography can then be arranged and definitive care planned.

Documentation

It is vital that there is thorough recording of the history and examination in all cases of injury. The details may be required by the police service, lawyers or the Criminal Injuries Compensation Board at some stage.

Children

While most injuries are quite innocent, it is important to consider the possibility of non-accidental injury (NAI) when presented with an injured child. Signs suggestive of NAI are:

- injuries sustained are not consistent with history provided by parent
- delayed presentation
- apparent lack of concern or apparently over-anxious parent
- clinical or radiological evidence of multiple injuries especially if of different ages
- fraenal tears in child less than 1 year old
- withdrawn or frightened child.

The situation must be dealt with very delicately if there is the suspicion of NAI and it is better not to involve the parents in any discussion at this early stage. It may be useful to arrange admission of the child to hospital and discuss suspicions with a paediatrician. When presentation and management take place in an accident and emergency (A&E) department, the dentist may request a check of the local child protection register, best done via the nominated lead nurse or clinician for child protection procedures.

Adult domestic violence

The face is a common target in assault and consequently the dentist and dental care professional have a part to play in identifying domestic violence. Domestic violence is a term which refers to a wide range of physical, sexual, emotional and financial abuse of people who are, or have been, intimate partners – whether or not they are married or cohabiting. Although domestic violence can take place in any intimate relationship, including gay and lesbian partnerships, and whilst abuse of men by female partners does occur, the great majority and the most severe incidents of domestic violence, are perpetrated by men against women.

It is not the job of the dentist or dental care professional to give advice to someone experiencing domestic violence on what direct action they should take but rather to identify violence and provide information about where the individual can go for help.

8.2 Dental injuries

Dental injures are more common in children than adults. In children, they are frequently the result of falls and in adults they are commonly the consequence of sport without mouthguard protection. Increased overjet and incompetent lips are predisposing factors.

Definitions of a few basic terms are useful (Fig. 106).

Concussion. A traumatic event leads to damage to the periodontium without loosening or displacement of the tooth.

Subluxation. Damage to the periodontium leads to loosening of the tooth without overt displacement.

Luxation. This is the term given to dislocation of the tooth within its socket, leading to loosening and some degree of displacement. Luxation can be intrusive, extrusive or lateral in direction.

Avulsion. The tooth is completely displaced from its socket.

Management

Table 10 gives the management for injuries to primary and permanent teeth. Reassurance and analgesia are especially important for children. Patients will require regular review to assess development of late sequelae.

If there has been any loss of consciousness at the time of injury and a tooth or part of a tooth has been lost, then a chest radiograph should be arranged to confirm that this has not been inhaled.

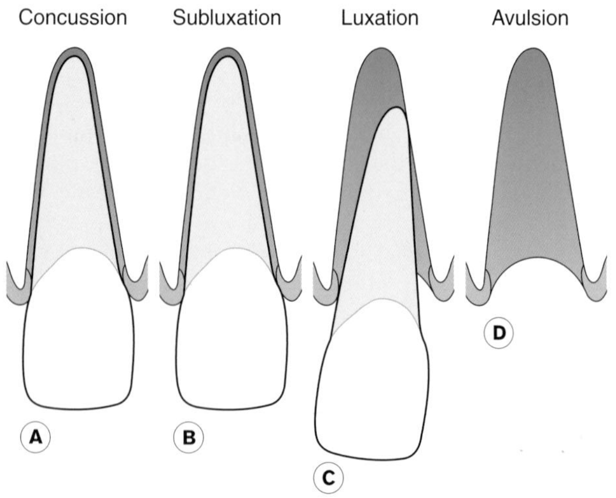

Splints can be directly constructed in the mouth of the patient or indirectly constructed on a model in a laboratory. Direct splints may be made from foil adapted over the teeth and cemented with zinc oxide eugenol or better with composite that is attached to the teeth over a wire using an acid-etch technique.

8.3 Facial soft-tissue injuries

Aetiology

Soft-tissue injury may result from interpersonal violence, road traffic accidents, falls, sport and industrial accident. Weapons may or may not be involved. Facial injury may also result from burns either as an isolated injury or in association with burns of the trunk or other part of the body.

Clinical presentation

Lacerations and wounds may involve anatomical structures such as the facial nerve, resulting in facial paralysis, the parotid salivary gland duct, resulting in a salivary fistula, or arteries, resulting in significant blood loss. They may be 'clean' or obviously contaminated. Burns are described according to their depth and extent. They may be superficial (first-degree burn), partial thickness (second-degree burn) or full thickness (third-degree burn). The 'rule of nines' may be used to describe the total body surface area affected by burn: 9% for each arm and the head, 18% for each leg, front and back of trunk and 1% for the external genitalia. The rule is modified for children who have a relatively larger head and face. The estimation is important for calculating fluid replacement.

Radiology

Radiographs of the soft tissues may be necessary to locate glass or other foreign body in a wound or to exclude an underlying bony injury. Soft-tissue radiographs are taken with reduced exposure to avoid 'burn-out' of low-density debris, and using intra-oral films wherever possible for greatest detail.

Surgical management of lacerations

Small, straightforward lacerations may be managed by accident and emergency physicians or senior nurses. Lacerations involving the vermilion border of the lip, intra-oral lacerations, other more serious lacerations and gunshot wounds will be referred on to an oral and maxillofacial surgeon. General dentists may undertake management of intra-oral lacerations in a primary care situation.

Concussion   Subluxation   Luxation   Avulsion

(A)   (B)   (C)   (D)

Fig. 106 Examples of some dental injuries.

Table 10 Management of tooth injuries

Injury	Management
Primary teeth	
Concussion	Soft diet
Crown fracture	Smooth or restore (when root canal treatment may be necessary) or extract depending on extent
Root fracture	Soft diet or extract if causing crown mobility
Luxation	Soft diet
Intrusion	Leave to erupt (when may require later pulp treatment) or extract if radiograph suggests underlying permanent follicle involved
Extrusion	Extract if more than 2 mm
Avulsion	Do not re-implant
Permanent teeth	
Concussion	Soft diet
Enamel fracture	Smooth or restore
Fracture involving dentine	Protect dentine and restore
Fracture involving pulp	Pulp cap (<1 mm exposure) or pulpotomy (>1 mm exposure) when the apex is open; pulp cap (if immediate presentation) or pulpectomy (if later presentation) when apex is closed
Root fracture	Splint (2 weeks minimum) if mobile
	Apical or middle third: root treat to fracture line
	Coronal third: extract coronal part of tooth and restore root after gingivectomy or orthodontic extrusion
	Vertical: extract
Luxation	Reposition tooth manually under local anaesthesia and splint (2 weeks) followed by root treatment as necessary
Intrusion	Leave to erupt when the apex is open or use orthodontic extrusion if apex closed, followed by root treatment as necessary
Extrusion	Reposition tooth manually under local anaesthesia and splint (2 weeks) followed by root treatment as necessary
Avulsion	Less than 1 hour since avulsion: irrigate with saline and re-implant (tooth should have been stored in saliva, milk or water preferably); compress alveolus to reduce any fracture of the socket; splint (for approximately 7 days) and prescribe antibiotics and chlorhexidine mouthwash; root treat as necessary
	Tooth avulsed for more than 30 minutes or apex closed; root treat with calcium hydroxide

Small lacerations can usually be sutured under local anaesthesia unless the patient is a young child, in which case general anaesthesia is indicated. Thorough cleaning is necessary before wound closure. Skin lacerations are closed with absorbable material such as polyglactin (Vicryl) placed deep if necessary and then the overlying skin closed with fine non-absorbable material such as 6/0 Prolene or Ethilon. Intra-oral wounds may be closed with Vicryl or silk. It is important when repairing a lip laceration which involves the vermilion border that it is accurately lined up to avoid an ugly step on healing.

Alternate skin sutures should ideally be removed at 4 days and the remaining sutures at 5 days to minimise scarring while maintaining wound support.

Antibiotics are prescribed to reduce the risk of wound infection: flucloxacillin for skin lacerations and amoxicillin for intra-oral wounds, unless contraindicated. Tetanus prophylaxis should be recommended if immunisation is not up to date.

Surgical management of burns

Initial management according to ATLS. There could be late threat to airway due to scar contracture. During the initial 48 hours the patient is hypovolaemic due to pericapillary tissue exhudation and tissue oedema. After 48 hours the patient becomes diuretic and fluid replacement demands reduce.

Analgesia is required and prevention of wound infection with antibiotics and dressings. The area of burn may require excision. Partial thickness burns may be best left exposed to the air when epithelialisation may start at 12 days. Reconstruction may be with skin grafts or microvascular free tissue transfer.

Evidence of carbon deposits in the mouth, pharynx or sputum are important signs of smoke inhalation that may lead to respiratory distress.

8.4 Facial fractures

Learning objectives

You should:
- know how to identify facial fractures clinically and radiologically
- know the principles of management of the different facial fractures
- know the techniques used to fix facial fractures.

Aetiology

Facial fractures may result from interpersonal violence, road traffic accidents, falls, sport and industrial accident or from pathology resulting in weakness of a bony region. There is a decline in the number of injuries following road traffic accidents, mainly because of the wearing of seat belts, although this has not been as great as hoped because drivers choose to drive at greater speeds because they feel safer. There is a rise in the number of facial fractures following assault. Facial injuries incurred through domestic violence are being increasingly recognised. The commonest fracture is that of the mandible.

Clinical presentation

Examination consists of the palpation of bony margins of the facial skeleton starting with the supra-orbital rims and progressing down to the lower border of the mandible, comparing right and left sides. The eyes are examined for double vision (diplopia), any restriction of movement and subconjunctival haemorrhage. The condyles of the mandible are palpated and movements of the mandible checked. Swelling, bruising and lacerations are noted together with any areas of altered sensation that may have resulted because of damage to branches of the trigeminal nerve. Any evidence of cerebrospinal fluid leaking from the nose or ears is noted, as this is an important feature of a fracture of the base of the skull. An intra-oral examination is then carried out, looking particularly for alterations to the occlusion (Fig. 107), a step in the occlusion (Fig. 108), fractured or displaced teeth, lacerations and bruises. The stability of the maxilla is checked by bimanual palpation,

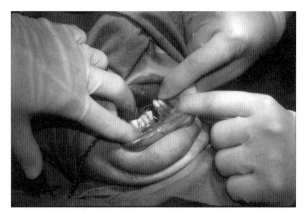

Fig. 108 A step in the occlusion observed in a fracture of the body of the mandible.

one hand attempting to mobilise the maxilla by grasping it from an intra-oral approach, and the other noting any movement at extra-oral sites such as nasal, zygomatic-frontal and infra-orbital. Features that suggest the fracture of a particular part of the facial skeleton are:

- mandible
  - pain and swelling
  - deranged occlusion
  - paraesthesia in distribution area of inferior alveolar nerve
  - floor-of-mouth haematoma
- zygoma
  - clinical flattening of the cheekbone prominence
  - paraesthesia in distribution area of infra-orbital nerve
  - diplopia, restricted eye movements, subconjunctival haemorrhage (Fig. 109)
  - limited lateral excursions of mandibular movements
  - palpable step in infra-orbital bony margin
- orbit: diplopia, restricted eye movements, subconjunctival haemorrhage
- maxilla
  - maxilla mobile
  - deranged occlusion
  - gross swelling if high-level fracture

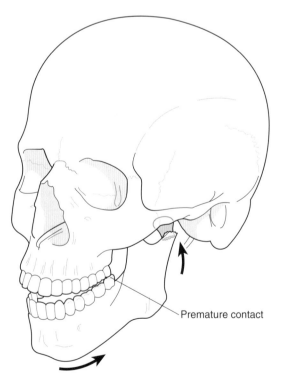

Fig. 107 Altered occlusion observed in a fracture of the condyle of the mandible.

Premature contact

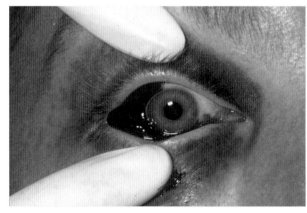

Fig. 109 Subconjunctival haemorrhage associated with a fracture of the zygomatic complex.

– bilateral circumorbital bruising
– subconjunctival haemorrhage
– cerebrospinal fluid leaking from nose (rhinorrhoea) or ear (otorrhoea)
• nasal/nasoethmoidal
– swelling
– bilateral circumorbital bruising
– clinical deviation or depression of nasal bridge
– nose bleed (epistaxis).

Radiological examination

At least two views are usually needed to demonstrate a fracture adequately.

Teeth. Periapical view is supplemented by another intra-oral view from an oblique angle, e.g. oblique occlusal or bisecting-angle periapical.

Dento-alveolar fracture. Periapical(s) and oblique occlusal views.

Mandible. Panoramic film and postero-anterior (PA) of mandible are the basic views. A reverse Towne's (modified PA) is useful for suspected condylar fractures. True occlusal views of a fracture in the body or symphysis are helpful.

Zygoma (or malar) fractures. Occipitomental (OM) and OM30° views are required.

Maxillary fractures. OM, OM30° views of true lateral facial bones and computed tomographic scans are helpful for complicated fractures.

Nasal fractures. True lateral nasal bones, sometimes with the addition of superoinferior nasal bones: both are taken using occlusal films.

Nasoethmoidal fractures. Views are as for maxillary fractures.

Principles of facial fracture management

Good bony healing of fractures requires close apposition of the fragments and immobility for a period of about 6 weeks. This period may be shorter in children and longer in elderly patients. Mobility of the fracture site will lead to fibrous union. The principles of fracture management are, therefore, those of reduction and fixation.

There are many different techniques for fixation of facial fractures and these may be described as rigid, semi-rigid or non-rigid. The fracture site may be surgically opened and fixation such as plates applied directly, or left closed and indirect fixation applied. There has been a move in the developed world towards greater use of direct fixation of fractures rather than the indirect, but the latter does still have particular indications.

Dento-alveolar fractures

Fractures of the tooth-bearing part of the mandible or maxilla are reduced and then immobilised by one of many methods. All techniques involve fixing the teeth involved in the fracture to adjacent teeth, and this may be achieved by means of wiring, arch bars, acid-etch-retained composite splinting, orthodontic banding or cement-retained acrylic splints. Splinting is required for a minimum of 4 weeks.

Mandibular fractures

Fractures are classified according to their site: dentoalveolar, symphyseal, parasymphyseal, body, angle, ramus, coronoid and condyle (Fig. 110). They may be compound, involving the mouth (including via the periodontal membrane of teeth) or skin, or may be simple or comminuted. It is more unusual to describe fractures as favourable or unfavourable according to whether they resist the pull of attached muscles. The standard treatment is open reduction and internal fixation (ORIF) with mini-plates. This approach has revolutionised the management of mandibular fractures and also other facial fractures. A fracture of the mandible in a dentate patient may typically be reduced and fixed with intermaxillary fixation (IMF) achieved by placement of arch bars (see below). The fracture site is then surgically opened and fixed with a mini-plate, the wound closed and the intraoperative IMF released. The occlusion is, therefore, utilised for accurate reduction of the fracture but the postoperative disadvantages of IMF avoided.

If there is a partly erupted or erupted tooth in the line of a fracture, one should consider whether it ought to be removed to avoid predisposing to later infection of the fracture site or whether it could remain. Most surgeons would leave the tooth in situ unless it is fractured, grossly carious or has periapical pathology.

Fractures of the condyle not interfering with the occlusion are frequently managed conservatively, that is with soft diet and regular review. A 2-week period of IMF rather than ORIF is a common treatment choice if the occlusion is deranged.

Zygoma (or malar) fractures

Zygoma fractures are most commonly reduced by elevation via a Gillies' temporal approach. A Rowe's elevator is placed beneath the deep temporal fascia, slid under the zygoma and lifted without levering on the temporal bone (Fig. 111). Alternative methods include an intra-oral approach and direct lifting of the zygoma with a hook placed through the skin of the cheek. The zygoma may or may not need fixation depending on its stability. When needed, titanium mini-plates may be placed at the zygomatic-frontal, infra-orbital and buttress regions as necessary (Fig. 112).

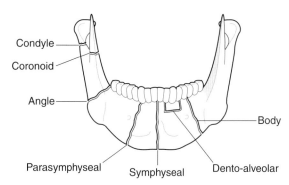

Fig. 110 Common sites of fracture in the mandible.

Condyle
Coronoid
Angle
Body
Parasymphyseal
Symphyseal
Dento-alveolar

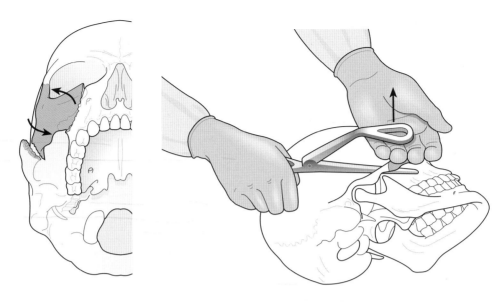

Fig. 111 Gillies' temporal approach for the elevation of a depressed fracture's zygomatic complex.

Orbital fractures

Fractures of the zygomatic complex will necessarily involve the orbit, but it is also possible to sustain an isolated fracture of the orbit. This may tether the inferior rectus muscle, causing diplopia, or be large enough to permit herniation of orbital fat and muscle into the maxillary antrum. Such a 'blow-out' may be repaired with 'silastic' or titanium mesh materials or bone taken from another site, for example iliac crest of the hip or the cranium.

Maxillary fractures

Fractures of the maxilla are classified as Le Fort I, II or III (Fig. 113). Le Fort I is the lowest level of fracture, in which the tooth-bearing part of the maxilla is detached. Le Fort II or a pyramidal fracture of the maxilla involves the nasal bones and infra-orbital rims, while Le Fort III involves the nasal bones and zygomatic-frontal sutures and the whole of the maxilla is detached from the base of the skull. After reduction of the fracture, fixation may be achieved by a variety of means, including directly applied plates and indirect fixation such as an external frame made of stainless steel pins, rods and universal joints fixing the maxilla to the cranium. Intermaxillary fixation may also be required.

Nasal/nasoethmoidal fractures

Nasal bone fractures may be manipulated with the fingers or surgical instruments and then splinted with plaster of Paris or a specifically designed thermoplastic material. Nasoethmoidal fractures usually require open reduction and fixation with plates. The medial canthus may need fixing so that the distance between the eyes is corrected.

Techniques for facial fracture management

Closed reduction and indirect fixation in the mandible

Acrylic splints. Hard acrylic splints applied with dental cement are useful for dento-alveolar fractures. Similar splints constructed from metal (cast silver) were popular in the past for the definitive management of mandibular fractures.

Intermaxillary fixation. Fixation of the mandible and maxilla together (mandibular-maxillary fixation) is commonly referred to as IMF. The teeth are used to check the correct reduction of the fracture and then used for fixation. The occlusion will, therefore, be accurately re-established and the technique is straightforward, although it would be described as producing non-rigid fixation. Intermaxillary fixation may be achieved through a variety of means:

- *Direct interdental wiring:* simple rapid immobilisation of jaws is achieved with stainless steel wire placed about the neck of tooth and the two ends twisted together to produce a tail, which in turn can be twisted with another tail of the opposing arch to effect IMF. Rarely used today.
- *Eyelet wiring:* pre-prepared wires with loops, to facilitate placement of separate IMF tie wires, are applied to pairs of teeth.
- *Arch bars:* these may be commercially produced bars that are cut to length and bent to shape or custom-made arch bars can be prepared for the individual patient from dental impressions. The bars have cleats that facilitate IMF tie wires. They also allow the ready placement of elastic traction should that be required, which is not

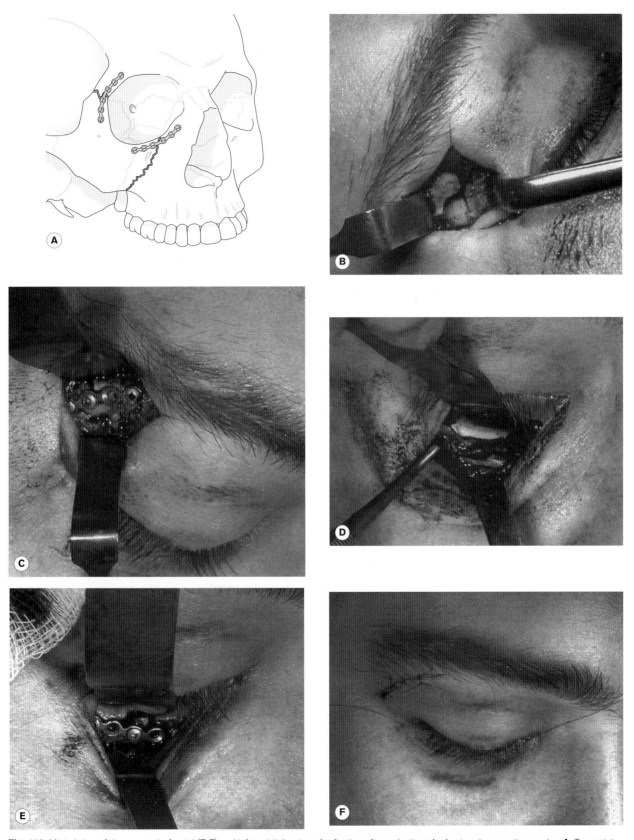

Fig. 112 Mini-plating of the zygomatic-frontal (Z-F) and infra-orbital regions for fixation after reduction of a fractured zygomatic complex. **A.** Two-point fixation of fractured zygomatic complex. **B.** Fracture of Z-F. **C.** Reduced and plated Z-F. **D.** Fracture of infra-orbital rim. **E.** Reduced and plated infra-orbital rim. **F.** Wound closure.

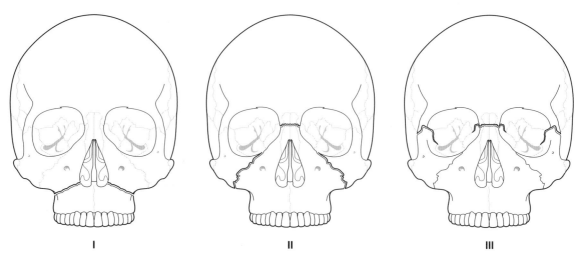

| I | II | III |

Fig. 113 Le Fort classification of fractures to the maxilla.

possible with direct interdental wiring or eyelets. The bars are fixed to the teeth by interdental wiring.

- *Bonded brackets:* brackets bonded to teeth result in less soft-tissue trauma; such trauma can potentially be a postoperative problem with dental wires and arch bars.

Disadvantages of IMF fixation:

- The airway is partially compromised and is at increased risk in the event of postoperative swelling, regurgitation or vomiting. Opioid analgesia and other central nervous system depressants should be avoided to minimise respiratory depression and nausea.
- There is reduced tidal volume.
- Patients are unable to take solid diet. Patients should receive 3 litres of fluid and 2500 calories each day, and some encouragement will be required initially to achieve this when a patient is in IMF.
- It is difficult to maintain good oral hygiene. Toothbrushing of lingual aspects of teeth is not possible; therefore, the patient must compensate with copious mouthrinsing and the use of a chlorhexidine rinse.
- There is poor patient tolerance of IMF fixation.
- Post-treatment stiffness of the temporomandibular joint can occur and there is a risk of ankylosis.
- Inhalers for asthma therapy are difficult to use.

Peralveolar and circumandibular wiring. Stainless steel wire is passed through the alveolar bone of the maxilla or around the body or anterior mandible by means of an awl. The wire may be used for fixation of a fracture or to hold a Gunning-type splint in place.

Gunning-type splints. These splints are used for immobilisation of fractures of the edentulous mandible. They may be constructed by modifying the patient's dentures. Accurate positioning of the bone fragments is difficult; consequently, this technique is now less frequently used. Figure 114 indicates how difficult it could be to reposition fragments.

Closed reduction and indirect fixation in the maxilla

Suspension wires. Stainless steel wire is placed through prepared holes in the frontal bone just above the frontozygomatic suture or the pyriform fossa. These can then be attached to the mandible or maxilla, usually via an arch bar. Wire may be suspended from the zygomatic arch by passing the wire around it, and no holes need be drilled. An awl is used to direct the wire. This method is not popular now because it can inadvertently shorten the facial height.

Extra-oral craniomandibular fixation. Halo and box frames are used for fractures of maxilla and are fixed between the cranium and the mandible. The frames are cumbersome and unsightly and are rarely used now.

Pin fixation. Introduced during World War II, metal pins are placed through the skin into the bone beneath. The fracture is reduced and then the pins are rigidly united by rods and universal joints or fast-setting acrylic.

Open reduction and direct fixation in the mandible and maxilla

The direct visualisation of a fracture site after surgical exposure so that it may be reduced and immobilised with fixation such as plates has superseded the more traditional

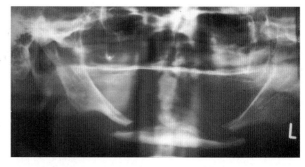

Fig. 114 Radiograph showing bilateral severely displaced fractures of an edentulous mandible.

methods of management. It provides a more accurate anatomical repositioning of the fractured bone. However, it is more costly and not, therefore, available in many parts of the world. Also, this technique may be contraindicated where there is significant comminution or infection and in children where unerupted teeth are present in the jaws.

Plating with mini- and micro-plating systems. These plate systems are sometimes referred to as rigid osteosynthesis, although they technically produce only semi-rigid fixation. The slight micro-movement permitted has been associated with preferential healing, a view disputed by the advocates of totally rigid compression plates. Titanium plates are now used rather than stainless steel. The plate is bent to conform accurately to the bone surface across the fracture site (Fig. 115). A water-cooled drill is used for placement of screws, which are left in place indefinitely unless they cause a problem such as ulceration of overlying thin soft tissue, in which case they are removed. This is a technique that is commonly used in the developed world.

Titanium mesh. This has greater coverage and may be applied to the bone surface and secured with screws.

Biodegradable plates and screws. Plates and screws that resorb following bony healing have recently become available for use.

Transosseous and intra-osseous wiring. Direct wiring is placed through drilled holes either side of fracture site. Intra-osseous wire such as Kirschner wire is placed with a power drill within bone.

Bone screws. Screws can be placed through both outer cortex and inner cortex of bone. Lag screws are specially designed to compress the fracture segments together.

8.5 Gunshot wounds

Learning objective

You should:
- understand the particular management of injury resulting from gunshot.

Weapons

Shotguns. Usually do not inflict deeply penetrating injuries but may discharge multiple pellets and if at close range may be deep.

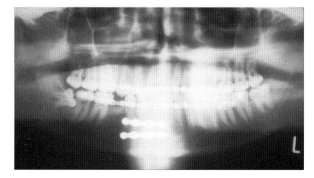

Fig. 115 Mini-plating of a fractured mandible.

Military semi-automatic. Designed for maximum effect with small entry point but extensive tissue damage in the track of the projectile.

Other. Specialised projectiles such as soft-tipped or explosive-tipped bullets.

Management

Initial. The usual ATLS management. Screening for other injuries is particularly important.

Imaging. Radiography and CT scanning to identify and locate position of projectiles or fragments in addition to assessing tissue damage.

Soft tissues. Superficial removal of pellets and thorough irrigation for low-velocity injuries. Wounds inflicted by high-velocity projectiles should be opened widely for removal of bullets and debridement.

Hard tissues. Fractures are likely to be comminuted and infected.

8.6 Complications of facial injury

Learning objective

You should:
- understand the complications that can arise from injuries to teeth, and the face.

Complications of dental injury

Primary teeth

- Grey discoloration of teeth after trauma suggests pulp death, while yellowing may suggest calcification. At the earliest sign of pulpal death, the tooth should undergo root treatment or extraction.
- Ankylosis is the fusion of the cementum to the surrounding alveolar bone. While its exact pathogenesis is unknown, it occurs whenever periodontal tissue is lost and cementum/dentine come into direct contact with the alveolar bone. It is, therefore, sometimes the consequence of trauma, which may cause inflammation or destruction of the periodontal membrane.
- An underlying developing permanent tooth may be damaged when primary teeth are involved in trauma.

Permanent teeth

- Re-implanted teeth have a high incidence of developing external (surface) resorption. The incidence is related to the length of time between avulsion and re-implantation. Internal (inflammatory) resorption may also occur, although early removal of the pulp after injury can prevent its development.
- Re-implanted teeth are also subject to ankylosis if not lost by external resorption.

Complications of facial soft-tissue injury

- Scarring is inevitable but should be minimised by good surgical technique, including thorough removal of any foreign body such as dirt, good wound apposition and eversion of wound margins.

- Scars may be thickened and result in functional deformity as well as an unacceptable cosmetic appearance. Hypertrophic scars (elevated above skin surface) occur more commonly than keloids (extend beyond original wound margins).

Complications of facial fractures

- If serious nerve damage was caused by the initial injury, then long-term paraesthesia in the relevant region may result.
- Infection at the fracture site may delay healing or result in non-union. Inadequate reduction or fixation may also result in non-union or malunion.

- Retrobulbar haemorrhage is a rare complication that may occur after fracture of a zygomatic complex or its surgical management. It may lead to blindness if the haemorrhage in the muscle cone of the orbit is not surgically decompressed urgently.
- Loss of smell (anosmia) may follow olfactory nerve damage in high-level maxillary fractures.
- Orbit fractures may result in diplopia or backward displacement of the globe (enophthalmus) if there has been significant loss of the orbital fat and muscle into the antrum.

Self-assessment: questions

Multiple choice questions

1. Fractures involving the orbit:
   a. May increase the volume of the orbit
   b. Are described either as 'blow-out' or as 'blow-in' fractures
   c. May be complicated by blindness
   d. Always require surgical repair
   e. May cause subconjunctival haemorrhage

2. Fractures of the maxilla:
   a. Are less frequent if seat belts are worn
   b. May cause limited opening of the mandible
   c. May be suspected if there is intra-oral bruising
   d. May result in severe haemorrhage
   e. Can result from less force than required to fracture the mandible

Extended matching items

EMI 1. Theme: Facial fractures

Options:

A Fracture of the alveolus of the mandible
B Fracture of body of mandible
C Fracture of right and left mandibular condyle
D Fracture of mandibular symphysis
E Comminuted fracture of the mandible
F Pathological fracture of the mandible
G Fracture of the zygomatic complex
H Le Fort I fracture of the maxilla
I Fracture of the orbital floor
J Nasoethmoidal fracture

Lead in: Select the most likely type of facial fracture from the list above for each of the following cases. Each option can be used once, more than once or not at all.

1. A 19-year-old male is unable to close his front teeth together and has a laceration to his chin.
2. On examination of a patient involved in a road traffic accident the upper dentition together with alveolus and palate are found to be mobile relative to the upper maxilla.
3. A 22-year-old patient presents with a left enophthalmus 6 months after an alleged assault in which he sustained facial injuries.
4. A patient requires intermaxillary fixation rather than open reduction and direct fixation with titanium mini-plates.
5. A 55-year-old man suffers a sharp pain in his jaw when eating breakfast and then notices that his teeth don't meet properly.

EMI 2. Theme: Facial injury

Options:

A Interdental wires
B Peralveolar wires
C Suspension wires
D Intra-osseous wires
E Acrylic dental splint
F Circumferential wires
G Extra-oral craniomandibular fixation
H Intermaxillary fixation
I Arch bars
J Titanium plates

Lead in: Select the most likely technique to be of use from the list above for each of the following cases. Each option can be used once, more than once or not at all.

1. An 8-year-old boy is involved in a cycle accident and suffers a fracture of his premaxilla which is quite mobile. Figure 116 shows the radiograph.
2. The anterior mandibular teeth of a 35-year-old male are found to be mobile following an alleged assault. Radiographs show that he has a dentoalveolar fracture.
3. A 28-year-old male has a Le Fort level I fracture of his maxilla and a comminuted fracture of his right zygomatic complex.
4. A 45-year-old female who is fit and well suffers bilateral mandibular body fractures in a domestic violence incident.
5. An elderly edentulous female with osteoporosis falls and fractures her mandible. Her general health contraindicates general anaesthesia.

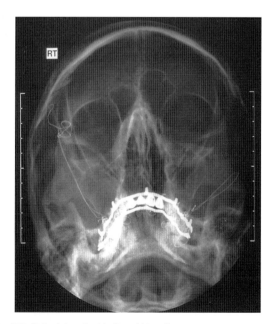

Fig. 116 Patient described in Case history 3.

Case history questions

Case history 1

A 4-year-old child has fallen against a climbing frame while running in a park. She has lacerated her upper lip and loosened two upper front teeth.

1. List the key points of the history and examination.
2. Describe the principles of management.

Case history 2

A 21-year-old man arrives in the accident and emergency department with facial injuries following an alleged assault with a baseball bat.

1. List the patient management priorities.
2. Describe specifically the method for oral and maxillofacial assessment including special investigations.

Case history 3

The patient shown in Figure 117 was brought to the accident and emergency department following an alleged assault in which he sustained facial injuries.

What anatomical structures may be particularly relevant to this injury and require evaluation?

Case history 4

The patient in Figure 118 has undergone treatment for a fracture to his mandible.

Describe the advantages and disadvantages of this method of management and also of the more usual alternative treatment.

Viva questions

1. What surgical techniques are available for the management of fractures to the mandible?
2. What are some of the complications that may arise during mandibular fracture management?
3. How may dento-alveolar fractures be managed?
4. Describe the management of a laceration to the tongue.
5. Why is placement of a nasogastric tube sometimes contraindicated in a patient with a midface fracture?

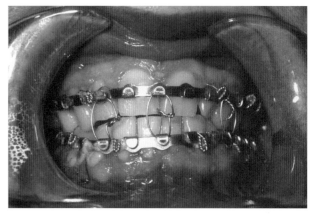

Fig. 118 Postoperative radiograph of the case described in EMQ 2 part 3.

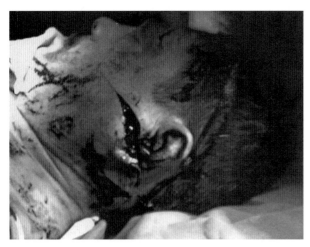

Fig. 117 Patient described in Case history 4.

Self-assessment: answers

Multiple choice answers

1. a. **True.** The normal volume of an orbit is about 30 ml. Fractures may increase or decrease this volume. A computed tomographic scan may report a significantly increased orbital volume on the suspected fracture side relative to the uninjured side. This is clinically significant because there is more room for the globe in the orbit and its position may change.
    b. **False.** While some orbital fractures may be described as 'blow-out' or 'blow-in', there are many more common fractures that are not described in these terms. For example, fractures of the zygomatic complex will involve the orbit as this bone contributes to the anatomy of the orbit (unless there is an isolated fracture of the zygomatic arch).
    c. **True.** A haemorrhage within the muscle cone of the globe from rupture of one or more of the posterior short ciliary arteries may result in a retrobulbar haemorrhage. This may follow injury or more often after surgical reduction of a fracture, although in less than 1% of cases. Urgent surgical decompression is required. High-dose steroids and diuretics are used while theatre is arranged.
    d. **False.** Not all orbital fractures require repair although this is controversial. If the fracture results in a small defect and no clinical eye signs, then it may not be necessary; however, a larger defect will need to be repaired, even if there are no signs, as a late sinking back of the globe (enophthalmos) may develop.
    e. **True.** Fractures of the orbit usually, but not always, result in a subconjunctival haemorrhage. There may also be an associated circumorbital ecchymosis, the classic black eye.

2. a. **True.** The wearing of seat belts significantly reduces the incidence of facial injury. However, drivers may feel a sense of greater security when wearing a belt and drive at greater speeds, thus resulting in more serious injuries when accidents do occur.
    b. **True.** Displaced fractures of the maxilla can result in lengthening of the midface so that the patient believes that they have restricted mouth opening when in fact the mandible has been forced open by the maxilla and, therefore, cannot open any more. On examination 'gagging' of the posterior teeth will be observed.
    c. **True.** Haematoma present in the upper buccal sulcus is a sign of maxillary fracture.
    d. **True.** Rupture of the maxillary artery in facial trauma is rare, but when it does occur, it results in severe haemorrhage into the nasopharynx. Urgent placement of anterior and posterior nasal packs is one method used to control this haemorrhage.
    e. **True.** The maxilla is very fragile in an antero-posterior direction but has strong struts transmitting the forces of mastication up to the base of the skull. The force from an injury that is directed in a horizontal direction can cause serious damage to the maxilla. The direction of the force is, therefore, important, and a lesser force than that necessary to fracture the mandible may result in fracture of the maxilla.

Extended matching items answers

EMI 1

1. **C.** A fall onto the chin resulting in bilateral fractured mandibular condyles has been described as a 'guardman's' fracture because these military personal may faint and fall forward, suffering such an injury after standing still for lengthy periods of time.
2. **H.** If there is movement between the upper and lower parts of the maxilla, the fracture is likely to be at the Le Fort I level.
3. **I.** Fracture of the orbital floor may permit herniation of the orbital soft tissue into the maxillary sinus. The consequent reduction in orbital volume leads to the globe (eyeball) moving backwards into the socket (enopthalmus) giving an unattractive sunken appearance to the eye.
4. **E.** If a fracture is severely comminuted, then it may be unwise to raise the periostium from the bony fragments to facilitate plating as this will reduce their blood supply. It may also be difficult to plate very small fragments of bone. In this situation consideration should be given to intermaxillary fixation.
5. **F.** Pathological fracture of the mandible can arise when the jaw bone is severely weakened by a pathological process or lesion (such as a dentigerous cyst).

EMI 2

1. **E.** As the fracture is mobile, the displacement must be reduced and fixation will be required. A full coverage acrylic dental splint made to a dental impression and model is likely to be all that is required for fixation in a young child where healing is good.
2. **E.** A full coverage acrylic splint is useful to stabilise dentoalveolar fractures. Alternatively the teeth either side of the fracture segments could be wired together (interdental wires) but this doesn't usually offer the same three-dimensional stability and may cause extrusion of teeth from their sockets.
3. **C.** Suspension wires can be used to maintain the vertical position of the fracture segments and are wired into an archbar. In this case a transzygomatic wire was used on the left side and a frontal wire on the right (Fig. 116 shows the postoperative radiograph). This method has been superseded by contemporary plating techniques when possible to provide improved three-dimensional stability of bone fragments.

4. **I.** Semi-rigid osteosyntheis with titanium plates and screws is the contemporary technique of choice if there are no contraindications for fixation of facial fractures.
5. **F.** If the fracture is displaced then it will require reduction and fixation but if it really is not possible to arrange for general anesthesia, then it may be possible to attempt placement of a Gunning type splint secured with circumferential wires about the mandible.

Case history answers

Case history 1

1. A complete history is required but it is also important to find out the time of the accident; any loss of consciousness or headache, nausea or vomiting since the accident; last food and drink, in case a general anaesthetic is required; and tetanus status as the injury occurred outside. The usual oral and facial examination is required plus any evidence of an injury other than facial (facial bony margins, eyes, bruising, etc.), depth of lip laceration and involvement of vermilion border, any missing teeth or tooth fragments, degree of mobility of involved teeth and any interference with occlusion.
2. The first stage in management will be reassurance of the child and parents. Wound cleaning and closure is likely to need general anaesthesia given the age of the patient, who should, therefore, be admitted to hospital. Attempt to use resorbable sutures to avoid difficulty of removal. If the primary teeth are sufficiently mobile to be a threat to the airway when the child is sleeping, or if they are interfering with the occlusion, then they should be extracted at the same time as the laceration is sutured. Otherwise, no treatment is indicated other than recommending a soft diet and prescribing analgesia.

Case history 2

1. Patient management priorities are according to the Advanced Trauma Life Support (ATLS) protocol. The patient is simultaneously resuscitated and examined during the primary survey (airway, breathing, circulation, disability and exposure). Essential radiographs (cervical spine, chest and pelvis) are then taken. Once the patient is stable, a thorough examination and assessment of the patient is undertaken, which is described as the secondary survey.
2. The oral and maxillofacial assessment will consist of a thorough examination of the head and neck and, in particular, the orofacial region. This will include bony margins, condylar movement, eyes, ears, any leakage of cerebrospinal fluid, lacerations, bruising, altered sensation and intra-oral examination. Facial radiographs will be requested and possibly a computed tomographic scan, depending on the clinical findings.

Case history 3

Cheek lacerations may involve several vital structures including the superficial temporal and facial arteries,

parotid salivary gland and duct and the facial nerve. As the external ear is also involved in this injury, the pinna, external auditory canal and tympanic membrane need to be examined. The hearing should also be evaluated.

Case history 4

The patient in Figure 118 has been treated with intermaxillary fixation (IMF). The more usual alternative is open reduction and internal fixation (ORIF).

Advantages of indirect fixation with IMF. It is an uncomplicated technique requiring minimal and cheap equipment and can be used in severely comminuted infected fractures.

Disadvantages of indirect fixation with IMF. There is no direct visualisation of the fracture site and fragments may not, therefore, be as closely apposed. Some movement may occur about the fracture site and this can increase the incidence of fibrous tissue and non-union. Other important factors are: longer hospitalisation is required until the patient can take on adequate oral intake, compromised oral hygiene, normal speech compromised, potential airway compromise, poor patient acceptance and delayed return to work.

Advantages of ORIF. These are essentially the opposite to the disadvantages of IMF.

Disadvantages of ORIF. Specialised, expensive equipment is necessary and it is possible to damage tooth roots or nerves. ORIF cannot be used in a severely comminuted or infected fracture.

Viva answers

1. The principles are of reduction and fixation. Reduction may be closed and indirect or open for direct fixation, usually with mini-plates.
2. The most common complications that arise during mandibular fracture management are infection, delayed union or non-union (usually as a consequence of infection or inadequate fixation), malocclusion, alveolar nerve damage, wound dehiscence and damage to teeth.
3. Fractures of the alveolar bone are managed according to the principles of reduction and fixation. Finger pressure is used to reduce the fractured fragments and fixation is by suturing of the associated soft tissues as necessary and splinting of the teeth.
4. The tongue has a rich blood supply and heals well. Very small lacerations do not need any treatment and heal quickly. Antibiotics should be prescribed. Closure of other lacerations is undertaken under local anaesthesia or general anaesthesia in a small child. This is done in layers using resorbable material. One should consider the airway, which may become compromised by haematoma or oedema, if the wound is large. Radiographic examination may be necessary to identify foreign bodies such as tooth fragments.
5. Fractures of the midface may extend through the nasal cavity and result in tearing of the soft tissue in the nasopharynx. Attempting to place a nasogastric feeding tube may further tear these soft tissues or a tube could potentially enter the cranium if there is a skull fracture.

Dentofacial and craniofacial anomalies

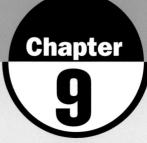

Overview

Abnormalities of the jaws, face and cranium may be the consequence of faulty development or acquired as a consequence of trauma, tumour, fibrous dysplasia or surgery for neoplastic disease. Dentofacial clefting is the most common of the congenital anomalies but hundreds of others are recognised. Dentofacial and craniofacial anomalies frequently require combined orthodontic and surgical management for their correction.

9.1 Congenital anomalies

Learning objectives

You should:
- be aware of the aetiology of congenital abnormalities
- be able to conduct a clinical examination and choose suitable further investigations
- be able to make a diagnosis and prepare a treatment plan.

Aetiology

The embryology of the face has been studied in detail and has provided insight into the cause of dentofacial anomalies. Advances in medical and dental genetics are now providing further insight. Various growth factors induce formation of 'growth centres', and malformation may occur because these centres are defective or there is a lack of coordination between them.

Cleft lip is more common in Mongoloid races and rare in Negroids. A family history exists in 12–20% of complete cleft cases. The gene responsible for the expression of transforming growth factor beta 3 has been implicated in human cleft palate. A genetic predisposition to anomalies such as clefting may reach a threshold after which environmental factors come into play. There is, for example, an association between the anticonvulsant phenytoin and

cleft disease. Excess vitamin A is similarly associated, whilst folic acid is important in the prevention of cleft disease. Infections in the mother such as rubella have also been implicated in cleft formation in the infant.

Cleft lip and palate disease ranges from a submucous cleft or bifid uvula to complete bilateral cleft lip and palate. The incidence is given in Box 10.

The craniosynostoses result from premature fusion of the craniofacial sutures and may arise sporadically when a single suture is involved or are inherited in the more complex syndromes. The diagnosis may be made according to the clinical presentation alone or involve molecular biological techniques to provide a genetic diagnosis now that access to such testing is more widely available.

Clinical management

Clinical management consists of the following phases:

1. history
2. clinical examination
3. investigations
4. diagnosis
5. treatment plan.

History

It is important to establish what is of concern to the patient. There may be difficulty in eating or problems with speech or the appearance of the teeth or face. Patients may be reluctant to discuss dissatisfaction with their appearance and feel that it is more acceptable to present a functional problem to the clinician. They should, therefore, be reassured of the legitimacy of describing their aesthetic problem and the effect it has on them. Family members may underestimate the significance of abnormality to the patient and inhibit the patient in this discussion.

Children with abnormal appearance of teeth or face may suffer nicknames and teasing from other children, and this can affect their psychological development. The

Box 10 Incidence of dentofacial clefting	
Submucous cleft	1:1200
Bifid uvula	1:100
Isolated cleft lip	1:1000 (either unilateral or bilateral)
Isolated cleft palate	1:2200
Complete cleft	1:1800

development of emotional attachment between child and parents can also be adversely affected. In adulthood, many subtle influences come into play. Attractiveness has been shown to be related to social advantage, so that more attractive individuals are, for example, more likely to find a partner and more likely to be successful in the work environment. The general public have difficulty in accepting facial disfigurement and prefer to look away or ignore the individual concerned. Correction of abnormality can be very beneficial to the patient and this benefit can be displayed in many ways, such as improved peer relationships and social confidence.

Occasionally, a patient may present requesting surgery for improvement of a small or non-existent physical defect. The clinician should arrange referral to a liaison psychiatrist in this situation in case the patient is suffering from body dysmorphic disorder (BDD). Similarly, clinical neurosis and frank psychosis should be excluded before surgery. Patients with these conditions will not be satisfied with the outcome and may have very severe postoperative problems.

The patient will need to be motivated if they are going to pursue lengthy orthodontic treatment and major surgery. They also need to be well informed so that they may provide valid consent.

The family history and even obstetric history may be relevant particularly when syndromic features are present.

Clinical examination

The clinical examination should include observation of the following:

- skull shape and size
- orbits and eyes
- ears
- facial height
- asymmetry
- lip and tongue morphology and function
- lateral relationship of mandible and maxilla to skull
- nose and chin.
  The intra-oral examination will look at:
- teeth present and missing
- centre line
- occlusion, including the use of wooden spatula between upper and lower teeth to check the level of the occlusal plane
- crowding/spacing
- overbite and overjet
- tongue size
- any cleft and site.

Figure 119 shows the occlusion of a patient with severe asymmetry owing to overgrowth of her left mandible.

Investigations

Investigations include:

- imaging
- dental study models
- intra-oral and facial photography
- cephalometric analysis.

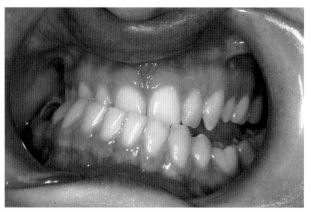

Fig. 119 Deranged occlusion in a patient with severe asymmetry caused by overgrowth of the left mandible.

Imaging

Appropriate imaging is selected on an individual basis, including:

- lateral and postero-anterior cephalometric radiographs
- computed tomographic scanning, with consideration given to using three-dimensional reconstruction of images
- other imaging: requirements will be tailored to individual needs.

Cephalometric analysis

Lateral skull tracing for cephalometric measurements may be carried out manually with tracing paper and pencil or digitised tracing may be performed for computer-assisted analysis and operation planning. Radiographic landmarks are shown in Figure 120 and also the lines that are then drawn between some of these landmarks. The angles between these can then be compared with standard values to indicate facial skeletal variations from normal. Digital photographic images may also be superimposed on the radiographic images and surgical predications carried out with the computer software.

Typical Caucasian measurements are:

SNA $\quad 81 \pm 3°$
SNB $\quad 78 \pm 3°$
ANB $\quad\;\; 3 \pm 2°$

An ANB difference in a Negroid patient of 5° is acceptable whereas in Oriental patients 3° or less is normal.

Diagnosis

For dentofacial anomalies, the diagnosis will describe the maxillary and mandibular base relationship relative to the skull together with a description of the dental occlusion and comments about general condition of the dentition and oral hygiene. The mandible and maxilla may be described as prognathic, hypoplastic or asymmetrical. The effect of these may be to produce a long face, open bite or short face. The chin may also be described using various classifications of excess (macrogenia), hypoplasia (microgenia) and asymmetry. For craniofacial anomalies,

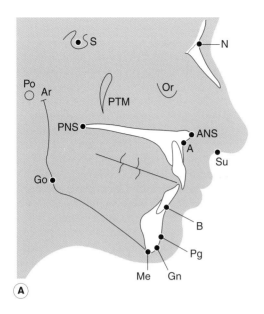

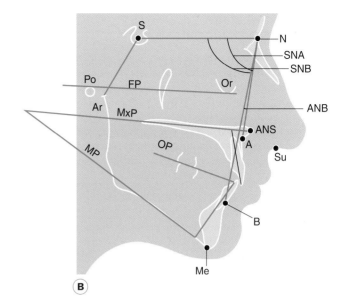

S	Sella	A	Point A
N	Nasion	B	Point B
Po	Porion	Gn	Gnathion
Ar	Articulare	Go	Gonion
PTM	Pterygomaxillary fissure	Me	Menton
Or	Orbitale	Pg	Pogonion
PNS	Posterior nasal spine	Su	Subnasale
ANS	Anterior nasal spine		

Fig. 120 Cephalometric landmarks and lines for Caucasians.

the diagnosis will also describe the orbits, eyes, ears and other features and may suggest various syndromes in a differential diagnosis.

Clinical box Typical diagnosis for a dentofacial anomaly

Class III skeletal relationship owing to both prognathic mandible and hypoplastic maxilla. Lower facial height increased. Competent lips and large tongue. Prominent nose and normal ears.

Class III occlusal relationship with spaced lower incisors. Narrow maxillary intercanine width.

All first molar teeth restored. No other restorations.

Oral hygiene poor.

Treatment planning

Treatment planning usually consists of:

1. Preoperative orthodontic management to move teeth into a position for the best possible occlusion at operation. This may involve relief of crowding, flattening of the occlusal plane or other treatment.
2. Surgery. Osteodistraction rather than traditional surgical techniques may have an increasingly prominent role in the future for

some types of dentofacial and craniofacial anomaly.
3. Postoperative orthodontic management.

9.2 Orthognathic surgery

Learning objectives

You should:
- be able to describe a preoperative care plan and preparatory treatment
- know the surgical options available
- understand the essentials of postoperative care and after care.

Orthognathic surgery involves the correction of occlusal and facial disharmony. Such surgery may play a part in gender reassignment treatment to produce a more feminine or masculine face. Surgery carried out to change racial characteristics or the facial characteristics in conditions such as Down syndrome is controversial. The majority of patients who undergo orthognathic surgery are referred by their general dental practitioner either directly or via an orthodontist because they have a malocclusion that is beyond the scope of orthodontic management alone. Advances in orthodontic treatment and surgical management has led to predictable outcomes from orthognathic surgery.

Preoperative stage
Preoperative planning
1. A surgical plan is made to correct the abnormality described by the lateral cephalometric tracing. The surgically predicted outcome may be produced readily by computer software packages designed for this use and visualised on screen.
2. Model surgery is carried out on duplicate models and dental splints (occlusal wafers) are constructed for use during the operation to position correctly the bony fragments once osteotomised.

Preoperative care

- A full blood count and haemoglobin are measured.
- Blood is grouped and saved if a bimaxillary osteotomy is intended as blood transfusion may be required. This is usually unnecessary for surgery to the mandible alone.
- A coagulation screen carried out.
- Antibiotic prophylaxis.

Treatment
Mandibular surgery
There are many surgical techniques for the correction of the mandibular position. The sagittal split osteotomy is the most popular technique (Fig. 121). It enables the body of mandible to be moved forwards or backwards by sliding the split ramus and angle and thus providing a large amount of bone overlap for healing. The buccal and retromolar cortex of the mandible is sectioned with burs and the cancellous bone carefully split with chisels and osteotomes, avoiding damage to the inferior alveolar bundle. After repositioning, the mandibular fixation is achieved directly with screws or mini-plates, or indirectly with intermaxillary fixation (IMF).

Genioplasty
The chin may be reduced or undergo augmentation as an isolated procedure or as part of a mandibular or maxillary orthognathic operation. Genioplasty may be undertaken via an intra-oral approach and fixation with mini-plates is usual (Fig. 122).

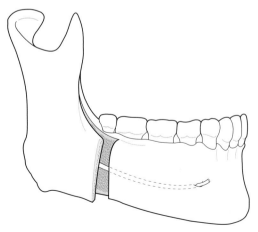

Fig. 121 Sagittal split mandibular osteotomy technique.

Maxillary surgery
The surgical techniques used for maxillary surgery are generally described by the Le Fort classification used for fracture description (Ch. 8). The higher-level osteotomies are obviously more complicated surgical operations. The most common maxillary osteotomy is the Le Fort I (Fig. 123). This operation is very versatile and enables movement of maxilla in any direction. Access is by an intra-oral approach and bone cuts are made with a saw and chisels. Fixation is with mini-plates. Higher-level maxillary osteotomies may require access via discrete skin incisions about the face or these may be avoided by a bicoronal approach. In the latter, a scalp incision is made across the vertex of the skull from ear to ear. This approach provides excellent access to the upper facial skeleton and a scar that is concealed beneath hair unless the patient develops hair loss.

Bone grafting may be required with harvesting from the iliac crest of cancellous bone to place into osteotomy sites.

Postoperative care
Postoperative care involves:

- airway management
- analgesia
- liquid or soft diet
- oral hygiene: may be aided with chlorhexidine mouthrinses
- antibiotics: usually continued for several days
- steroids in reducing doses
- the occlusion may require support with intermaxillary elastics.

Airway management
Surgical airway management with a tracheostomy is usually unnecessary for orthognathic surgery other than high-level maxillary procedures. However, close clinical and electromechanical observation with pulse oximetry is necessary to check that the patient does not become hypoxic as the result of soft-tissue swelling following surgery. The level of nursing supervision required means that the first postoperative 24 hours are usually spent in a high-dependency or intensive care unit. A nasopharyngeal airway is well tolerated in conscious patients and may be left in situ postoperatively to safeguard the airway during the first night. This will require frequent suction to maintain a clot-free patent airway.

Analgesia
Analgesia is essential for all postoperative patients. Bolus doses of opioids are best avoided because of the risk of respiratory depression in a patient with potential airway compromise. However, titration of opioids to the point of analgesia will ensure the dose is below that causing respiratory depression. Similarly, patient-controlled analgesia (PCA) with an opioid is useful in the initial postoperative stage. Otherwise, non-steroidal anti-inflammatory analgesics (NSAIDs) are the drugs of choice for surgical inflammatory pain.

Follow-up
Relapse is a possibility following orthognathic surgery. This is largely caused by muscle pull, especially the

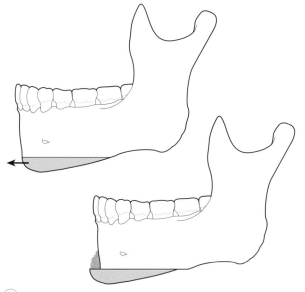

(A) Chin augmentation with sliding genioplasty

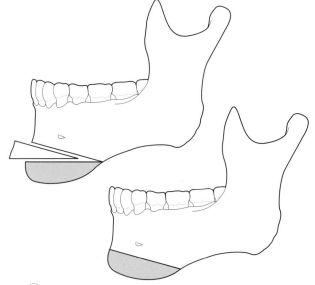

(B) Chin reduction by removal of a wedge of bone

Fig. 122 Examples of genioplasty techniques.

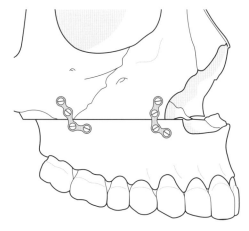

Fig. 123 Le Fort I osteotomy technique for advancement of the maxilla.

masseteric pterygoid muscle sling about the posterior mandible. Joint orthodontic and surgical review appointments are arranged to provide monitoring.

9.3 Cleft lip and palate surgery

Learning objective

You should:
- know the sequence of treatment for children with cleft lip and palate.

The spectrum of disease severity is wide. A team approach to management of cleft lip and palate is important; this may include the oral and maxillofacial surgeon, orthodontist, paedodontist, speech therapist, audiologist, otolaryngologist, nurses and midwives. Table 11 shows the sequence of treatment.

Table 11 Typical sequence of treatment for patients with cleft lip and palate

Age	Treatment
Birth	Initial assessment; presurgical orthodontics is no longer carried out
3 months	Primary lip repair surgery; Millard and Delaire are two commonly used surgical techniques
9–18 months	Surgical repair of palate, which is good for speech development but is associated with impaired growth of the maxilla; von Langenbeck and Delaire are two commonly used surgical techniques
2 years	Speech assessment
3–5 years	Lip revision surgery
8–9 years	Pre-bone graft orthodontic treatment; speech therapy
10 years	Alveolar augmentation with cancellous bone from ileac crest, which allows maxillary canines to erupt and provides support for alar base
12–14 years	Definitive orthodontics
16 years	Nose revision surgery
17–20 years	Advanced conservation treatment; orthognathic surgery to correct hypoplastic maxilla

- Surgical repair of the lip and palate is required and a variety of techniques using soft-tissue flaps are described. The Millard rotation advancement flap is common with the Delaire flap gaining in popularity for lip closure. Velopharyngeal incompetence is also corrected with flap surgery.

- Alveolar bone grafting is undertaken during the mixed dentition phase and is a well-established procedure. Bone is most commonly harvested from the anterior superior iliac crest by open operation or trephine. Grafting of the alveolar cleft allows union of the alveolar segments to occur and provides an intact alveolus for the maturation of the dentition, in particular, the eruption of the canine teeth.
- Orthognathic surgery is usually required to correct the maxillary hypoplasia and class III malocclusion.
- Nose: correction of the columella, alar cartilages and bony nasal skeleton may be required and rhinoplasty is becoming more common for adult patients.

Palatal clefts may be acquired as a result of trauma, especially gunshot wounds or because of tumour.

9.4 Craniofacial surgery and osteodistraction

Learning objectives

You should:
- know the indications for craniofacial surgery and its objectives
- understand the technique of osteodistraction.

The general aim of craniofacial surgery may be to facilitate normal assimilation into society, as is the case for much orthognathic surgery, but there may be secondary objectives such as the prevention of visual impairment, reduction of intracranial pressure or alleviation of respiratory impairment, which may prompt urgent surgery.

The team is likely to be larger than that involved in the management of patients undergoing orthognathic surgery or cleft lip and palate surgery, described above. In addition, the following specialities may be involved: neurosurgery, clinical genetics, psychology, ophthalmology and anaesthesia.

Craniofacial surgery is undertaken at a limited number of specialist centres to permit a high level of expertise to develop in the management of these rare and complex disorders. Advances in paediatric anaesthesia and imaging techniques have contributed to the evolution of this type of surgery. The craniofacial skeleton has an excellent healing potential and this allows large soft-tissue flaps with periosteum to be raised without detriment. The bicoronal flap or unilateral fronto-temporal scalp flap are standard techniques that provide good access to the cranial vault. Additional access may be required to the upper facial skeleton using transconjunctival, blepharoplasty, paranasal or intra-oral incisions.

Osteodistraction techniques

Osteodistraction or distraction osteogenesis was first described in 1905 but was little used until the Russian orthopaedic surgeon Ilizarov developed its use for the elongation of tubular bones. The technique is applicable to many areas of the skeleton and has more recently been used in oral and maxillofacial surgery. Osteodistraction is now used in the surgical correction of many types of anomaly ranging from defects of the alveolus to the craniosynostoses.

The process involves the gradual, controlled displacement of a surgical fracture. The displacement process is referred to as transport; the gap created during the displacement of the bone segment fills with immature non-calcified bone. It is this callus that is distracted and then matures during a subsequent fixation period. The adjacent soft tissues are expanded as the bone segment is transported and this unique ability to expand soft tissues simultaneously with bone makes this technique invaluable.

Technique

1. Osteotomy and placement of distraction device.
2. Latency period (about 1 week) after which the distraction device is activated.
3. Distraction period until the desired transport is achieved.
4. Fixation period (about 4 weeks) during which the distraction device is passive and after which it is removed.

Figure 124 shows an alveolar distraction device.

9.5 Cosmetic facial surgery

Learning objective

You should:
- know the more common techniques.

The demand for cosmetic surgery is increasing in the developed world. The need for surgery is sometimes controversial when it is seen to be entirely to produce an improved aesthetic rather than functional outcome. A rhinoplasty for a patient who has already undergone surgical correction for a cleft lip and palate may be more acceptable than for an individual who wishes to change a racial characteristic. Similarly surgery to maintain a more youthful appearance may be criticised. As for all surgery, the risks and benefits must be carefully considered.

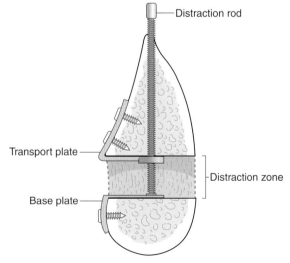

Fig. 124 Alveolar osteodistraction device.

Scar revision. Various 'Z' and 'W' plasties and local flap techniques may be used to disguise facial scars.

Dermabrasion. Used to remove superfically embedded foreign bodies from dirty facial abrasions and allow to heal without tatooing. Also used to treat acne scarring.

Laser resurfacing and ablation. Used to treat acne scarring and remove tatoos.

Collagen augmentation. To improve lip profile.

Liposuction. To remove excess subdermal fat and improve facial contour.

Rhytidectomy. To remove wrinkles by dissecting above the superficial musculoaponeurotic system (SMAS), stretching and closure after excision of excess tissue. Dissection at this plane preserves the facial nerve beneath. Procedure also known as 'face-lift'.

Blepharoplasty. Corrects periorbital skin wrinkling and orbital fat herniation.

Pinnaplasty. Corrects prominent ear lobes or pinnae. Pressure bandage required for 5–7 days to prevent haematoma that could lead to hyperplastic pinnae or 'cauliflower ears'.

Brow lifts. Undertaken via eyebrow, mid brow incision or endoscopic approach.

Self-assessment: questions

Multiple choice questions

1. Mandibular orthognathic surgery:
   a. Is always undertaken via an intra-oral approach
   b. Is usually associated with nerve damage following sagittal split technique
   c. Causes facial swelling that can be reduced with systemic steroids
   d. Requires both preoperative and postoperative orthodontics
   e. Should be discussed with appropriate patients by the general dental practitioner

2. In patients with cleft lip and palate:
   a. Dental abnormalities may include missing teeth
   b. Speech may be described as hypernasal
   c. There may be eustachian tube dysfunction
   d. Osseointegrated implants are contraindicated
   e. Childhood surgery prevents the need for later orthognathic surgery

3. The craniofacial anomaly of craniosynostosis:
   a. Includes the syndromes of Crouzon and Apert
   b. Does not require surgical treatment until the patient has reached adult age
   c. May require surgery on more than one occasion
   d. Results in disturbed growth of the mandible
   e. Requires management by a large multidisciplinary team

Extended matching items

Theme: Orthognathic surgery

Options:

A Hemifacial microsomia
B Mandibular asymmetry
C Cleft lip and palate
D Mandibular condylar trauma
E Anterior open bite
F Occlusal cant
G Nasomaxillary hypoplasia
H Maxillary hypoplasia
I Infra-orbital deficiency
J Pseudo-proptosis

Lead in: Select the most appropriate condition from the list above for each of the following cases. Each option can be used once, more than once or not at all.

1. Construction of a feeding appliance may be necessary to permit bottle feeding during infancy.
2. This condition may be caused by digit sucking in children but may self-correct if the habit stops sufficiently early.
3. Branchial arch syndromes such as first and second arch syndromes are associated with this condition.
4. Adults may acquire this condition if they develop a habit of pen sucking. The pen may act as an orthodontic appliance.
5. Patients with class III malocclusion frequently have this condition in addition to a prognathic mandible.

Viva questions

1. Describe the clinical features of mandibular prognathism.
2. Describe the clinical features of hemimandibular hyperplasia.
3. What are the potential complications of mandibular orthognathic surgery?
4. What is a submucous cleft?
5. What is a Millard flap?
6. Can distraction osteogenesis be used in place of all conventional orthognathic surgical techniques?

Self-assessment: answers

Multiple choice answers

1. a. **False.** While the sagittal split osteotomy is undertaken via an intra-oral approach, some types of operation may use an extra-oral approach. The vertical subsigmoid (VSS or vertical ramus) osteotomy is such a procedure (Fig. 125). This operation is less technically difficult and less time consuming than the sagittal split osteotomy and results in less inferior nerve damage. It can be performed via an intra- or extra-oral approach and the choice is determined by the ease of access for the type of fixation to be used in a particular case. Usually the extra-oral approach is favoured so that mini-plates can be used, and incisions are made in the submandibular or retromandibular area. This operation is less versatile than the sagittal split but useful for correction of asymmetry and lengthening or shortening of the vertical part of the ramus.

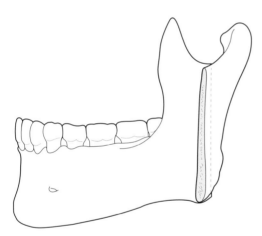

Fig. 125 Vertical subsigmoid osteotomy technique.

b. **True.** The inferior alveolar nerve is at significant risk during the sagittal split operation. Reports suggest that about 80% of patients experience mental paraesthesia in the immediate postoperative phase. A large proportion of these recover sensation, and reports of long-term paraesthesia vary between 0 and 24%. The incidence is increased in older patients.

c. **True.** Many surgeons use systemic steroids such as dexamethasone to help to reduce postoperative swelling. These are given intravenously during the surgery and in reducing doses over the postoperative days.

d. **True.** It is usual for mandibular and maxillary orthognathic surgery to require orthodontic treatment to move the teeth into positions to ensure a good occlusion at operation. Postoperative orthodontic treatment will facilitate minor adjustments and ensure stability. Other specialists such as a restorative dentist or periodontist may also be involved in the management of the patient requiring orthognathic surgery.

e. **True.** Patients with obvious facial skeletal discrepancies should be advised by the dentist that surgery may be an option with the potential to improve eating, speaking or the appearance. The patient should then be referred to an oral and maxillofacial surgeon for further investigation. Patients with lesser discrepancies are likely to be referred for orthodontic treatment and then, if the discrepancy is beyond the means of such treatment, the orthodontist will arrange a joint consultation with the surgeon.

2. a. **True.**

b. **True.** A surgical procedure called a pharyngoplasty may be beneficial to reduce hypernasal speech by narrowing the velopharyngeal opening.

c. **True.** Insertion of grommets is usually required because of eustachian tube dysfunction.

d. **False.** Dental implants may well form a part of comprehensive restorative management in the adult patient. Although the aim of childhood surgery and orthodontics treatment is to avoid the need for later restorative treatment, there may still be the need to replace missing teeth or the retention of obturators to close oronasal for some patients.

e. **False.** Adult patients with cleft lip and palate commonly have a hypoplastic maxilla, causing a class III skeletal base and dental occlusion with cross-bite. This may require correction with orthodontic expansion followed by an osteotomy to advance the maxilla. The aim of childhood surgery is to prevent the need for adult orthognathic surgery by facilitating the normal growth and development of the maxilla. However, such secondary surgery is still sometimes required. In Europe, almost as many surgical techniques as surgical specialist units have been practised. Some childhood surgical techniques may offer superior outcomes over others, and current randomised clinical trials evaluating the long-term results will provide us with more informed choices in the future.

3. a. **True.** Crouzon and Apert syndromes are both familial types of craniosynostosis with an autosomal dominant inheritance. They are described as among the more common craniosynostoses, although all are rare. Premature fusion of the cranial and base of skull sutures results in characteristic head and face morphology.

b. **False.** The growing brain causes an increase in intracranial pressure because of the limited growth of the skull. Early surgery is indicated to allow normal brain development. Headaches are a common early sign. It is not unusual for surgery to be undertaken at 5 to 7 years of age. This has the advantage of the child starting school with an improved appearance.

c. **True.** Following suture release and skull reshaping, the child is observed. Further reshaping may be required and is carried out if any increase in cranial pressure is noted. The cranial vault and orbits are normally about 90% of their adult size around the time of eruption of the maxillary first molar teeth at about 7 years of age, and so this is a good age for surgery. An example of a surgical procedure to enlarge the cranium and orbits is shown in Figure 126. Orthognathic surgery in late teenage years may be indicated.

d. **False.** The mandible develops in the normal way. The maxilla does not have the same growth potential and a class III skeletal base develops with class III dental occlusion. A maxillary advancement osteotomy may, therefore, be necessary.

e. **True.** Craniosynostoses are rare. Health services are organised so that a few centres treat more patients; this allows expertise to develop and the effectiveness of treatment types can be evaluated.

Extended matching items answers

1. **C.** Palatal obturation or a feeding appliance may be required to facilitate feeding in infancy.
2. **E.** Digit sucking is common and particularly damaging to the developing occlusion. Prolongation of the habit may result in severe, potentially irreversible derangement of dental occlusion.

3. **A.** First and second arch syndromes exhibit variable degrees of disturbed development of ear, midfacial, infratemporal and mandibular structures.
4. **E.** Anterior open bite may be acquired in adulthood with a habit of pen or instrument sucking.
5. **H.** Patients with class III facial skeletons frequently have a hypoplastic maxilla in addition to a prognathic mandible and consequently require a bimaxillary osteotomy rather than mandibular surgery alone.

Viva answers

1. Mandibular prognathism in isolation is rare. There is a frequent association with maxillary deficiency. The features of mandibular prognathism are exaggerated when part of a bimaxillary anomaly. The chin and lower lip are relatively forward of the upper lip. The occlusal class III relationship may not appear to be as severe as the skeletal bone discrepancy because of compensations such as the proclined maxillary anterior teeth and upright mandibular anterior teeth. The mandibular body and mandibular angle are well defined.
2. Hemimandibular hyperplasia typically causes a gradually developing asymmetry of the dental occlusion and lower face during puberty. It is sometimes described as a condylar hyperplasia but the effects are seen as far forward as the midline (Fig. 127). A lateral open bite develops and the ramus and body increase significantly in size. The growth carries the neurovascular bundle down to the lower border. The lateral open bite may close by compensatory overgrowth of the alveolus of both the mandible and maxilla. The occlusal plane is, therefore, tilted down to the affected side, as seen in Figure 119.
3. Complications of mandibular orthognathic surgery include early relapse because of inaccurate positioning of the mandibular condyles in the glenoid fossa (difficult in an unconscious patient) before fixation was applied or movement of the bone segments if they were not adequately immobilised, and late relapse caused by muscle pull. Other complications include unfavourable bone splits, extrusion of teeth, periodontal defects, temporomandibular joint dysfunction, alveolar nerve injury, infection and non-union.

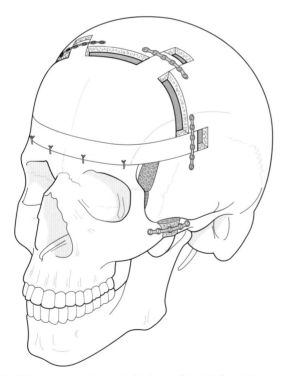

Fig. 126 An example of a surgical technique (Monobloc) used for the management of some craniosynostoses.

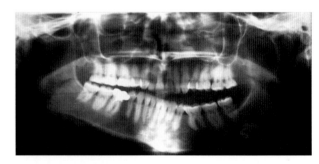

Fig. 127 Digital panoramic topographic radiograph showing effects of hemimandibular hyperplasia.
(This is the radiograph of the patient shown in Fig. 123.)

4. The Millard rotation-advancement flap is a commonly used method of cleft lip repair. It is a modified Z-plasty placed at the top of the cleft so that the area of greatest tension is positioned at the alar base. It is used for complete, incomplete and narrow and wide cleft repairs. The scar closely resembles the philtrum of the lip on the cleft side.

5. Distraction osteogenesis is a relatively new technique introduced to manage orthognathic discrepancies. There is a need for further investigation of this technique, in particular for randomised controlled trials where possible to compare effectiveness and morbidity of the traditional surgery with this new technique. Distraction osteogenesis cannot be used in situations where a reduction in prognathism is required.

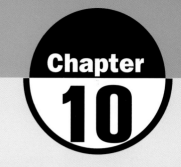
Overview

The first part of this chapter deals with the different types of cyst that can occur in the orofacial area. The general features by which cysts are identified and their investigation are covered together with the specific features of some types of cyst. This section closes with the surgical management of cysts. The second part of this chapter deals with odontogenic tumours. It starts by considering their origin and classification. The different types of tumour, according to the tissue of origin, are discussed in turn. Finally, the chapter ends by looking at surgical management of odontogenic tumours.

10.1 General features

Learning objectives

You should:
- know the types of cyst that can occur
- the origins of the different types of cyst.

A cyst is a pathological cavity, not formed by the accumulation of pus, with fluid or semi-fluid contents.

Cyst growth

Several mechanisms are described for cyst growth, including:

- epithelial proliferation
- internal hydraulic pressure
- bone resorption.

Classification of cysts

Cysts can be classified on the basis of:

- location
  - jaw
  - maxillary antrum
  - soft tissues of face and neck
- cell type
  - epithelial
  - non-epithelial
- pathogenesis
  - developmental
  - inflammatory.

Box 11 lists the cysts found in the orofacial region using these groups.

Other cysts

Cysts associated with the maxillary antrum

- Benign mucosal cyst of the maxillary antrum
- Postoperative maxillary cyst (surgical ciliated cyst of the maxilla).

Cysts of the soft tissues of the mouth, face and neck

- Dermoid and epidermoid cysts
- Lymphoepithelial (branchial cleft) cyst
- Thyroglossal duct cyst
- Cysts of the salivary glands: mucous extravasation cyst, mucous retention cyst, ranula.

Odontogenic cysts

Odontogenic cysts are lined with epithelium derived from the following tooth development structures:

- rests of Malassez: radicular cyst, residual cyst
- reduced enamel epithelium: dentigerous cyst, eruption cyst
- remnants of the dental lamina: odontogenic keratocyst, lateral periodontal cyst, gingival cyst of adult, glandular odontogenic cyst
- unclassified: paradental cyst.

10.2 Examination

Learning objectives

You should:
- know the clinical signs and symptoms of cysts
- understand the radiological appearance of cysts and the features that need to be noted.

Based on the World Health Organization 1992 classification.

Epithelial cysts

Developmental odontogenic cysts
- Odontogenic keratocyst
- Dentigerous cyst (follicular cyst)
- Eruption cyst
- Lateral periodontal cyst
- Gingival cyst of adults
- Glandular odontogenic cyst (sialo-odontogenic)

Inflammatory odontogenic cysts
- Radicular cyst (apical and lateral)
- Residual cyst
- Paradental cyst

Non-odontogenic cysts
- Nasopalatine cyst
- Nasolabial cyst

Non-epithelial cysts (not true cysts)
- Solitary bone cyst
- Aneurysmal bone cyst

General clinical features

Cysts may be detected because of clinical symptoms or signs (Table 12). Occasionally an asymptomatic cyst may be discovered on a radiograph taken for another purpose. Symptoms may include:

- swelling (Fig. 128)
- displacement or loosening of teeth
- pain (if infected).

The most important clinical sign is expansion of bone. In some instances, this may result in an eggshell-like layer of periosteal new bone overlying the cyst (Fig. 129). This can break on palpation, giving rise to the clinical sign of 'eggshell cracking'. If the cyst lies within soft tissue or has perforated the overlying bone, then the sign of fluctuance may be elicited by palpating with fingertips on each side of the swelling in two positions at right angles to each other.

If a cyst becomes infected, the clinical presentation may be that of an abscess, the underlying cystic lesion only becoming apparent on radiographic examination.

Radiological examination: general principles

As a basic principle, radiological examination should commence with intra-oral films of the affected region; for small cystic lesions, intra-oral films may be all that is needed for diagnosis, while for all cysts the fine detail of intra-oral radiography will help to clarify the relationship between lesion and teeth. For larger lesions, more extensive radiography is appropriate. Selection of films should take account of the value of having two views with differing perspectives (preferably at right angles to each other; Fig. 129).

Table 12 Clinical features of cysts

Cyst type	Typical age (decade at presentation)	Sex distribution	Commonest site	Common clinical signs
Radicular	3rd and 4th	M > F	Tooth-bearing areas of jaws especially anterior maxilla; most common odontogenic cyst	Slowly enlarging swellings, frequently symptomless and discovered by radiography of non-vital teeth
Residual	4th and 5th	M > F	Mandibular premolar area	Slowly enlarging swellings, frequently symptomless
Keratocyst	2nd and 3rd	M > F	Angle of mandible	Frequently symptomless and discovered on dental examination or radiography; tooth displacement and occasional paraesthesia lower lip
Dentigerous	3rd and 4th	M > F	Mandibular 3rd molar followed by maxillary canine	Like keratocyst may grow to large size before diagnosed; most discovered on radiograph taken because of tooth eruption failure
Eruption	1st and 2nd	M > F	Deciduous and permanent teeth, most frequently anterior to first permanent molar	Smooth swelling of normal or blue-coloured mucosa over erupting tooth
Nasopalatine	4th, 5th and 6th	M > F	Nasopalatine canal	Swelling anterior palate or floor of nose
Nasolabial	4th and 5th	F > M	Nasolabial fold	Swelling in soft tissue
Solitary	2nd	M = F	Mandible	Discovered on radiograph
Aneurysmal	2nd	F > M	Posterior mandible	Firm swelling, rapidly expanding

F, female; M, male.

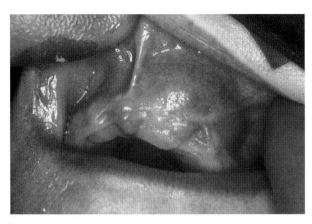

Fig. 128 Photograph showing buccal swelling caused by residual cyst in maxilla.

Maxilla. Suitable views are:

- periapicals and oblique occlusals
- panoramic radiograph or lateral oblique
- occipitomental (OM)
- true lateral (anterior maxilla)

Mandible. Suitable views are:

- periapicals and true occlusals
- panoramic radiograph or lateral oblique
- postero-anterior (PA) of mandible.

Computed tomography (CT) may be useful in planning surgery of large cysts, particularly in the posterior maxilla.

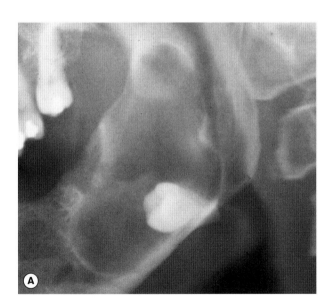

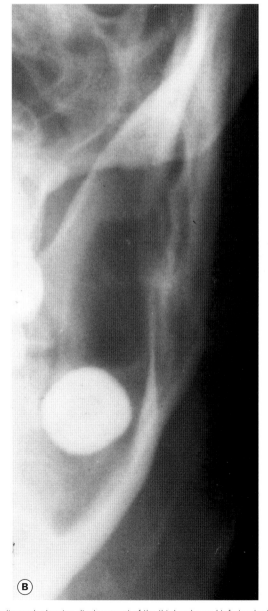

Fig. 129 An odontogenic keratocyst of the left mandible. **A.** Part of a panoramic radiograph showing displacement of the third molar and inferior dental canal to the lower border of the mandible. **B.** Part of a postero-anterior radiograph of the same lesion.

Radiological signs

Classically, cysts appear as well-defined round or ovoid radiolucencies, surrounded by a well-defined margin.

Margins. Peripheral cortication (radio-opaque margin) is usual except in solitary bone cysts. 'Scalloped' margins are seen in larger lesions, particularly keratocysts. Infection of a cyst tends to cause loss of the well-defined margin.

Shape. Most cysts grow by hydrostatic mechanisms, resulting in the round shape. Odontogenic keratocysts and solitary bone cysts do not grow in this manner and have a tendency to grow through the medullary bone rather than to expand the jaw.

Locularity. True locularity (multiple cavities) is seen occasionally in odontogenic keratocysts. However, larger cysts of most types may have a multilocular appearance because of ridges in the bony wall.

Effects upon adjacent structures. Where a lesion abuts another structure, such as a tooth or the inferior dental canal, it may cause displacement. Roots of teeth may be resorbed. When a cyst reaches a certain size, the cortex of the bone often becomes thinned and expanded. In posterior maxillary lesions the antral floor may be raised. Perforation of the cortical plates may be recognised as a localised area of greater radiolucency overlying the lesion.

Effect on unerupted teeth. Unerupted teeth may become enveloped by any cyst, a feature which may lead to erroneous diagnosis as a dentigerous cyst.

10.3 Specific cysts

Learning objectives

You should:
- know the radiographic appearance of the more common cysts affecting the jaw
- understand the pathology of these cysts.

Radicular cyst

Radiology

A well-defined, round or ovoid radiolucency is associated with the root apex or, less commonly in the lateral position, of a heavily restored or grossly carious tooth. A corticated margin is continuous with the lamina dura of the root of the affected tooth. The appearances are similar to those of an apical granuloma, but lesions with a diameter exceeding 10 mm are more likely to be cystic (Fig. 130).

Pathology

The cyst lumen is lined by a layer of simple squamous epithelium of variable thickness, which may display areas of discontinuity where it is replaced by granulation tissue. Arcades and strands of epithelium may extend into the cyst capsule, which is composed of granulation tissue infiltrated by a mixture of acute and chronic inflammatory cells. This infiltrate reduces in intensity as the more peripheral areas of the cyst capsule are approached, where mature fibrous tissue replaces the granulation tissue (Fig. 131).

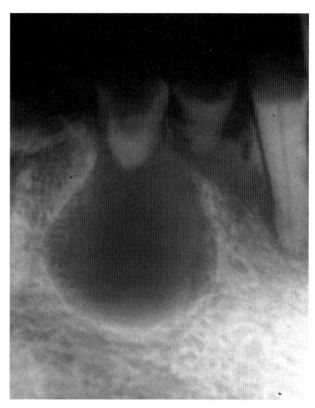

Fig. 130 A radicular cyst related to a retained root of a mandibular premolar. It is easy to imagine how the cyst has developed from the periodontal ligament and that its corticated margin is an extension of the lamina dura on either side of the root.

Several features associated with inflammatory odontogenic cysts may be present in the cyst lumen, lining and capsule: cholesterol clefts, foamy macrophages, haemosiderin and Rushton's bodies. *indicate odontogenic origin*

Residual cyst

Radiology

The residual cyst has a well-defined, round/ovoid radiolucency in an edentulous area. Occasionally flecks of calcification may be seen.

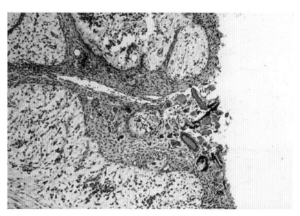

Fig. 131 Photomicrograph of a radicular cyst.

Pathology

The lining and capsule are similar to the radicular cyst; however, both appear more mature, with the former lacking the arcades and strands of epithelium extending into the capsule.

Odontogenic keratocyst

Radiology

There is a well-defined radiolucency in odontogenic keratocysts, often with densely corticated margins. The shape margins may be 'scalloped' in shape. Occasionally, there is a multilocular appearance. Expansion typically limited, with a propensity to grow along the medullary cavity (Fig. 132).

Pathology

The cyst is lined by a continuous layer of stratified squamous epithelium of even thickness (5–10 cells) the surface of which is corrugated. The basal-cell layer is well defined, being composed of cuboidal or columnar cells that display palisading. This epithelium is most commonly parakeratinising, although orthokeratosis may be observed. The lumen of the cyst is filled with shed squames. The cyst capsule is composed of rather delicate fibrous tissue and is, classically, free from inflammation (Fig. 133). However, should the cyst become infected then an inflammatory infiltrate may be seen and the characteristic features of the epithelial lining will be lost.

The presence of daughter cysts within the capsule is a well-recognised finding, particularly in those odontogenic keratocysts arising as a component of the basal-cell naevus syndrome.

Dentigerous cyst

Radiology

In dentigerous cysts, there is a pericoronal radiolucency greater than 3–4 mm in width that is suggestive of cyst

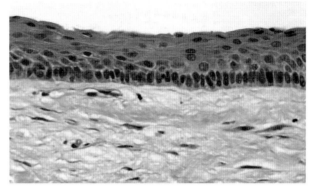

Fig. 133 Photomicrograph of a keratocyst.

formation in a dental follicle. The well-defined, corticated radiolucency is associated with the crown of an unerupted tooth. Classically the associated crown of the tooth lies centrally within the cyst, but lateral types occur (Fig. 134).

Pathology

The defining feature of a dentigerous cyst is the site of attachment of the cyst to the involved tooth. This must be at the level of the amelocemental junction. The lining of the cyst is composed of a thin layer of epithelium, either cuboidal or squamous in nature, some 2–5 cells thick (Fig. 135). This lining is of even thickness and may include mucous cells along with focal areas of keratinisation of the superficial epithelial cells. The cyst capsule is, classically, free from inflammation. However, in common with the odontogenic

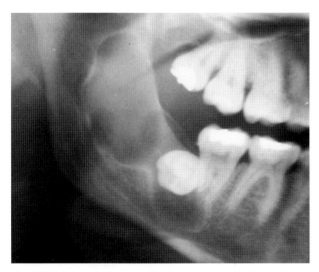

Fig. 132 Odontogenic keratocyst. The lesion is very well defined with a corticated margin. The wisdom tooth appears displaced, as does the inferior dental canal, visible at the inferior and posterior aspects of the cyst. The shape is not round or ovoid, but rather irregular with a separate locule below the crown of the wisdom tooth.

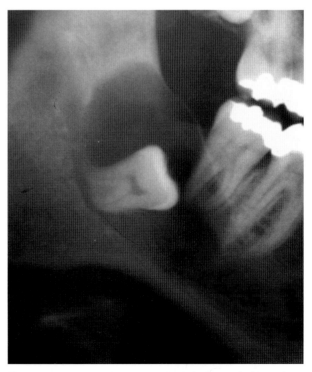

Fig. 134 A dentigerous cyst associated with the lower right third molar. The radiolucency is located pericoronally. Note that both the tooth and inferior dental canal appear to have been displaced inferiorly by the lesion.

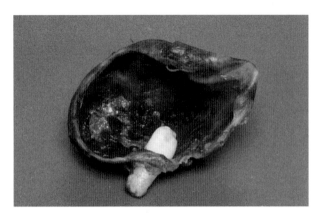

Fig. 135 Dentigerous cyst showing origin from the amelocemental junction.

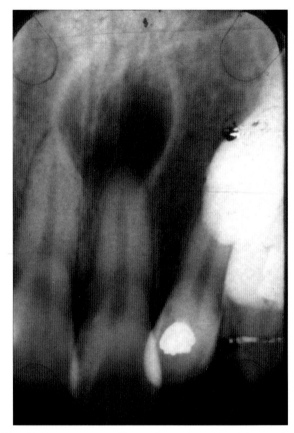

Fig. 136 Nasopalatine cyst. This small example could easily be mistaken for a radicular cyst, but the presence of the lamina dura of the incisors indicates that this is not the case.

keratocyst, the normal features of the epithelial lining may be distorted when an inflammatory infiltrate is present.

Eruption cyst

Radiology

The extra-bony position of the eruption cyst means that the only radiological sign is likely to be a soft-tissue mass.

Pathology

An eruption cyst is basically a dentigerous cyst in soft tissue over an erupting tooth. The histological features are similar to those of the dentigerous cyst, though reduced enamel epithelium is often seen.

Gingival cysts

Gingival cysts are commonly found in neonates but are rarely encountered after 3 months of age. Many appear to undergo spontaneous resolution. White keratinous nodules are seen on the gingivae and these are referred to as Bohn's nodules or Epstein's pearls. Gingival cysts arise from the dental lamina and histologically are keratin containing. Many open into the oral cavity forming clefts from which the keratin exudes. Gingival cysts are lined by stratified squamous parakeratotic epithelium. In neonates and infants, the cysts are typically between 2 and 5 mm in diameter. They do not involve bone and no treatment is required.

Gingival cysts of adults are much less common and are found mainly in the buccal gingivae in the mandibular premolar–canine region. The cyst typically presents as a solitary soft blue swelling within the attached gingivae, seldom larger than 5 mm in diameter. Gingival cysts of adults are lined by a thin cuboidal or flattened epithelium resembling dental follicle. They do not extend into bone although they may rest in a shallow depression in the cortex. They are usually removed by excision biopsy for diagnosis.

Nasopalatine cyst

Radiology

The nasopalatine cyst appears as a well-defined, round radiolucency in the midline of the anterior maxilla (Fig. 136). Sometimes it appears to be 'heart-shaped' because of superimposition of the anterior nasal spine. Radiological assessment should include examination of the lamina dura of the

central incisors (to exclude a radicular cyst) and assessment of size (the nasopalatine foramen may reach a width of as much as 10 mm).

Pathology

The cyst is lined by a layer of pseudostratified ciliated columnar epithelium and/or stratified squamous epithelium. The capsule of the cyst is fibrous and may include the incisive canal neurovascular bundle.

Nasolabial cyst

Radiology

As the nasolabial cyst is a soft-tissue lesion, radiography may reveal nothing. However, radiography will be performed to exclude other causes of the swelling. 'Bowing' inwards of the anterolateral margin of the nasal cavity has been recorded as a feature. Ultrasound examination would be an appropriate investigation.

Pathology

The nasolabial cyst is lined by non-ciliated pseudostratified columnar epithelium, which is often rich in mucous cells.

Solitary bone cyst

Radiology

The solitary bone cyst appears as a well-defined but non-corticated radiolucency. Typically, it has little effect on

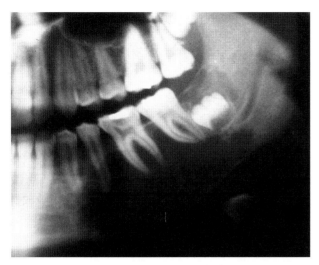

Fig. 137 Solitary bone cyst. There is a large radiolucency in the body of the mandible that arches up between the roots of the teeth, which appear otherwise unaffected. The lower border cortex is very thin. The inferior dental canal is not displaced but appears to stop abruptly at the posterior end of the lesion.

adjacent structures and 'arches' up between the roots of teeth (Fig. 137). The inferior dental canal may not be displaced, but the cortical margins of the canal may be lost where it overlies the lesion. Expansion is rare.

Pathology

The cyst is lined by fibrovascular tissue that often includes haemosiderin and multinucleate giant cells.

Aneurysmal bone cyst
Radiology

The aneurysmal bone cyst typically presents as a fairly well-defined radiolucency. Sometimes it has a multilocular appearance because of the occurrence of internal bony septa and opacification. Marked expansion is a feature.

Pathology

The predominant feature of an aneurysmal bone cyst is the presence of blood-filled spaces of variable size lying in a stroma rich in fibroblasts, multinucleate giant cells and haemosiderin. Deposits of osteoid are also seen.

10.4 Surgical management of cysts

Learning objectives

You should:
- know the general management of cysts
- know the specific approach for the more common cysts of the jaw.

Surgical management of cysts generally implies enucleation, but occasionally marsupialisation is the technique of choice. Some small radicular cysts do not require surgery and regress once the root canal of the associated tooth has been effectively cleaned and filled. Antibiotic therapy

may be required if a cyst has become infected. Aspiration of fluid from a pathological cavity may be helpful in confirming the presence of cyst rather than maxillary sinus (air) or tumour (solid). Biochemical analysis of the aspirate indicating protein content of less than $40\,g/l$ and cytology showing parakeratinised squames suggests an odontogenic keratocyst.

Enucleation

Enucleation of a cyst involves the removal of the whole cyst, including the epithelial and capsular layers from the bony walls of the cavity. This permits histopathological examination and ensures that no pathological tissue remains. A large mucoperiosteal flap, usually buccal, is raised to ensure that closure will be over adjacent sound tissues and not the bony cavity. Primary closure is nearly always undertaken unless the cyst is very infected, in which case this may be delayed and the cavity initially dressed with Bismuth Iodoform Paraffin Paste (BIPP) on ribbon gauze.

Enucleation of a nasopalatine cyst will require the raising of a palatal flap to provide surgical access and cyst removal. This inevitably damages the nasopalatine nerves and vessels and results in a small area of paraesthesia, which usually does not cause concern to the patient.

Marsupialisation

Marsupialisation is a simple operation that may be performed under local anaesthesia in which a window is cut and removed from the cyst lining. This allows decompression of the cyst, which then slowly heals by bone deposition in the base of the cavity. However, this technique permits histopathological examination of only a small and possibly non-representative sample of tissue. Primary closure is not undertaken but rather the cyst lining is sutured to the oral mucosa to keep the cavity open (Fig. 138). The cavity must be filled with a dressing such as BIPP, which must be frequently replaced, to prevent food debris trapping during the many months the cavity may take to heal. Alternatively, an extension may be added to a denture to protect the cavity, which becomes reduced in size as the cavity heals.

Marsupialisation is advocated when the cyst is so large that jaw fracture is the likely outcome of enucleation,

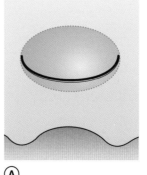
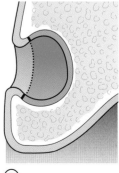

Fig. 138 Marsupialisation. **A.** An incision is made over a large cystic lesion in the maxillary alveolus. **B.** The flap is sutured to the margins of the cyst lining following excision of a window of tissue for pathological examination.

although enucleation and simultaneous bone grafting may be preferable. The technique may also be useful if there are associated structures, such as the inferior alveolar nerve, maxillary antrum or nose, that are at risk of damage during enucleation. Similarly, marsupialisation of an eruption cyst will allow the eruption of a tooth without it being damaged by enucleation.

Surgical management of particular cysts

Radicular cysts

Large radicular cysts, or small ones that do not resolve following conventional endodontic treatment, require enucleation and surgical endodontic management to seal the root canal of the associated tooth.

Access for apical surgery is gained via a three-sided or a semi-lunar mucoperiosteal flap (Fig. 139). The latter avoids involvement of the gingival margin, which may be important where the tooth is restored with a crown, but does not offer adequate access or permit closure over bone for larger cysts. Bone is removed with a rosehead bur over the tooth root apex, which is then divided with a fissure bur and removed so that the root face may be readily visualised from the buccal aspect (Fig. 139C). The cyst is enucleated in the usual way and sent for histopathological examination. An access cavity is prepared in the root face and restored with filler – the retrograde root filling – to seal the root canal of the tooth. Following irrigation of the surgical site, wound closure is achieved with an appropriate suture material that will provide adequate wound support. If the suture material is absorbed too early, semi-lunar flaps are likely to show dehiscence and three-sided flaps may cause gingival recession. Follow-up with radiography to check bony healing is indicated. See also Chapter 5.

Keratocyst

High recurrence rates are reported (up to 60%) because of technical difficulty in removing all of the cyst lining, including projections into cancellous bone. Enucleation must be thorough. Some advocate irrigating the cyst cavity with chemical fixatives to cause necrosis of any

remaining remnants, and others suggest excision to include a bone margin about the cyst. Annual radiographic review is recommended.

Eruption cysts

Reassurance of the parents is usually the only management required as these cysts frequently fenestrate spontaneously and require no surgical intervention. Occasionally, however, they may require marsupialisation to expose the tooth.

Solitary bone cyst

These bone cysts are often incidental findings on radiographs. Aspiration may reveal clear fluid or air indicating that no further intervention is necessary.

Aneurysmal bone cyst

These cysts benefit from curretage. However, they may be associated with a second pathological lesion such as a vascular malformation which may lead to profound haemorrhage. Patients with this cyst need to be managed in hospital.

10.5 Odontogenic tumours: origin, behaviour and classification

Learning objectives

You should:
- understand the developmental origin of the cells that give rise to odontogenic tumours
- have knowledge of the WHO scheme of classification of odontogenic tumours.

During fetal development, epithelium from the dental lamina invades the future jaw bones in order to form teeth and their associated supporting structures. Odontogenic cells are derived from the ectoderm of the first branchial arch and the ectomesenchyme of the neural crest. Formation of dental hard tissues requires their interaction. Odontogenic tumours are mostly derived from tooth-forming cells that remain in the jaws after tooth

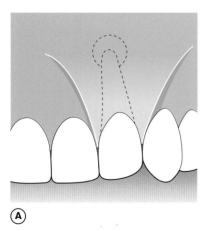

(A)

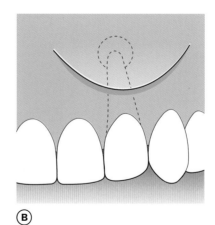

(B)

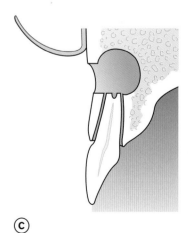

(C)

Fig. 139 Enucleation of a radicular cyst. **A.** A three-sided incision. **B.** A semi-lunar incision to gain access to a radicular cyst associated with a maxillary lateral incisor. **C.** Oblique sectioning of the apical root to permit good access to seal the root canal with amalgam.

formation. Sometimes an odontogenic tumour forms in place of a tooth. The biological behaviour of odontogenic tumours ranges from benign developmental anomaly to malignant. An unusual feature of **ameloblastoma** (the most common odontogenic neoplasm) is that it is locally invasive but does not metastasise. This property is shared with some other odontogenic tumours and is explained by the biological ability of odontogenic ectodermal cells to invade bone in order to form teeth.

Many classification schemes have been proposed. The current WHO classification is based on whether the tumour is **epithelial** (ectodermal origin), **mesenchymal** (ectomesenchymal origin) or **mixed** (Box 12). Only the mixed group

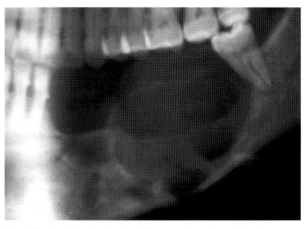

Fig. 140 Ameloblastoma in the left lower molar region, displaying multilocularity and expansion of the bone. Note that the upper margin of the lesion is in contact with the occlusal surfaces of the maxillary teeth.

Box 12 Odontogenic tumours

Benign tumours
Odontogenic epithelium with mature, fibrous stroma without odontogenic mesenchyme
- Ameloblastoma, solid/multicystic type
- Ameloblastoma, extra-osseous/peripheral type
- Ameloblastoma, desmoplastic type
- Amelobastoma, unicystic type
- Squamous odontogenic tumour
- Calcifying epithelial odontogenic tumour
- Adenomatoid odontogenic tumour
- Keratocystic odontogenic tumour

Odontogenic epithelium with odontogenic mesenchyme, with or without hard-tissue formation
- Ameloblastic fibroma
- Ameloblastic fibrodentinoma
- Odontoma, complex type
- Odontoma, compound type
- Odontoameloblastoma
- Calcifying cystic odontogenic tumour
- Dentinogenic ghost-cell tumour

Mesenchyme and/or odontogenic ectomesenchyme with or without odontogenic epithelium
- Odontogenic fibroma
- Odontogenic myxoma
- Cementoblastoma

Malignant tumours
Odontogenic carcinomas
- Metastasising (malignant) ameloblastoma
- Ameloblastic carcinoma – primary type
- Ameloblastic carcinoma – secondary type
- Ameloblastic carcinoma – secondary type (dedifferentiated), peripheral
- Primary intra-osseous squamous-cell carcinoma – solid type
- Primary intra-osseous squamous-cell carcinoma derived from keratocystic odontogenic tumour
- Primary intra-osseous squamous-cell carcinoma derived from odontogenic cysts
- Clear-cell odontogenic carcinoma
- Ghost-cell odontogenic carcinoma

Odontogenic sarcomas
- Ameloblastic fibrosarcoma
- Ameloblastic fibrodentinoma and fibro-odontosarcoma

---

can contain enamel or dentine because both cell types need to interact for dental hard tissue to form.

10.6 Specific odontogenic tumours

Learning objectives

You should:
- have a good knowledge of ameloblastoma, the most common odontogenic tumour
- be aware of the other odontigenic tumours.

Odontogenic epithelial tumours

Ameloblastoma is the most common odontogenic neoplasm. It arises mostly in the posterior mandible but can also occur in the posterior maxilla and less commonly at other sites in the jaws. The pattern of disease varies in populations. Ameloblastoma is most frequent in black Africans. The midline mandible is often involved which is a rare site in Caucasian people. Ameloblastoma is slow growing and typically expands the jaw. Expansion of the lingual plate is a helpful diagnostic sign in the mandible, because cysts rarely expand the plate. Adjacent teeth may be displaced or the roots may undergo resorption. Pain may be a presenting feature. A multilocular ('soap-bubble') radiolucent cystic lesion is typically found on radiographs (Fig. 140). Pathologically ameloblastomas often show extensive cystic change and biopsy of a solid area in the wall of the tumour is essential for diagnosis. In the microscope ameloblastoma contains islands of odontogenic epithelium. Columnar cells resembling pre-ameloblasts are found at the periphery of the islands. The nuclei are polarised away from the basement membrane and there is abundant cytoplasm. Stellate reticulum-like cells are present in the centre of the islands. Cystic and microcystic changes are seen microscopically. Follicular and plexiform patterns are seen; often both patterns are present.

Variants of ameloblastoma are recognised. The unicystic type is noteworthy because if no extramural islands are

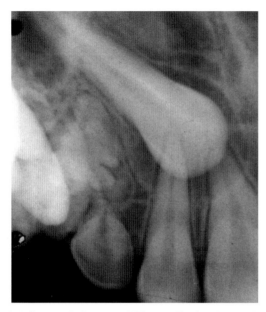

Fig. 141 Compound odontome in UR3 region. This has the typical radiological appearance of a small (1 cm diameter or less), well-defined mass of radio-opaque 'denticles' with a radiolucent periphery. These are often identified by radiography when investigating unerupted teeth, as in this case.

present it behaves as a cyst and can be treated by enucleation rather than resection.

Mixed epithelial and ectomesenchymal odontogenic tumours

Some tumours in this group form enamel, dentine and cementum. **Odontomes** are benign malformations rather than true neoplasms and are very common affecting up to 2% of the population. Typical presenting signs are failure of eruption of nearby permanent teeth or acute infection resembling a dental abscess. Two types are recognised:

- complex odontome: a disorganised mass of dental hard tissue, usually found in the posterior mandible
- compound odontome: separate rudimentary teeth (denticles) in a sac, usually found in anterior maxilla (Fig. 141).

Soft-tissue mixed odontogenic tumours are less common. Diagnosis is based on biopsy and radiographic features. Surgery is the treatment of choice and depends on precise diagnosis.

Mesenchymal odontogenic tumours

Odontogenic myxoma most often occurs in the mandible and is characterised by a destructive radiolucent lesion. Biopsy shows loose myxoid tissue with variable fibrosis. Surgical excision is needed. Cementoblastoma is a true neoplasm of cementum. It is found most often around the roots of the first mandibular molar. The associated tooth may be extruded and can become painful, but remains vital. On radiographs there is a characteristic radiodense central nidus surrounded by radiolucent rim. The lesion must be removed surgically along with the tooth. Cementoblastoma may recur following removal and patients should be warned of that risk.

Malignant odontogenic tumours

These are extremely rare. Intra-osseous squamous-cell carcinoma arises from epithelial inclusions in the jaw and has a poor prognosis. Malignant odontogenic neoplasms present with expansion of the jaw, destruction of adjacent tissue, displacement of teeth and sometimes pathological fracture. Secondary deposits of cancer in the jaw are more common than primary odontogenic cancer.

10.7 Surgical management of odontogenic tumours

Learning objectives

You should:
- have knowledge of the surgical methods appropriate to odontogenic tumour management.

Ameloblastoma is treated by surgery with the aim of removing the entire neoplasm with a small margin of surrounding normal tissue (block resection). The inferior border of the mandible may be preserved if not penetrated but for large ameloblastomas, hemimandibulectomy or hemimaxillectomy may be required. Surgery is required because ameloblastomas are relatively radioresistant. Unicystic types may be enucleated without taking a margin of surrounding tissue.

Odontomes are managed by surgical enucleation as they are generally well encapsulated and fairly well separated from surrounding bone.

Odontogenic myxoma requires block resection in most cases rather than local enucleation. Cementoblastoma requires the removal of the associated tooth but generally is well encapsulated so enucleates well.

Treatment for malignant odontogenic tumours is usually aggressive and may involve regional neck dissection followed by radiotherapy and chemotherapy.

Self-assessment: questions

Multiple choice questions

1. Odontogenic keratocysts:
   a. The soluble protein content is greater than 40 g/l
   b. May be a feature in patients with mutation in the gene *APC*
   c. Are thought to enlarge by hydrostatic pressure
   d. Are most common in the anterior maxilla
   e. Contain creamy-white, semi-fluid material

2. Dentigerous cyst:
   a. Is thought to arise from cystic degeneration between the inner and outer dental epithelial layers
   b. The lining typically attaches to a tooth at the amelocemental junction
   c. May be associated with displacement of teeth
   d. Is lined by a thin layer of epithelium, which often exhibits mucous metaplasia
   e. May expand the mandibular cortex resulting in eggshell cracking

3. Nasopalatine duct cyst:
   a. Is typically lined by keratinising stratified squamous epithelium
   b. Results in a salty taste in the mouth, which is a recognised presenting sign
   c. Has a capsule that often enmeshes a neurovascular bundle
   d. May cause tilting of the roots of the maxillary central incisor teeth
   e. Has a typical recurrence rate of 20%

4. Among the intra-osseous cysts in the jaws:
   a. Thinning of the bone cortex is responsible for the sign known as eggshell cracking
   b. Determination of tooth vitality is essential for diagnosis when any cystic lesion is related to root apices
   c. The maxillary sinus, Staphne's cavity, giant-cell granuloma, odontogenic tumours and metastatic deposits of cancer may all present radiographically as cysts
   d. Odontogenic keratocysts tend to form an hour-glass shape at the angle of the mandible while radicular cysts tend to be more rounded in shape
   e. Both ameloblastoma and odontogenic keratocyst may be detected as multilocular radiolucent lesions at the angle of the mandible, while the odontogenic keratocyst is less likely to cause lingual plate expansion

5. Gingival cysts:
   a. Are most common in the mandibular premolar region in adults
   b. May be multiple in neonates and are referred to as Epstein's pearls or Bohr's nodules
   c. Typically range between 1 and 3 cm in diameter
   d. Are typically lined by keratinising squamous epithelium
   e. May extend into the underlying septal bone

6. Among the cysts of the soft tissues:
   a. Mucous retention mucocoele occurs more commonly in the upper labial submucosa than in the lower labial submucosa
   b. Ranulae occur principally in the floor of mouth and soft palate
   c. Dermoid cysts in the orofacial region tend to occur in the midline, mainly either superior or inferior to the mylohyoid muscle
   d. Lymphoepithelial cysts occur mainly in the cervical region just below the anterior margin of the sternocleidomastoid muscle
   e. Thyroglossal tract cysts in the neck tend to elevate when the patient swallows

7. Among the bone and antral cysts:
   a. The Staphne cavity is an enclosed intra-osseous cavity located below the inferior alveolar nerve canal
   b. Aneurysmal bone cyst does not have an epithelial lining
   c. Solitary bone cyst is unlikely to involve interdental septa in the mandible
   d. Mucosal cysts in the maxillary sinus tend to enlarge progressively and usually require surgical removal
   e. Hyperthyroidism may result in multiple giant-cell lesions resembling cysts radiographically in the jaws

8. Eruption cyst:
   a. Is a dentigerous cyst in soft tissue
   b. Typically presents as a symptomless, blue, fluctuant swelling on the alveolar ridge
   c. Must be surgically fenestrated to permit eruption of the associated tooth
   d. Is lined by keratinising stratified squamous epithelium
   e. Usually involves multiple adjacent teeth

9. The paradental cyst:
   a. Is also called the cyst of Craig
   b. Occurs on the lateral aspect of third molars
   c. Is stimulated by pericoronitis
   d. Arises from the epithelial rests of Malassez
   e. Has a communication with oral cavity

10. Radicular cyst:
    a. Alternative terms are apical inflammatory periodontal cyst, periapical cyst, dental cyst, lateral inflammatory periodontal cyst
    b. Rushton's bodies may be found in the lining, particularly in residual radicular cysts
    c. Cholesterol crystals are commonly found in the cyst fluid, which appears to shimmer on aspiration as a result
    d. Is thought to enlarge by hydrostatic pressure
    e. Occurs more commonly in relation to the root of the maxillary central rather than lateral incisor tooth

Extended matching items

EMI 1. Theme: Pathology of cysts in the oro-facial region

Options:

A Radicular cyst
B Odontogenic keratocyst
C Nasopalatine duct cyst
D Stafne cavity
E Dentigerous cyst
F Paradental cyst of Craig
G Gingival cyst
H Botryoid cyst
I Aneurysmal bone cyst
J Solitary bone cyst

Lead in: Match the description from the list below that is most appropriate for each diagnosis above.

1. A radiolucent lesion found incidentally on a dental panoramic radiograph in a 30-year-old man. The cyst was located in the lower premolar and molar area above the inferior alveolar canal and showing a scalloped outline where it extended between the roots of the teeth. All teeth in the area were vital and the lamina dura was intact. Clear straw-coloured fluid was aspirated from the lesion.
2. A 26-year-old African patient presented with a rapidly growing lesion that expanded the maxilla. There was bone destruction on the radiograph and therefore malignancy was suspected. On biopsy the lesion was intra-osseous and was cavitated. There was profuse bleeding and a small biopsy of the lining was taken. The pathologist reported osteoclast-like giant cells and granulation tissue with blood clot.
3. A pear-shaped and well-circumscribed radiolucent lesion with a corticated outline was found on a radiograph related to the root of an upper central incisor. The tooth was not restored and proved vital on testing.
4. A cyst was enucleated from the posterior mandible of a 38-year-old man. The pathologist reported that the lining was composed of stratified squamous epithelium that showed parakeratosis and basal-cell palisading. Some areas were inflamed and cholesterol nodules were noted.
5. A cyst was removed along with an unerupted third molar tooth. The pathologist reported a fibrous capsule that was myxoid in places and that was lined by a thin layer of squamous and cuboidal epithelium. The cyst originated from the amelocemental junction.
6. A multilocular radiolucent lesion was found in the interdental bone between the lower first and second premolars. The teeth were vital and after enucleation the pathologist reported that the cyst had features of a developmental periodontal cyst lined by squamous epithelium with focal thickened areas.
7. A 1-week-old girl was referred by the paediatrician because of white nodules on her mandibular alveolar ridge.

8. A well-circumscribed radiolucent lesion with a corticated outline was found on a radiograph related to the root of an upper lateral incisor. The tooth was not restored but was slightly discoloured.
9. A radiolucent lesion found incidentally on a dental panoramic radiograph in a 30-year-old man. The cyst was located in the mandible below the inferior alveolar canal. It was roughly triangular in outline. Teeth in the area appeared vital.
10. A cyst was removed along with a partially erupted third molar tooth following three episodes of pericoronitis. The pathologist reported a heavily inflamed fibrous capsule that was lined by a layer of squamous epithelium that formed loops and arcades. The cyst originated from the buccal aspect of the molar furcation.

EMI 2. Theme: Pathology of soft-tissue cysts in the oro-facial region

Options:

A Dermoid cyst
B Thyroglossal tract cyst
C Branchial cyst
D Epidermal cyst
E Cystic hygroma

Lead in: Match the description from the list below that is most appropriate for each diagnosis above.

1. A 44-year-old man presented with a swelling in the midline floor of the mouth that elevated the floor of mouth and tongue. The mucosa over the cyst was yellowish in colour.
2. A 38-year-old man presented with a fluctuant swelling just anterior to the border of the sternocleidomastoid muscle.
3. A 25-year-old man presented with an anterior midline cystic swelling in the neck. When he protruded his tongue the cyst elevated.
4. A 2-week-old child had a slow-growing cystic cervical mass. The lesion had been diagnosed by ultrasound before the child was born.
5. A 54-year-old woman developed an unsightly cyst on the cheek skin which oozed cheesy material.

Case history questions

Case history 1

A 35-year-old man presents with painless expansion of the buccal aspect of the mandible in the third molar area. A dental panoramic radiograph reveals a multilocular radiolucent cystic lesion extending into the horizontal and ascending ramus. The third molar is absent.

1. What is the most likely diagnosis?
2. What advice might be given to the patient when seeking informed consent for surgical removal of this cyst?

3. Describe the cytological and biochemical features of the cyst content. What are the histological features of the lining epithelium?

Case history 2

An elderly man presents with a fluctuant blue cystic swelling in the anterior mandible. He wears complete dentures and recalls having had a cyst removed from the left side of his mandible many years ago. Radiographs showed that the residual bone in the anterior mandible is extremely thin.

1. It was felt appropriate to treat the cyst by marsupialisation. What are the indications for this in the above case?

The cyst lining is submitted for histopathological examination and is reported as consistent with residual cyst.

2. What features may be present in the biopsy tissue?
3. Is the history of this patient having had a previous jaw cyst significant?

Case history 3

A 22-year-old woman presented with a rapidly growing swelling expanding the ascending ramus of the mandible. The radiologist reported a destructive radiolucent lesion and was concerned that the lesion might be malignant. A biopsy was suggested. In theatre, there was profuse haemorrhage on opening the lesion and a small biopsy was taken before rapid closure was affected.

1. What is the most likely diagnosis?

The pathologist reported finding multinucleated giant cells, loose granulation tissue and areas of tissue resembling a fibro-osseous lesion.

2. What interpretation can be made of these appearances?
3. What approaches to treatment might be considered?

Short note questions

Write short notes on:

1. Imaging methods available for cysts of the jaw
2. Surgical treatment of periapical radiolucency
3. A radiolucency at the anterior of the maxilla
4. Marsupialisation as a surgical management for cysts

Essay questions

1. Give an account of odontogenic cysts
2. Discuss the clinical, histopathological and radiological differential diagnoses of a radiolucency at the angle of the jaw
3. Give a classification of cysts of the jaws and describe in detail the radiological and histopathological features of odontogenic keratocyst
4. An edentulous man aged 60 has a large cyst in his mandible requiring enucleation. Discuss the preoperative investigations that would be carried out, explaining the rationale for each, and describe the information that you would give the patient before he consents to the operation

Viva questions

1. What features of aspirates may help in the diagnosis of a suspected cyst?
2. How does an intra-osseous cyst cavity repair after enucleation?
3. What are the features of a branchial cyst?
4. Which odontogenic tumours may have similar presenting features to cysts in the jaws?
5. How do cysts enlarge?

Self-assessment: answers

Multiple choice answers

1. a. **False.** Soluble protein content may be greater than 40 g/l if the cyst is infected, with an inflammatory exudation, but levels of 40 g/l or less are typical of odontogenic keratocyst.
   b. **False.** Odontogenic keratocysts are found in basal-cell naevus syndrome, caused by alterations in the gene PCTH. Mutations in *APC* cause familial adenomatous polyposis.
   c. **False.** An odontogenic keratocyst enlarges by displacing medullary bone in a non-uniform growth pattern, suggesting that enlargement results from bone-resorbing factors released by the capsule.
   d. **False.** Two-thirds occur at the angle of the mandible.
   e. **True.** Odontogenic keratocysts contain keratotic squames and oily material, imparting a creamy-white semi-fluid texture.

2. a. **True.** Occurs after crown formation.
   b. **True.** This is an important diagnostic feature.
   c. **True.** Associated teeth may be grossly displaced.
   d. **True.** The epithelium is even, either cuboidal or squamous and resembles enamel epithelium.
   e. **True.** This is caused by breaking of the thin layer of periosteal bone that forms over the cyst.

3. a. **False.** The lining may be respiratory or stratified squamous in type, reflecting the oral/nasal cavity origin.
   b. **True.** Fluid leakage is thought to account for this peculiar sign.
   c. **True.** The nasopalatine neurovascular bundle may be damaged or even removed during enucleation. This causes little in the way of clinical problems.
   d. **True.** Tilting may cause 'butterfly' central incisors in children.
   e. **False.** Recurrence is very rare.

4. a. **True.** Expansion of bone to a thin layer prone to cracking is a clinical sign.
   b. **True.** Radicular cysts are associated with a non-vital tooth.
   c. **True.** All have distinct clinical features, however.
   d. **True.** Radicular cysts are thought to grow by hydrostatic pressure rather than through the intrinsic growth characteristics of the capsule.
   e. **True.** This is an important diagnostic clue; mandibular lesions producing buccal and lingual expansion are more likely to be neoplasms than cysts.

5. a. **True.** They occur in the buccal gingivae.
   b. **True.** They appear as white keratinous nodules.
   c. **False.** Gingival cysts rarely exceed 5 mm in diameter.
   d. **True.** Many contain keratin whorls.

e. **False.** In adults, they may rest in a shallow depression in the cortex but they do not extend into bone in neonates or adults.

6. a. **True.** Mucous extravasation mucocoeles are thought to arise from trauma that tears the minor salivary gland duct wall, allowing release of mucinous saliva into the surrounding tissue. They are very rare in the upper lip but are common in the lower lip, presumably because of trauma from the teeth. In general, it is wise to be suspicious that a persistent lump in the upper lip substance may be a tumour or mucous retention mucocoele. Biopsy is necessary to establish the diagnosis (see Ch. 13).
   b. **False.** The term ranula is applied to mucocoeles in the floor of mouth and not the palate (see Ch. 13).
   c. **True.** Dermoid cysts are derived from inclusions of skin in the midline tissues during embryological development. They are lined by stratified squamous epithelium and contain adnexal structures such as hair follicles, sweat glands and sebaceous glands in the capsule. They may elevate the tongue if located above the mylohyoid muscle or may occur as a submental swelling if situated below.
   d. **True.** Lymphoepithelial cyst is also commonly referred to as branchial cyst. (See also Viva question 3.)
   e. **True.** This is an important diagnostic sign. Thyroglossal tract cysts develop from the remnants of the hollow tube that extends from the anlage of the thyroid gland at the base of the tongue to the forming hyoid bone during embryological development. They often present in adult life and surgical removal is advised.

7. a. **False.** The 'cavity' is a depression related to development of the mandible around the submandibular gland.
   b. **True.** The lining is of fine granulation tissue, which may include multinucleated giant cells.
   c. **False.** Extension into the interdental septa is a typical feature.
   d. **False.** Often no treatment is required.
   e. **False.** Multiple giant-cell lesions ('brown tumours') are caused by hyperparathyroidism.

8. a. **True.** Radiological signs are only of a soft-tissue mass.
   b. **True.** It occurs over an erupting tooth.
   c. **False.** Often spontaneous resolution occurs, but fenestration may be necessary.
   d. **False.** The lining may be reduced enamel epithelium, stratified squamous or cuboidal in type, often with mucous metaplasia.
   e. **False.** It usually occurs over a single erupting tooth.

9. a. **True.** Inflammatory cysts developing on the lateral aspects of teeth as a result of proliferation of periodontal pocket lining are referred to as inflammatory collateral cysts. Craig described a cyst that developed on the lateral aspect of third molars as a result of pericoronitis. The inflammatory process is thought to stimulate the reduced enamel epithelium of the dental follicle. Often associated teeth possess buccal enamel spurs. The paradental cyst of Craig has been debated, particularly in relation to its pathogenesis and relation to the infected buccal mandibular cyst of childhood.
    b. **True.** See (a).
    c. **True.** See (a).
    d. **False.** It arises from pericoronal pocket lining, originating from the reduced enamel epithelium. Some authors do, however, favour origin from the epithelial rests of Malassez, but this seems unlikely as paradental cysts do not arise in a uniform distribution around the third molar.
    e. **True.** Paradental cysts often communicate with the pericoronal tissues and some oral pathologists do not regard them as true cysts but rather as 'pouches' of pericoronal collateral tissue.

10. a. **True.**
    b. **True.** Mucous metaphasia also occurs.
    c. **True.** The crystals appear as rhomboids with one 'corner' missing when viewed under the microscope.
    d. **True.** The protein content of the cyst fluid gives it a higher osmotic pressure than that of plasma.
    e. **False.** The maxillary lateral incisor appears to be more commonly involved with a radicular cyst than any other tooth.

Extended matching items answers

EMI 1

1. **J.** Solitary bone cyst is also known as haemorrhagic cyst and it probably arises from bleeding into the mandibular bone with destruction of trabeculae. Removal of the blood by natural processes leaves the cavity filled by air or clear fluid. No intervention is normally required after diagnosis by fine needle aspiration and imaging.
2. **I.** Aneurysmal bone cyst can be dramatic clinically due to rapid growth and attainment of large size. Bleeding can be so profuse at biopsy that transfusion is needed. The cysts often form around an underlying primary lesion such as a vascular malformation or bone tumour.
3. **C.** Nasopalatine duct cyst is a non-odontogenic cyst that arises from embryonic remnants anywhere along the naso-palatine tract. The lining typically shows both respiratory and squamous epithelium and a neurovascular bundle is often found in the capsule.
4. **B.** Odontogenic keratocyst lining shows basal-cell palisading, keratinisation, uniform thickness and the lumen is filled by keratinous material.

5. **E.** Dentigerous cysts form in relation to unerupted teeth from the follicle. The histological features are not defining and clinical features (particularly the origin from the amelo-cemental junction) aid diagnosis.
6. **H.** Botryoid ('like a bunch of grapes') cysts are typically small and develop from odontogenic epithelial remnants in the periodontal ligament, but are not driven by inflammation. Focally thickened epithelial plaques are often found microscopically.
7. **G.** Gingival cysts in a neonate are referred to as Epstein's pearls. Gingival cysts can also occur in adults.
8. **A.** Radicular cyst (periapical, apical or dental cyst) grows by osmotic pressure and is typically rounded and well circumscribed. The discolouration of the tooth suggests loss of vitality. Periapical inflammation is the stimulus. Radicular cyst occurs most frequently in relation to upper lateral incisor teeth.
9. **D.** Stafne cavity is in reality a developmental depression in the border of the mandible that can be confused with a cyst by the unwary.
10. **F.** This distinctive cyst forms in relation to pericoronitis and is often pouch like clinically.

EMI 2

1. **A.** Dermoid cysts arise from developmental midline skin inclusions. In the oral region they may be located above mylohyoid and bulge into the floor of mouth or below mylohyoid where they expand into submental soft tissue. Histological examination shows the lining to resemble epidermis and adnexal structures including hair follicles, sebaceous glands and smooth muscle are also present.
2. **C.** Branchial or lymphoepithelial cysts typically present in the second and third decades after slow enlargement. They are lined by squamous epithelium and have lymphoid tissue with prominent follicles in the wall. In older patients they may be confused with cystic metastatic squamous carcinoma in a lymph node. Metastatic thyroid cancer can also mimic branchial cyst. The cyst must be carefully examined by the pathologist.
3. **B.** Thyroglossal tract cysts develop at any point from the foramen caecum to the thyroid along the line of vestigal thyroglossal duct. Most occur below the level of the hyoid bone and in people under 30 years.
4. **E.** Lymphangiomatous malformations occur in the cervical region as cystic masses (cystic hygroma). The vast majority are diagnosed in the first 2 years of life.
5. **D.** Epidermal cysts are very common and occur anywhere on the head and neck skin and at other sites. They are lined by stratified squamous epithelium and contain oily keratinous material.

Case history answers

Case history 1

1. Odontogenic keratocyst.
2. The patient should be advised of the risks of possible damage to inferior dental nerve, jaw fracture and recurrence rates of up to 40%.

3. The cyst is expected to contain keratotic squames and the soluble protein content to be less than 40 g/l. The lining is a relatively uniform layer of parakeratinising stratified squamous epithelium 5–10 cells in thickness. The basal cells may be columnar or cuboidal and form a palisaded layer. Orthokeratotic variants are seen. Infection may alter both the biochemical and histological features.

Case history 2

1. Extreme atrophy of the mandible may predispose to fracture. The lower denture can be modified to maintain patency of the cyst opening after marsupialisation. Local analgesia may be used, avoiding the risk of general anaesthesia in the elderly.
2. Residual cysts are typically composed of a fibrous capsule lined internally by stratified squamous non-keratinising epithelium. Inflammation is often not a feature as the initiating inflammatory focus has been removed. The epithelial lining is variable in thickness but often lacks the arcades seen in developing cysts still related to a root apex. Residual cysts frequently contain Rushton's bodies, cholesterol and haemosiderin.
3. It has been suggested that some individuals are cyst-prone, i.e. have a tendency to form a cyst in response to periapical chronic inflammation.

Case history 3

1. The features suggest an aneurysmal bone cyst.
2. The loose granulation tissue and giant cells are consistent with aneurysmal bone cyst. Often such cysts form in relation to another lesion, in this case a fibro-osseous lesion. Other disorders associated with aneurysmal bone cyst in the jaws include haemangioma, giant-cell granuloma and bone tumours.
3. Feeding blood vessels might be identified and embolised, allowing the lesion to be removed and the bone curretted. The pathologist must search for a second pathology and all material removed should be submitted.

Short note answers

1. Intra-oral radiographs initially and then more extensive radiographs as necessary for large cysts. Give examples of radiographs for imaging maxillary and mandibular cysts. Mention that occasionally computed tomography is useful.
2. Necessity for surgery will depend on diagnosis, based on clinical presentation and radiography. Radicular cyst will require endodontic therapy with or without surgical enucleation and apicectomy with retrograde root filling. Describe the surgical procedure and follow-up.
3. The differential diagnosis of a radiolucency at the anterior of the maxilla includes: abscess, cyst, fibro-osseous lesion, benign and malignant bone tumour, odontogenic tumour and metastatic disease. Describe the clinical presentation and investigations, including vitality testing and radiography.

4. Define marsupialisation and then give the indications, surgical technique and the advantages and disadvantages.

Essay answers

For each question an essay plan can be made that would include the sections listed.

1. a. Introduction with definition
   b. Classification based on epithelial origins
   c. Clinical presentation
   d. Radiological and pathological features
   e. Surgical management
   f. Summary.

2. a. Introduction suggesting keratocyst, dentigerous cyst and ameloblastoma as most likely lesions responsible for radiolucency at angle of mandible
   b. Description of clinical presentation
   c. Histopathological description highlighting differences
   d. Radiological similarities and differences
   e. Summary discussing clinical importance of determining diagnosis.

3. a. WHO classification
   b. Odontogenic keratocyst defined and origins discussed
   c. Radiological features
   d. Histopathological features
   e. Summary commenting on the clinical importance of diagnosing this type of cyst because of the particular management required.

4. a. Introduction with definition of a cyst
   b. Investigations, including radiography and possibly aspiration for biochemistry and cytology
   c. General investigations appropriate to the general health of the patient if surgery is to be undertaken under general anaesthesia
   d. Surgical management options: enucleation or marsupialisation
   e. Information relevant to each of these options. Marsupialisation would include the need for long-term care and dressings/obturator. Enucleation would include altered mental sensation, recurrence, need for bone graft, fracture of mandible
   f. General information relevant to surgery: pain, swelling.

Viva answers

1. Usually air or fluid is aspirated:
   - air may be aspirated from the maxillary sinus or solitary bone cysts
   - brown, shimmering fluid containing cholesterol crystals is typical of radicular or residual cyst but may be seen in any cyst
   - creamy-white aspirate containing squames is typical of odontogenic keratocyst
   - when any type of cyst is infected, pus of similar appearance may be found
   - blood is aspirated from aneurysmal bone cysts.

If neither fluid nor air is aspirated, then a solid lesion must be suspected; a neoplasm must be excluded.

2. After enucleation, the cavity fills with blood. Granulation tissue from the endosteum and marrow spaces grows in. The blood clot is removed by macrophages and new woven bone trabeculae form on the cavity walls. These mineralise and remodel, showing up as new bone on radiographs. The corticated margin of the cyst wall also remodels and eventually the normal trabecular architecture is restored.

3. Branchial cysts tend to present as fluctuant swellings in the cervical region just below the upper anterior border of the sternocleidomastoid muscle. They are thought to arise from epithelial inclusions in lymph nodes. Often aspiration biopsy is performed to exclude the possibility of a metastatic cancer with central necrosis or an infective process. These cysts are referred to in pathology reports as lymphoepithelial cysts, as they contain lymphoid follicles in the capsules.

4. Ameloblastoma often presents as a multilocular cystic lesion and other less-common odontogenic tumours can also simulate cysts on radiographs. The adenomatoid odontogenic tumour often resembles a dentigerous cyst around the upper canine tooth.

5. Various mechanisms have been suggested. The radicular cyst grows by osmotic, hydrostatic pressure whereas odontogenic keratocysts and dentigerous cysts may enlarge because of the intrinsic properties of the cyst, which are thought to be similar to those of the follicle. The follicle enlarges naturally in development and this feature may be re-expressed. The aneurysmal bone cyst can enlarge dramatically because of the force of arterial blood. Cysts generally release bone-resorbing factors from their capsules. Often, reactive 'eggshell' bone is found around the capsule as a reaction to this process.

Mucosal diseases

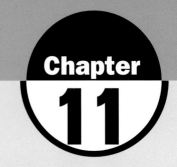

Overview

Oral mucosa shows considerable variation in its normal structure and can be affected by a wide range of conditions. The identification of oral mucosal abnormalities is important because they can be harmless, minor primary conditions and secondary indications of systemic disease. The situation is further complicated by the multiple causes for many mucosal lesions: for example ulceration can reflect simple trauma, a habit tic with psychiatric implications, lichen planus, infection, gastrointestinal disease such as Crohn's disease or a side-effect of a drug.

11.1 Normal oral mucosa

Learning objectives

You should:
- know the structure of the mucosa and what constitutes normal mucosal anatomy.

Three divisions of oral mucosa are recognised.

Masticatory. This is firm, pink and keratinised. It forms the hard palate and gingivae.

Lining. This division is extensible, red and non-keratinised. It forms the buccal and labial mucosa, vestibular, floor of mouth, ventral tongue and soft palate.

Specialised mucosa. This includes filiform, fungiform and circumvallate papillae of the dorsal tongue.

Normal structures

In order to be able to recognise mucosal abnormality it is necessary to be familiar with normal anatomical structures that patients may notice and become concerned about. These include:

- lingual papillae, especially circumvallate papillae
- incisive papilla and rugae, which are easily traumatised
- fordyce granules, which may be prominent in atrophic mucosa
- pterygoid hamulus, mandibular and palatal tori
- lingual veins
- parotid and submandibular duct openings
- mucogingival junction.

Leukoedema

Leukoedema is a variant of normal mucosa. It is a bilateral, diffuse, whitish translucency of the buccal mucosa found commonly in Black and variably in White people. It is caused by intracellular oedema of the prickle cell layer. Recognition of leukoedema is important because it may be mistaken for a clinically significant disorder.

11.2 Conditions related to friction or trauma

Learning objectives

You should:
- understand which diseases are caused by friction/trauma and can be treated by removal of the irritant
- be able to distinguish friction-related hyperplasia from neoplasia.

Frictional keratosis

Chronic mechanical, thermal or chemical trauma may induce a keratinising response in buccal mucosa (which is normally non-keratinising) and hyperkeratosis (excessive keratinisation) elsewhere (Fig. 142). This may occur through activation of keratin genes. The keratin becomes swollen, resulting in a spongy appearance. Diagnosis is clinical and treatment normally involves eliminating the cause and reviewing to ensure resolution. There may be a local cause such as a sharp tooth or it may be habit related. Biopsy is undertaken where doubt exists. The principal histopathological features are:

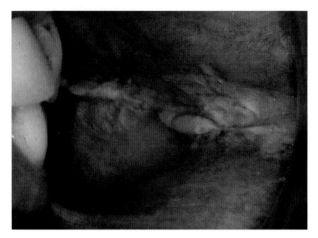

Fig. 142 Frictional keratosis in a patient who habitually chewed the buccal mucosa, particularly when stressed.

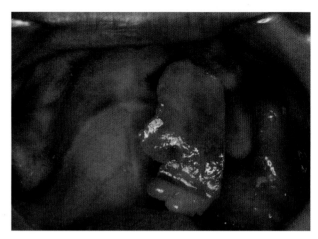

Fig. 143 Leaf-like fibrous hyperplasia of the palate caused by chronic irritation from an ill-fitting upper denture.

- regular epithelial maturation pattern
- hyperkeratosis, usually hyperparakeratosis
- parakeratin layer appears macerated and bacterial plaque is adherent
- acanthosis (widening of prickle cell layer).

Smoker's palatal keratosis

Smoker's palatal keratosis is also known as stomatitis nicotina. It is associated with any smoking habit but tends to be most florid in pipe smokers. The diagnosis is restricted to palatal lesions.

The principal features are:

- palatal mucosa appears white and crazed as a result of keratosis
- red spots occur through blockage of minor salivary gland ducts
- histopathology shows keratin plugs in duct openings
- reversible if smoking habit stopped
- not regarded as a potentially premalignant disorder.

Fibrous hyperplasia and neoplasia

Chronic irritation to the oral mucosa is common and often results in fibrous hyperplasia. Elimination of the cause of irritation may reverse the process, resulting in shrinkage or resolution. Many fibrous hyperplastic lesions are excised, however, because this is a simple and rapid method of treatment. All such tissue should be forwarded for histopathological examination to confirm the diagnosis.

Fibroepithelial polyp

A fibroepithelial polyp is typically a firm sessile or pedunculated polyp that arises most commonly on the labial and buccal mucosa as a result of mechanical trauma from the teeth or dentures (Fig. 143). It is easily excised under local analgesia but will recur unless the source of trauma is corrected.

Histopathologically there is a core of dense fibrous tissue covered by stratified squamous epithelium. The latter often shows keratinisation, reactive to trauma. Secondary ulceration may be seen.

Denture irritation hyperplasia

Denture irritation hyperplasia often forms in relation to denture flanges that have become overextended because of alveolar resorption. Folds of fibroepithelial tissue form in the vestibule. Papillary hyperplasia may be seen in the palatal mucosa covered by a poorly fitting denture.

Connective tissue neoplasms

Connective tissue neoplasms are uncommon in the oral mucosa, but benign tumours including lipoma, neuroma and fibroma may occur and mimic fibrous hyperplasia clinically. Malignant soft tissue neoplasms are extremely rare but may arise from any connective tissue in the oral cavity.

11.3 Ulceration

Learning objectives

You should:
- know the causes of ulceration
- know what drugs are likely to cause ulcers
- be aware of comorbid conditions associated with mouth ulcers
- understand the management of ulcers.

Oral ulceration is commonly caused by mechanical trauma. It is also associated with systemic diseases, drug side-effects and with infections (see Section 11.4).

Traumatic ulceration

An ulcer is a breach in the integrity of the covering epithelium. Traumatic ulceration is common in the oral cavity. The most frequent cause is mechanical injury from the teeth; such ulcers occur on the buccal mucosa, lateral tongue and lower lip in the occlusal plane. Ill-fitting dentures may also cause traumatic ulceration. Ulcers at other sites can be caused by habits (e.g. fingernail picking in children) or even deliberate self-harm. Sharp foodstuffs may cause traumatic ulceration of the palate. Thermal injuries are common at this site from over-hot drinks. Chemical causes of traumatic ulceration include placing aspirin in the vestibule, and rinsing with astringent chemicals. Traumatic ulcers are common on the lower lip and may follow mechanical or thermal injury after inferior alveolar nerve block.

Clinical features

On clinical examination, traumatic ulcers typically are painful and surrounded by erythema. The base is covered by fibrinous exudate and at a later stage by granulation tissue and regenerating epithelium (see Fig. 9, p. 14). Shape and location often give a clue as to the cause. On gentle palpation, traumatic ulcers lack induration and are tender.

Management

Management is to elicit an accurate history, document the features of the ulcer, eliminate the cause if possible, provide symptomatic treatment and review to ensure that healing takes place. Any ulcer that does not heal within 3 weeks should be considered as suspicious and fast-track referred for specialist opinion to exclude carcinoma.

Drug-related ulceration

An increasing number of drugs cause oral ulceration as an unwanted effect. Examples include nicorandil, indometacin (indomethacin) and phenytoin. These tend to produce solitary or multiple ulcers, often recurring at fixed sites. Often a lichenoid pattern is seen in biopsy specimens. Where such a drug reaction is suspected, the possibility of changing the medication believed to be responsible should be raised with the patient's general practitioner, who needs to balance any risks associated with such a change against the benefits to the patient. Cytotoxic drugs cause oral ulceration through toxicity to the rapidly turning over cell population in the oral epithelium. Direct application of legal and illegal drugs for extended periods to the oral mucosa can produce severe ulceration at the site.

Recurrent aphthous ulceration: aphthous stomatitis

Aphthous stomatitis or recurrent aphthous ulceration (RAU) is an extremely common disorder of the oral cavity, estimated to affect 20% of the population. There is some evidence of a familial tendency to RAU. The disorder first manifests in early childhood but more frequently is noticed at around the time of puberty. Three clinical patterns are recognised.

Minor RAU. Ulcers are up to 5 mm in diameter with a yellow–grey base and halo of erythema (Fig. 144). It affects only non-keratinised mucosa. Ulcers tend to occur in crops of two to three but variable patterns are seen, ranging from occasional single ulcers to over 20 at any one time. Individual ulcers heal without scarring in 10–14 days.

Herpetiform RAU. Pinhead-size ulcers occur in crops (Fig. 145). Typically, the ulcers become confluent and healing takes up to 40–50 days. Any mucosal site can be affected. The severity of symptoms is greater than in minor RAU, with some patients experiencing a continuous pattern of ulceration.

Major RAU. Ulcers progressively enlarge and can be up to 3 cm in diameter (Fig. 146). They can persist for up to 3 months and often heal with scarring. Any mucosal site can be involved; often the oropharynx is affected. This causes particularly severe symptoms, including pain on swallowing and gagging.

Aetiology

The aetiology of RAU is unknown, though there are strong associations with having a family history of RAU, stress, smoking cessation and haematinic deficiency. RAU is also seen in gastrointestinal disease, particularly Crohn's disease (which may involve the oral mucosa directly or induce oral ulceration secondary to malabsorption), coeliac disease and other disorders of malabsorption. Oral ulceration is additionally observed in immunological disorders. Behçet's disease is a multisystem autoimmune disorder for which RAU is one of the major diagnostic criteria. Classically, it is accompanied by genital ulceration and eye lesions (e.g. uveitis); however, the skin, joints, gastrointestinal tract, blood vessels and central nervous system may also be affected in various combinations. Severe unusual RAU is a recognised manifestation of infection with the human immunodeficiency virus (HIV).

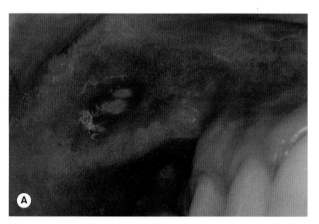

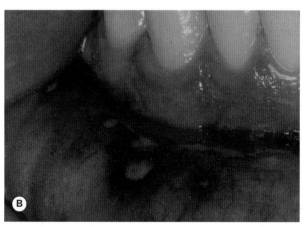

Fig. 144 Minor recurrent aphthous ulceration. Crops of ulcers up to 5 mm in diameter may involve the lining mucosa.

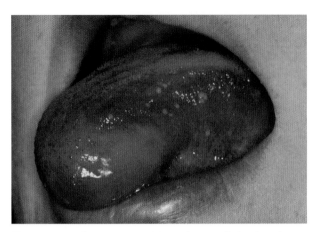

Fig. 145 Herpetiform recurrent aphthous ulceration. Pinhead-sized ulcers tend to become confluent with time.

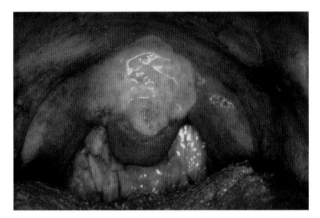

Fig. 146 Major recurrent aphthous ulceration. Ulcers tend to occur in the posterior part of the oral cavity and oropharynx.

Diagnosis

The diagnosis of RAU is made on clinical grounds. Because of its association with disease of the gastrointestinal tract, specific enquiry should be made into signs and symptoms of gastrointestinal problems. Similarly, the possibility of Behçet's disease leads to enquiry concerning the presence of other signs and symptoms of this disease. A full blood count and haematinics (serum vitamin B_{12}, ferritin (an iron-binding protein), folate and red blood cell folate) should be carried out. Where vitamin B_{12} deficiency is detected, the possibility of pernicious anaemia should be investigated by checking the blood for antibodies to intrinsic factor. Low levels of folate, often accompanied by low ferritin, are suggestive of coeliac disease (even in childhood) and the patient's blood should be checked for the presence of endomyseal or transglutaminase antibody. An increasing number of adult RAU patients with mild coeliac disease are identified nowadays. Other causes of folate deficiency (e.g. alcoholism) and vitamin B_{12} deficiency (e.g. diet) should also be considered. The most common cause of a low ferritin level is chronic blood loss. While correction of haematinic deficiencies can bring about resolution or improvement of the patient's oral ulceration this is pointless if the underlying cause of the deficiency is not addressed.

Management

It is difficult to prevent ulceration from occurring in susceptible individuals; however, limiting trauma to the oral mucosa by eliminating sharp foods, in particular crisps, from the diet can be of benefit. Similarly, where trauma from the teeth as a result of parafunctional habits is suspected, the provision of a soft bite guard for night-time wear may help. Unfortunately, the treatment of RAU lacks a robust evidence base. In terms of medication, some relief of symptoms may be obtained by the use of benzydamine mouthwash or spray. Both chlorhexidine and tetracycline mouthwashes can be of benefit; the latter seems to be of particular value in the treatment of herpetiform ulceration. Topical steroid preparations are widely used (see Section 11.5) and hydrocortisone lozenges seem to be particularly effective, if used on a daily basis, when episodes of ulceration are frequent. For severe cases, systemic medication is indicated, for example thalidomide, colchicine or systemic steroids; such agents should only be prescribed by a hospital-based specialist.

11.4 Infections

Learning objectives

You should:
- know the bacterial, viral and fungal infections that affect the oral mucosa
- be aware of the lesions associated with human immunodeficiency virus (HIV)
- understand the features of oral candidiasis.

Bacterial infections

Bacterial infections of the oral mucosa are rare. *Treponema pallidum* causes syphilis and mucosal lesions include primary chancres, secondary snail track ulcers and tertiary areas of focal necrosis (termed gumma). Syphilitic leukoplakia may also result. Tuberculosis infection is usually secondary to pulmonary lesions and presents as granular ulceration of the posterior palate and dorsal tongue. Raised red–white mucosal plaques termed lepromas are seen in established leprosy.

Viral infections

Herpes simplex

Oral involvement in herpes simplex (HSV) infection is commonly encountered, especially in children, and is most often due to HHV-1 (Fig. 147).

Primary herpetic gingivostomatitis

Initial infection results in primary herpetic gingivostomatitis. Grey blisters, which rapidly break down to form small ulcers, may be present anywhere on the oral mucosa and most frequently involve the gingivae. Crusted blisters may also appear on the circumoral skin. Infection is usually accompanied by a febrile illness, and bilateral tender cervical lymphadenopathy is frequently present. Infection

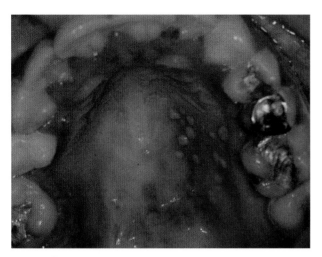

Fig. 147 Primary herpetic gingivostomatitis, showing vesicles and erythema of the palatal mucosa and gingivae.

can be spread to the fingers and conjunctiva by direct contact with the oral lesions, and advice should be given to avoid this. Resolution occurs within 2 to 3 weeks. Rest, maintaining fluid intake, chlorhexidine mouthwash to prevent secondary infection of the oral lesions and advice about cross-infection risks should be given. Infants under 6 months are at special risk of developing central nervous system infection and contact with infected siblings should be avoided. Prescription of systemic acyclovir is only of benefit in the early stages of the infection; a reasonable guide to this is the presence of intact vesicles. Diagnosis is usually made on clinical grounds, where doubt exists, serology performed on samples of acute and convalescent (2–3 weeks after onset of symptoms) blood should reveal a significant rise (of the order of fourfold or greater) in IgG antibodies against HSV in the later sample. Swabs, for culture or identification of viral DNA by polymerase chain reaction (PCR), and smears for cytology (showing ballooning of epithelial nuclei and/or multinucleate epithelial cells) may be useful but usually only if taken early in the course of the disease, ideally from an intact vesicle.

Herpes labialis (cold sores)

After primary infection, HHV-1 may remain in the trigeminal ganglion and low levels of virus are shed into the axoplasm thereafter. Local factors, such as exposure of the lip to intense sunlight, and systemic factors, such as depressed general immunity, result in herpes labialis (cold sores) in about 20–30% of individuals. Crusted vesicular patches appear on the lips, nose and circumoral skin. Acyclovir or pencyclovir cream applied immediately to new sores is an effective therapy. In a small number of individuals, recurrent intra-oral HSV infection may occur, lesions most commonly affect the hard palate and attached gingivae. Severe recurrent HSV infection may occur in the immunocompromised and further investigation to exclude this possibility should be performed.

Herpes zoster

Herpes zoster (HHV-3), the causative agent of chickenpox and shingles (Ch. 14), may involve the oral mucosa. Shingles tends to affect one or more dermatomes of the trigeminal nerve and is an important cause of facial pain. In the oral mucosa, rashes of grey vesicles restricted to the distribution of the sensory nerves are seen. High-dose systemic acyclovir or famcyclovir is usually prescribed.

Coxsackievirus

Coxsackieviruses cause hand, foot and mouth disease and herpangina. These manifest as vesicular eruptions and the management is conservative. Lifelong immunity is normally conferred.

Epstein–Barr virus

Epstein–Barr virus (HHV-4) causes hairy leukoplakia (see below).

Human papillomavirus

Human papillomaviruses produce focal proliferative lesions referred to as squamous papillomas (warts). They may be sessile or show finger-like projections. Histologically, fronds of keratotic squamous epithelium are supported by delicate fibrovascular stroma. Papillomas on the fingers can be the source of human papillomavirus, particularly for lesions on the lips and circumoral skin. Orogenital transmission is also possible. Intra-oral papillomas can be readily excised under local analgesia. HPV types 16 and 18 are an important cause of oral and particularly oro-pharyngeal carcinoma (see Ch. 12).

Human immunodeficiency virus

Initial infection by HIV may be asymptomatic or may cause a febrile illness with diarrhoea. An oral eruption clinically similar to primary herpetic stomatitis may occur at this time.

Numerous manifestations of established HIV infection are recognised. There are several with strong associated oral manifestations.

Kaposi's sarcoma. This is caused by human herpesvirus 8 (HHV-8), which is endemic in Mediterranean regions. Initial mucosal lesions are flat brown spots, which show haemosiderin deposition and vascular proliferation on biopsy. They progress into raised plaques and then nodular purple–red lesions, most often found on the palate, retromolar areas and gingivae. Oral lesions may precede the appearance of skin lesions.

Hairy leukoplakia. This lesion has been associated with progression from HIV infection to AIDS (acquired immunodeficiency syndrome) as the CD4 T lymphocyte count falls. It is caused by proliferation of Epstein–Barr virus (HHV-4) in the lateral tongue epithelium and rarely elsewhere in the oral cavity. Warty ridged or smooth white plaques are typical: sometimes extended papillary projections are seen. The lesion is also found in HIV-negative immunosuppressed patients, for example in renal transplant recipients. No treatment is required and the lesion is not premalignant.

Erythematous candidiasis. This is a frequent manifestation of HIV infection. It presents as white speckles on an erythematous background. Tongue and palate are frequently affected. Treatment can be a problem because of the development of resistant fungal strains in some patients. Hyperplastic and pseudomembranous forms of candidiasis are also common in HIV infection.

HIV-related gingivitis. This may resemble acute necrotising ulcerative gingivitis or present as a red lesion, termed linear gingival erythema.

HIV-related periodontitis. This manifests as unusual focal alveolar destruction. Severe alveolitis and osteomyelitis with sequestration of teeth and surrounding tissue may be seen in patients with advanced AIDS.

Other mucosal manifestations in HIV infection. Purpura results from thrombocytopaenia; bacillary angiomatosis, atypical ulceration, melanotic pigmentation, unusual infections and multiple viral papillomas are also seen.

Fungal infections

Candida albicans is the most common cause of fungal infection in the oral cavity (Fig. 148). It is a commensal organism carried by roughly half the population and disease is caused by opportunistic overgrowth. Oral candidiasis has been described as the 'disease of the diseased'. Local or

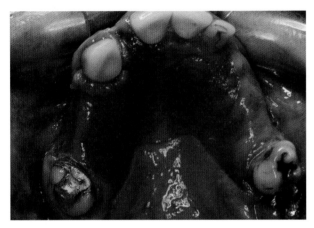

Fig. 148 Denture-related stomatitis. The oral mucosa of the denture-bearing area is erythematous, oedematous and hyperplastic. *Candida albicans* was recovered from the fitting surface of the denture.

systemic predisposing factors should be identified and corrected whenever possible (Table 13). Diagnosis is generally based on clinical features and can be confirmed by laboratory methods using material from oral swabs, smears or rinses. Where quantification is required, saliva samples, the oral rinse or the imprint culture techniques may be used. Other *Candida* sp. may also cause oral infection, particularly in the immunocompromised.

Treatment is based on the use of topical antifungal agents. Amphotericin is available in the form of lozenges and nystatin in the form of a suspension. Patients suffering from **xerostomia** may find the latter or miconazole gel more pleasant to use; similarly this gel is convenient for the treatment of denture-induced stomatitis as it can be applied directly to the fitting surface of the denture. In addition to the use of an antifungal agent, the patient should be advised to leave the denture out at night. Acrylic dentures should be soaked overnight in a 0.1% solution of hypochlorite. If a cobalt chromium denture is worn, it should be soaked for 15 minutes twice daily in chlorhexidine. These measures should eradicate those microorganisms adherent to the denture, which may be more heavily colonised than the mucosa.

Systemic antifungal agents (e.g. fluconazole) should be reserved for those cases of oral candidiasis where topical antifungal agents are not appropriate. There are an increasing number of reports of resistance to azole antifungal drugs. These drugs play a significant role in the treatment of candidal infections in the immunocompromised. In contrast to nystatin and amphotericin triazole or imidazole antifungal agents, including miconazole, are readily absorbed via the gastrointestinal tract thus care should be taken to check for possible drug interactions.

Angular cheilitis

Candida sp. alone, bacteria alone or a combination of *Candida* and bacteria (*Staphylococcus aureus*, β-haemolytic

Table 13 Classification of *Candida*-related oral lesions

Lesion	Characteristics
Thrush (acute pseudomembranous candidiasis)	Friable white plaques that can be scraped off; often involves oropharynx; affects infants, elderly and immunosuppressed adults
Antibiotic sore mouth	Generalised erythematous and sore oral mucosa; caused by elimination of bacterial competition; related to prolonged use of wide-spectrum antibiotics
Denture-induced candidiasis	Related to continuous wearing of acrylic dentures; mucosa over fitting surface appears erythematous and oedematous; patient should improve denture hygiene and leave dentures out at night
Chronic hyperplastic candidiasis	Fixed, white, folded plaques, commonly behind the angle of the mouth; smoking and poor denture hygiene are common predisposing factors; candidal hyphae invade the parakeratin layer
Erythematous candidiasis	Red patchy areas, typically on palate and dorsum of tongue; associated with low CD4-cell counts, particularly in HIV infection; may be a cause of linear gingival erythema
Angular cheilitis	Crusted cracked lesions at the angle of the mouth; may be infected by *Candida* sp. or *Staphylococcus aureus*; predisposing factors include anaemia and saliva spreading to skin
Median rhomboid glossitis	Lozenge-shaped erythematous patch on the midline dorsal tongue; usually symptomless; epithelial hyperplasia with neutrophils in the parakeratin layer
Mucocutaneous candidiasis	Generalised chronic oral candidiasis resulting in fixed mucosal white patches; immune defect may be detected but sometimes idiopathic; some types associated with endocrine or thymus disease; nails often affected, other mucosal sites may also be involved

streptococci) may cause angular stomatitis. Unless the classic golden yellow crusts associated with *S. aureus* are present, treatment should be commenced with antifungal drugs, e.g. a combined miconazole/hydrocortisone cream (miconazole has some antibacterial properties). When clinical features indicate *S. aureus* infection, fusidic acid cream is appropriate. If intra-oral candidiasis is present, this must be treated concurrently or recurrence of the angular stomatitis will occur. Iron deficiency is a significant aetiological factor in angular cheilitis.

Aspergillosis

Aspergillus sp. infection is sometimes encountered in the maxillary sinus in severe immunosuppression or in association with zinc-containing endodontic material inappropriately extruded through the roots of maxillary molars.

Chronic hyperplastic candidiasis

Oral white and red lesions may be seen in oral infections with *C. albicans*. Chronic hyperplastic candidiasis is a particular form of candidiasis that presents as a persistent white plaque that cannot be scraped off. Smoking and continuous denture wearing are the main predisposing factors, although the condition may also be associated with reduced immunity.

Clinical features

- Dense white rough or nodular patch
- Typically found on the buccal mucosa adjacent to the angle of the mouth
- Often bilateral, may be multifocal
- Associated with smoking and poor denture hygiene habits.

Histopathological features

- Epithelial acanthosis and parakeratosis resulting in broad, blunt rete processes
- Candidal pseudohyphae penetrate the parakeratin layer
- Neutrophils form microabscesses in the parakeratin layer
- Intense diffuse chronic inflammatory infiltrate present in the lamina propria
- May regress following elimination of local predisposing factors and antifungal therapy (often systemic antifungal drugs are used)
- If microscopic dysplasia found (~40% cases) then the lesion may be clinically classified as **candidal leukoplakia**.

Median rhomboid glossitis

Median rhomboid glossitis is an abnormality of the midline dorsal tongue where a lozenge-shaped, smooth or nodular red flecked area of depapillated mucosa is found. A corresponding area of erythema may be present on the palate. It is often (but not always) associated with candidal infection and *Candida* can often be recovered. Further investigation and treatment are usually unnecessary. Treatment, with topical antifungal agents, is only normally indicated if the lesion gives rise to discomfort.

11.5 Lichen planus

Learning objectives

You should:
- know the types of lesion that can occur
- know how to diagnose lichen planus
- understand the possible aetiology and, therefore, the management.

Lichen planus is a common condition affecting around 1% of the population and involving skin and mucous membranes. The peak incidence is in the third to sixth decades, 60% in females.

Clinical features

Oral lesions

Oral lesions are classically bilateral and affect the buccal mucosa and lateral aspects of tongue; gingivae may show red atrophic appearance ('desquamative gingivitis'). The palatal mucosa is usually spared. Atypical distribution of lesions is suggestive of a lichenoid reaction; the possibility of lupus erythematosus should also be considered in these circumstances. Three clinical variants of oral lichen planus are recognised:

- non-erosive type: most common, typically painless
- minor erosive type: areas of redness and superficial ulceration
- major erosive type: atrophy, redness and extensive ulceration.

Oral lesions of various types may occur in any of the variants of lichen planus:

- reticular lesions: network or linear white bands (Fig. 149)
- plaque lesions: white patches
- papular lesions: small white spots, which may join up
- annular lesions: circular arrays of white lines
- atrophic lesions: diffuse red areas
- erosive lesions: extreme atrophy leading to ulceration (Fig. 150)
- bullous lesions: blood-filled blisters, rare type.

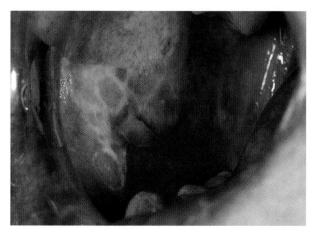

Fig. 149 Lichen planus, showing typical reticular lesions.

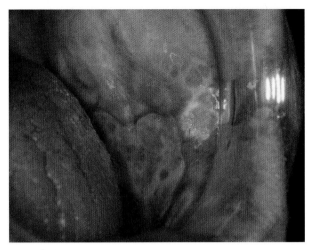

Fig. 150 Lichen planus showing erosive and superficially ulcerated lesions.

Skin lesions

Skin lesions are classically violaceous, itchy macules and papules on the flexor surfaces. The papules show distinctive white lines, termed Wickham's striae. They may be more widespread on the trunk. Fingernails may be ridged or atrophied. The scalp may be involved, leading to hair loss. In females, the vulva and, far less commonly, the vagina may be affected.

Lichenoid mucositis

Lichenoid mucositis is a clinical term for conditions that have similar clinical features, such as lichenoid reaction (drugs and restorative materials), lupus erythematosus and graft-versus-host disease. Lichenoid reaction due to amalgam is increasingly recognised clinically where restorations are in direct contact with the oral mucosa.

Histopathological features

Appearances vary and successful diagnosis depends on adequate biopsy from a representative site (Fig. 151):

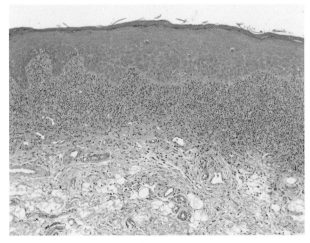

Fig. 151 Lichen planus, showing the subepithelial band of lymphohistiocytic infiltrate and basal-cell degeneration.

- epithelium varies in thickness and may show keratosis or atrophy
- subepithelial band of T lymphocytes and histiocytes
- T lymphocytes 'cross' the basement membrane into epithelium
- basal-cell liquefaction and degeneration
- apoptosis of basal cells results in Civatte (colloid) bodies
- 'sawtooth' rete processes, typical of skin lesions, not always seen.

Ulceration may alter the characteristic features.

Aetiology

The cause of lichen planus is not known, though it has been linked with hepatitis C infection in southern European peoples. Skin lesions tend to be transitory, while oral lesions are more persistent. Non-erosive lichen planus is often not symptomatic. Biopsy is required, however, to establish a tissue diagnosis. Erosive lichen planus is also considered as a premalignant condition and appropriate advice about alcohol, paan and tobacco as risk factors for oral cancer should be given. Regular review may be required in some cases.

Management

Treatment is indicated for those patients who experience oral discomfort. It is important that patients appreciate that such treatment should alleviate their symptoms but will not 'cure' the condition, which may persist for several years. Treatment should be adjusted to match the fluctuations in disease severity that characterise oral lichen planus. Modification of diet by avoiding foods that are acidic, spicy, salty or that have a rough texture can reduce discomfort at meal times, and changing to a bland toothpaste makes good oral hygiene easier to maintain. The latter is particularly important when the gingivae are involved as plaque and calculus act as aggravating factors. Mild symptoms may be controlled by the use of an analgesic mouthwash or spray such as benzydamine hydrochloride; however, topical steroids are often required. These are available as:

- pastes, e.g. triamcinolone dental paste
- lozenges to be dissolved in the mouth, e.g. hydrocortisone lozenges
- soluble tablets used to make up a mouthwash, not to be swallowed, e.g. betamethasone sodium phosphate
- inhalers sprayed onto the affected areas, e.g. beclomethasone diproprionate.

If the latter two types of preparation are felt to be necessary, a specialist oral medicine opinion should be sought prior to their prescription.

Choice of medication is determined by disease severity and the sites involved. If the painful lesions are localised to one or two areas that are easily accessible to the patient, then triamcinolone paste is a reasonable choice. If, however, the lesions are generalised, then a steroid mouthwash would be more appropriate. For severe cases, systemic medication is indicated, for example systemic steroids in combination with the immunosuppressant azathioprine, which should only be prescribed by a hospital-based specialist.

Where a lichenoid drug reaction is suspected, the possibility of changing the medication believed to be responsible should be raised with the patient's general practitioner, who needs to balance any risks associated with such a change against the benefits to the patient. Patch testing to restorative materials can be carried out but may not always be indicated if there is a close anatomical relationship between the restorations and the patient's lesions. Again the decision to replace any restoration must take into account the possible benefits to the patient.

11.6 Pigmented lesions

Pigmentation of the oral mucosa can be extrinsic or intrinsic. Extrinsic pigmentation is usually easily recognised and common causes are regular chlorhexidine rinsing and paan chewing, which produces an orange–brown discoloration. Natural racial oral pigmentation is prominent in dark-skinned races and sometimes can be a confusing finding in individuals of mixed race.

Black hairy tongue

Black hairy tongue is caused by overgrowth of filiform papillae accompanied by bacterial pigmentation from commensal flora. In reality, it is often brown in colour and, although harmless, may cause anxiety for the patient. Increasing friction to the dorsal mucosa by gentle rubbing with a toothbrush or sucking a peach stone can be effective remedies.

Amalgam tattoos

Amalgam tattoo presents as an area of grey–black discoloration of the mucosa (Fig. 152). It is caused by entry of dental amalgam into the mucosa at the time of placement of amalgam restorations or during dental extractions. As the amalgam corrodes, particles are taken up by macrophages and collagen fibres become stained by the silver component. The lesion may appear to enlarge clinically.

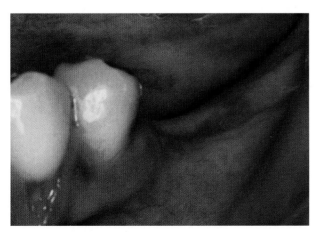

Fig. 152 An amalgam tattoo on the alveolar ridge.

Radiographs will usually reveal amalgam particles in the tissue, but sometimes excision biopsy is performed to exclude a melanotic lesion.

Melanotic lesions

Melanotic lesions can be focal or diffuse.

Discrete melanin-pigmented lesions. Intra-oral pigmented naevi or oral focal melanosis are discrete lesions. Multiple pigmented oral and circumoral macules can be a manifestation of Peutz–Jeghers syndrome. Oral and nail pigmentation is found in Laugier–Hunziker syndrome.

Malignant melanoma. This is a diffuse lesion, presenting mostly on the palate or gingivae as a spreading area of pigmentation, which may evolve into a nodular ulcerated tumour. Early diagnosis can lead to excision and cure but nodular lesions have a poor prognosis.

Diffuse oral melanosis. A diffuse melanosis can be seen in melanin incontinence. This is caused by increased release of melanin in response to chronic irritation, such as smoking, or chronic inflammatory disease involving the oral mucosa. Increased adrenocorticotrophic hormone secretion in Addison's disease may cause diffuse mucosal pigmentation particularly in areas subject to chronic low-grade trauma, e.g buccal mucosa at and around the level of the occlusal plane. Drugs and heavy metal exposure can cause increased oral pigmentation.

Other lesions

Drugs, HIV infection and ingestion of heavy metals can cause oral pigmentation. Blood breakdown products may be deposited in the oral mucosa in jaundice and haemochromatosis.

11.7 Vesiculo-bullous lesions

A vesicle is a small fluid-filled lesion (blister) affecting skin or mucosa; larger fluid-filled lesions are referred to as bullae. Vesiculo-bullous lesions involving the oral mucosa may be seen in:

- viral infections
- traumatic injury
- drug reactions
- genetic disorders
- autoimmune conditions.

Immune-mediated conditions

Benign mucous membrane pemphigoid

Benign mucous membrane pemphigoid (cicatricial pemphigoid) is an autoimmune disease, characterised by blisters and erythematous lesions affecting the oral mucosa, conjunctiva and vulvovaginal region. The oral mucosa may be the only site affected clinically but

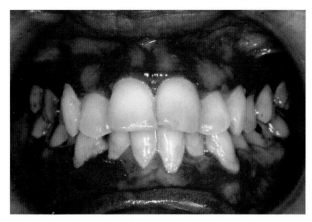

Fig. 153 Desquamative gingivitis. The atrophic, erythematous appearance can be caused by a number of diseases. This example is cicatricial pemphigoid.

examination by an ophthalmologist is always indicated. Pemphigoid may present as desquamative gingivitis (Fig. 153), though other disorders such as lichen planus may also cause red, shiny, tender attached gingivae. Autoantibodies, most commonly IgG, react with a variety of targets around the basement membrane causing loss of adherence of epithelial hemidesmosomes, and formation of a **subepithelial blister**. Laminin V is a common antigenic target, but molecular heterogeneity is recognised and accounts for the variations in clinical features. Diagnosis is based on direct immunofluorescence testing of a fresh biopsy of perilesional mucosa. Circulating autoantibodies may be detected but only if a sensitive indirect immunofluorescence technique is used employing salt-split skin. Specialist referral is necessary when this diagnosis is suspected, particularly in view of the scarring, which may lead to blindness if there is conjunctival involvement. Where oral involvement alone is present, topical steroid treatment may be sufficient to control the disease. As with lichen planus, the maintenance of good oral hygiene is an important adjunct to treatment when desquamative gingivitis is present. When oral lesions are unresponsive to topical steroids, or present in conjunction with other manifestations of the disease, systemic treatment is appropriate. There is evidence for the efficacy of dapsone and drugs drawn from the sulphonamide group of antibiotics, such as sulfapyridine and sulfamethoxypyridazine.

Pemphigus vulgaris

Pemphigus vulgaris is a less common autoimmune vesiculo-bullous disease with life-threatening potential. In approximately 50%, blisters appear first in the oral cavity, but the skin may be involved at the outset or later. The oral mucosa is painful, and blisters appear readily at sites of minor injury. Sloughing may occur and the appearances can resemble a burn. Autoantibodies, most commonly IgG, react with a component of desmosomes called desmogleins, in particular desmogleins 3 and 1. This causes stearic hindrance within the desmosomal attachment and the suprabasal oral epithelial cells separate, forming an **intra-epithelial blister**. Separation in

this way is known as acantholysis. Diagnosis is made by direct immunofluorescence on fresh biopsy or cytological material. Referral to a specialist is essential when this diagnosis is suspected. The use of topical steroids may be of benefit for oral lesions but is only an adjunct to systemic treatment, most commonly with steroids and a steroid-sparing immunosuppressant such as azathioprine.

Other autoimmune conditions

Bullous pemphigoid, linear IgA disease, dermatitis herpetiformis and epidermolysis bullosa acquisita are characterised by the presence of skin lesions but oral involvement is often reported in each.

Erythema multiforme

Erythema multiforme is typified by recurrent bullous eruptions. Crusted haemorrhagic bullae are often seen on the lips, the oral mucosa, eyes and genital area. Target lesions sometimes occur on the skin. Sites may be affected in isolation or in combination. In rare severe disease, there may be febrile illness and hospital admission may be needed. Diagnosis is primarily made on clinical grounds, although the oral lesions may mimic primary herpetic gingivostomatitis. The disorder is believed to be an immunologically mediated hypersensitivity reaction. Attacks may be triggered by recurrent herpetic lesions, drugs or chemicals. During the acute phase, systemic steroids may be prescribed if not contraindicated, and it is important to ensure that fluid intake is maintained. Antiseptic mouthrinses may be used to prevent secondary infection. It is then important to establish the cause and prevent exposure to the causative agent if possible. Prophylactic acyclovir is generally prescribed to prevent herpetic-induced attacks.

Genetic disorders

Genetic disorders where there is derangement of the components of the mucosa may cause oral blisters. An example is one form of epidermolysis bullosa, where there is a mutation of the collagen VII gene resulting in defective anchoring fibrils.

Angina bullosa haemorrhagica

Angina bullosa haemorrhagica is characterised by the appearance of recurrent blood blisters in the oral mucosa. The most commonly affected site is the posterior hard and soft palate, where the blood-filled blisters suddenly appear and may reach 2 cm in diameter. Other sites in the oral cavity can be affected. It is necessary to exclude bleeding disorders and autoimmune diseases, but then patients can be reassured that the condition is harmless. Associations with the use of steroid inhalers applied without a nebuliser, the eating of rough foodstuffs and the taking of very hot drinks have been reported, and these risk factors should be considered in providing advice. Some clinicians advise pricking any fresh lesions with a sterilised needle to release the blood and speed healing. If discomfort is experienced the use of an analgesic mouthwash such as benzydamine hydrochloride may be of benefit.

11.8 Granulomatous disorders

Learning objectives

You should:
- know what a granuloma is and how to investigate it
- know the potential causes of granuloma.

A granuloma is a collection of macrophages in tissue and granulomas are found in a number of local and systemic disorders of the oral mucosa.

Investigation

A deep mucosal biopsy is needed for diagnosis because granulomas may only be seen in the underlying muscle. Granulomas are typically non-caseating and consist of mononuclear macrophages, epithelioid macrophages and Langhans giant cells. Lymphoedema, dilated lymphatic channels and scattered chronic inflammatory cells are also found in the lamina propria, often around small vascular channels. When patients present with the oral features of Crohn's disease, referral to a gastroenterologist or other specialist is necessary.

Causes of granulomas

Foreign body

Foreign-body granulomas can form around implanted materials such as retained sutures, restorative materials and even vegetable pulses, the last sometimes resulting in a proliferative periostitis.

Orofacial granulomatosis

Orofacial granulomatosis is a generic and rather imprecise term used to describe a number of disorders characterised by the presence of granulomas in the oral mucosa. It has been associated with food allergies, such as to benzoates and cinnamaldehydes used as preservatives or flavourings. Minor changes may be present in the gastrointestinal tract on endoscopy.

Crohn's disease

Crohn's disease is a chronic granulomatous disorder of the gastrointestinal tract. Lesions are most common in the terminal ileum. Skip lesions are characteristic. The oral manifestations (Fig. 154) are:

- diffuse swelling of the lips and cheeks
- cobblestone mucosa
- mucosal tags and folds resembling irritation hyperplasia
- angular cheilitis
- aphthous or deep slit-like non-healing ulcers
- granular gingivitis
- glossitis, related to haematinic deficiency.

Sarcoidosis

Sarcoidosis is a multisystem chronic granulomatous disorder affecting predominantly young adults. Pulmonary, lymph node, skin, salivary and eye lesions are most common. Oral lesions present as submucosal nodules, erythema, or granular gingival patches.

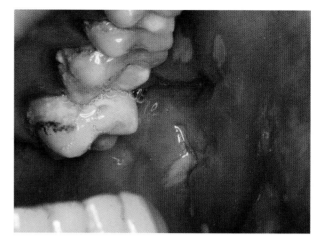

Fig. 154 Crohn's disease, showing cobblestone mucosa and slit-like fissure ulcers.

Wegener's granulomatosis

Wegener's granulomatosis is an autoimmune vasculitic disorder. Strawberry hyperplastic gingival lesions, palatal ulceration and delayed healing may all be presenting signs. Antineutrophil cytoplasmic antibodies (ANCA) can be detected in the circulation. Histopathologically, fibrinoid necrosis of vessels, dense active chronic inflammatory infiltrate and multinucleated giant cells may be found.

11.9 Other mucosal conditions

Learning objectives

You should:
- know how to identify white sponge naevus
- know how to identify geographic tongue
- know how to identify epulides
- be able to differentiate the harmless or minor conditions from potentially serious diseases with similar appearance.

There are a number of harmless or minor conditions that give rise to mucosal lesions very similar to those associated with serious disorders. Some of these have been covered earlier in the chapter in association with the diseases of similar appearance:

- leukoedema
- median rhomboid glossitis
- some pigmented lesions
- angina bullous haemorrhagica.

White sponge naevus

White sponge naevus is an autosomal dominant condition in which the oral mucosa is white, soft and shows irregular thickening (Fig. 155). Often, the entire oral cavity is affected, but the condition may manifest in patches. In some patients, the anus and genital mucosa is also affected.

Eleven

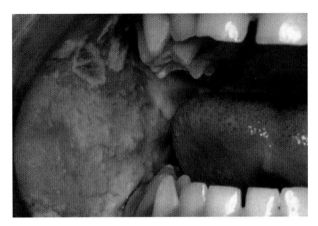

Fig. 155 White sponge naevus. The buccal mucosa appears folded and spongy.

Mutations in keratin genes 4 and 13 have been identified as a cause.

Diagnosis

Diagnosis is by family history and clinical features. The white areas are diffuse and characteristically folded.

Biopsy is only undertaken in cases of doubt; it shows epithelial hyperplasia, parakeratosis and typical 'basket-weave' appearance.

Management

No treatment is needed; patients can be reassured that there is no risk.

Geographic tongue

Geographic tongue is also known as erythema migrans. It is a common benign disorder of uncertain aetiology sometimes associated with soreness and discomfort of the tongue. Irregular smooth red areas with sharply defined edges appear on the dorsal surface of the tongue. These extend, heal and are then replaced by new lesions in other areas. Sometimes a pale white or yellow raised margin is seen. Rarely other areas of the mucosa may be affected.

Diagnosis

Diagnosis is usually based on clinical features alone; biopsy is only undertaken in cases of doubt. The histopathological appearances are of epithelial thinning and active chronic inflammatory inflammation, with neutrophils in the oral epithelium.

Management

Control of symptoms may be achieved by using an analgesic mouthwash such as benzydamine hydrochloride.

Epulides

An epulis is defined as a localised swelling on the gingivae. A variety of diseases may present as a localised gingival swelling, including primary and metastatic cancers and peripheral extensions of underlying bone lesions. For this reason, a radiograph should always form part of the investigations for an epulis and excised epulides should be examined by a histopathologist. Generally the term epulis is reserved for three common reactive lesions, which arise most often in the anterior part of the oral cavity.

Fibrous epulis. This is the equivalent of fibro-epithelial polyp arising on the gingiva. Chronic irritation, from calculus and defective restorations, is a common cause. Fibrous epulis has a core of dense collagenous tissue. Calcification and even ossification may be present and these features are linked with recurrence. The core is covered by epithelium, which may be ulcerated or keratotic.

Vascular epulis. This presents as a red, fleshy gingival swelling, which sometimes has a thick fibrinous crusted surface and a collar of regenerating epithelium at its base (Fig. 156). It is associated with hormonal changes in puberty and pregnancy but may arise as a result of local irritative factors. Growth is usually rapid and recurrence is possible, especially in pregnancy. It is the histopathological equivalent of pyogenic granuloma, being composed of a core of vascular granulation tissue with a variable chronic inflammatory infiltrate and fibrinous crust.

Giant-cell epulis (peripheral giant-cell granuloma). It arises as a red or brown–purple friable swelling. Histopathologically, there are foci of osteoclast-like multinucleated giant cells in a background of fibroblasts and mononuclear precursor cells. A rich vascular plexus composed of thin-walled channels is characteristic. The lesion is covered by mucosa. This lesion must be distinguished from central giant-cell granuloma and hyperparathyroidism; this can be achieved in the first instance radiographically with subsequent biochemical investigations if a central lesion is identified.

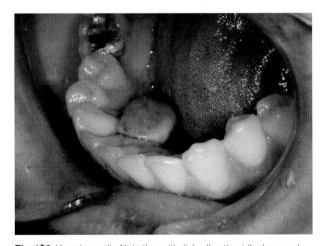

Fig. 156 Vascular epulis. Note the epithelial collarette at the base and ulcerated surface.

Self-assessment: questions

Multiple choice questions

1. In vesiculo-bullous disorders involving the oral cavity:
   a. A positive Nikolsky's sign is only found in pemphigus vulgaris
   b. Mucous membrane pemphigoid is typified by subepithelial bullae
   c. Circulating autoantibodies are present at a high titre in mucous membrane pemphigoid
   d. Mucous membrane pemphigoid (MMP) is the most common cause of desquamative gingivitis
   e. Prompt fixation of a mucosal biopsy is required for successful direct immunofluorescence testing

2. Recurrent aphthous ulceration (RAU):
   a. Affects up to 10% of the population
   b. Usually onsets during the first 2 years of life
   c. Is nearly always related to underlying iron, folate or vitamin B_{12} deficiency
   d. Herpetiform aphthae may involve the hard palate
   e. Severe aphthous stomatitis may be a feature of HIV infection

3. The oral lesions of lichen planus:
   a. Typically exhibit sawtooth rete ridges in biopsies
   b. On the gingiva are most commonly reticular in nature
   c. Are most commonly bilateral and often symmetrical
   d. Are typically associated with a subepithelial band of infiltrating B lymphocytes
   e. Often improve clinically with topical corticosteroid therapy

4. In oral candidiasis:
   a. Most pathogenic *Candida* species involving the oral cavity are dimorphic
   b. *Candida* species never invade the oral epithelium
   c. Diffuse chronic mucocutaneous candidiasis may be associated with endocrine abnormalities
   d. Miconazole can be absorbed systemically from its oral gel preparation (Daktarin oral gel)
   e. *Candida* carriage rates are higher in smokers than in non-smokers

5. Oral manifestations of human immunodeficiency virus (HIV) infection and the acquired immunodeficiency syndrome (AIDS):
   a. Initial infection is not associated with oral manifestations
   b. Hairy leukoplakia is an AIDS-defining lesion
   c. Kaposi's sarcoma is caused by cytomegalovirus
   d. HIV infection may result in salivary gland lesions
   e. Oral candidiasis is the most common oral manifestation of AIDS

6. Gingival enlargements:
   a. Generalised gingival overgrowth may be caused by tacrolimus
   b. An epulis may occur in any part of the oral cavity
   c. Chronic lymphatic leukaemia is the most frequent type of leukaemia associated with gingival enlargement
   d. May be caused by an autosomal dominant gene
   e. Excessive gingival overgrowth in transplant recipients should be trimmed away under local anaesthesia in the dental surgery

7. Mucosal manifestations of systemic disease:
   a. Coeliac-associated recurrent oral ulceration can be detected by testing for α-gliadin autoantibodies
   b. Cobblestone mucosa, fissure ulcers and mucosal tags are found exclusively in Crohn's disease
   c. Chronic iron deficiency may be linked to the finding of oral epithelial dysplasia in mucosal biopsies
   d. Pyostomatitis vegetans is a manifestation of ulcerative colitis
   e. Diffuse mucosal pigmentation may be seen in Addison's disease

8. Herpes virus infections of the oral mucosa:
   a. Herpes simplex virus type II infections may cause primary herpetic gingivostomatitis
   b. Acyclovir cream applied twice daily is the most appropriate treatment for recurrent intra-oral herpes simplex infection
   c. Herpes simplex is an RNA retrovirus
   d. Herpes simplex infection may rarely cause serious gastroenteritis in neonates
   e. Herpangina is a clinical variant of herpes simplex infection that results in painful vesicles affecting the soft palate and oropharynx.

9. White sponge naevus:
   a. Is an autosomal recessive disorder
   b. Is restricted to the oral mucosa
   c. Exhibits hyperparakeratosis, spongiosis and a basketweave appearance in biopsies
   d. Is caused by a mutation in the gene APC
   e. Is a premalignant condition

10. The tongue may:
    a. Become enlarged in amyloidosis
    b. Show migratory glossitis as an indicator of systemic disease
    c. Develop a lozenge-shaped red patch on the midline dorsal mucosa as a result of candidiasis
    d. Become smooth and red as a result of sickle cell anaemia
    e. Become covered by pigmented hyperkeratotic filiform papillae in Peutz–Jeghers syndrome.

Extended matching items

EMI 1. Theme: Pathology of gingival erythematous lesions

Options:

A Lichen planus
B Mucous membrane pemphigoid
C Erythroplakia
D Plasma-cell mucositis
E Pemphigus vulgaris
F Leukaemia

G Linear gingival erythema
H Primary herpetic gingivostomatitis
I Wegener's granulomatosis
J Peripheral giant-cell granuloma

Lead in: Match the case history from the list below that is most appropriate for each diagnosis above.

1. A 55-year-old woman presented with oral soreness progressively worsening over a 3-month period. The attached gingivae were brightly erythematous and small haemorrhagic blisters were seen in places. She also had redness of the conjunctiva and an ophthalmologist found that symblepharon was present.
2. A 60-year-old man presented with velvety red gingival patches. He smoked 10 cigarettes per day and drank 40 units of alcohol each week. An incisional biopsy was reported as showing basal-cell hyperplasia with formation of drop-shaped rete processes and moderate cellular atypia.
3. A 30-year-old woman developed enlarged gingival papillae that were strawberry red. Ulceration of the soft palate was present and she experienced nose bleeds. The cANCA test was positive and a biopsy of mucosal tissue showed vasculitis, multinucleated giant cells and accumulations of neutrophils.
4. A 50-year-old woman developed itchy red-purple raised and flat lesions on her wrists and ankles. Her dentist diagnosed desquamative gingivitis and referred her to an oral medicine specialist. Faint white striae were noticed on the buccal mucosa and a biopsy was performed.
5. A 26-year-old Yemeni man presented with widespread bright red granular lesions on the gingivae and palate. He chewed Khat (Qat) leaf, a habit that is popular in the Yemen. The lesions regressed when he abstained from chewing.
6. A 9-year-old child presented to the dentist with sore red gums, coated tongue, and tender cervical lymphadenopathy of 1 week's duration. On close examination a few recently ruptured vesicles were spotted on the hard palate.
7. A 25-year-old HIV positive man who was non-compliant with therapy presented with redness of the attached gingivae. A direct smear showed a tangled mass of *Candida albicans* pseudohyphae.
8. A 70-year-old man developed enlarged red gingival papillae, with continuous oozing of blood from the crevice. He also had been experiencing haematuria and had been unwell for 3 weeks.
9. A 53-year-old woman presented with an increasingly sore mouth over a 6-month period. The oral mucosa peeled away with light pressure and a biopsy showed suprabasal intra-epithelial splitting.
10. A 38-year-old man presented with an enlarged interdental papilla that was red-brown in colour. An excision biopsy was performed and the pathologist reported the presence of foci of multinucleated giant cells, haemosiderin, thin-walled vessels and red cells in the tissue.

EMI 2. Theme: Pathology of oral mucosa

Options:

A Hairy leukoplakia
B Minor aphthae
C White sponge naevus
D Haemangioma
E Nicorandil-related ulceration
F Smoker's keratosis
G Chronic hyperplastic candidosis
H Fordyce spots
I Amalgam tattoo
J Traumatic ulcerative granuloma with stromal eosinophils

Lead in: Match the case history from the list below that is most appropriate for each diagnosis above.

1. A 63-year-old man with severe angina complained of deep painful and persistent ulcers in the mouth.
2. A 29-year-old man who had had a renal transplant 2 years ago noticed bilateral white plaques and papillary lesions on the lateral borders of his tongue.
3. A 13-year-old boy complained of crops of ulcers affecting the buccal mucosa, vestibule and undersurface of tongue.
4. The parents of a 4-year-old child noticed that his entire oral lining had a white folded appearance. The child had not experienced any oral symptoms.
5. A 60-year-old man presented with an indurated ulcer on the lateral border of the tongue. He was a heavy smoker and a biopsy was taken to exclude squamous carcinoma.
6. A vocational trainee dentist noticed that one of her new patients had widespread areas of 1–2 mm yellowish lesions on the buccal mucosa on both sides of the oral cavity.
7. A 47-year-old patient was referred because the dentist was concerned about a pigmented patch on the alveolus that had increased in size since the patient's last visit.
8. White lesions with a crazy-paving appearance and red spots were noticed on the soft palate of a 53-year-old man. The patient said that he smoked in the past but had given up.
9. A 23-year-old woman complained of pigmented raised lumps on the tongue. On examination these were found to blanch under gentle pressure.
10. A 55-year-old complete denture wearer presented with white lesions on the buccal mucosa at behind the angle of the mouth. On biopsy the pathologist noted acanthosis, hyperrparakeratosis and broad blunt test-tube-shaped rete processes. Microabscesses were present in the parakeratin layer.

Case history questions

Case history 1

A 68-year-old woman developed severe mouth ulcers, some of which tended to recur at the same sites. Her medical history was clear apart from angina, which was poorly controlled. She took 75 mg aspirin daily and nicorandil.

1. How might the drug therapy relate to her oral ulceration?
2. What investigations should be undertaken?
3. Which agents might be prescribed for symptomatic relief?

Case history 2

A 46-year-old schoolteacher noticed white thickening of the buccal mucosa after reading about oral leukoplakia on a health website. He consulted his general dental practitioner who reassured him and referred him for specialist opinion. At the clinic, the specialist found that there were white bands at the level of the occlusal plane on the buccal mucosa and noted marked wear facets on the teeth.

1. What clinical diagnosis is most likely?
2. Why might the teeth show marked wear facets?
3. How could the diagnosis be established without recourse to mucosal biopsy?
4. If a biopsy of the buccal mucosa was taken, which features would you expect to be present?

Case history 3

A 36-year-old bank clerk was concerned about the sudden appearance of blood-filled blisters, which were occurring with increasing frequency on the roof of his mouth. Some reached to 2 cm across and were painful until they burst. He was medically fit and well and his asthma, present since childhood, was well controlled.

1. What is the most likely diagnosis?
2. What investigations should be undertaken?
3. What is the possible link with his asthma?
4. What advice should be given to prevent further lesions?

Case history 4

An 8-year-old boy presented with soreness and crusting at the angles of the mouth. Swabs and smears were taken which revealed *Candida* species and *Staphylococcus aureus* infection. The condition responded well to cream applied daily. One year later he returned with persistent swelling of the lips and on examination was found to have lobulated buccal mucosa, ulceration and red, granular gingivitis. A biopsy of the buccal mucosa was taken and he was subsequently referred to a paediatric gastroenterologist.

1. Suggest suitable creams which might be used to treat the initial complaint.
2. Which condition is present at re-presentation?
3. What might be seen in the biopsy?
4. Why was referral to a physician needed?

Case history 5

Figure 157 shows the buccal mucosa of an Italian member of the tifosi. He was otherwise fit and well although he felt stressed when his favourite motor racing team was losing, at which times his condition tended to flare up. His medical history was clear apart from his having had rheumatic fever and hepatitis C in childhood.

1. What lesions are present on the buccal mucosa?
2. List the features you would expect to see in a biopsy of the buccal mucosa.
3. What is the link with his medical history?

Viva questions

1. What are the common causes of diffuse oral pigmentation?
2. Which topical steroid preparations are available for use in the mouth? How would you advise patients to apply them?
3. What factors should you take into account when taking a mucosal biopsy to aid the pathologist?
4. Why are both swabs and smears taken for the diagnosis of suspected *Candida* infection?
5. How would you manage an elderly patient with submucous fibrosis?
6. What are the three common histological types of epulis?
7. Which mucosal lesions are strongly associated with HIV infection?
8. What are the possible oral manifestations of leukaemia?

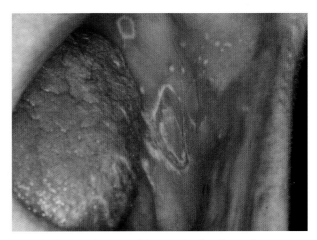

Fig. 157 The buccal mucosa of the patient in Case history 5.

Self-assessment: answers

Multiple choice answers

1. a. **False.** Nikolsky's sign is the formation of a blister when lateral pressure is applied to skin or mucosa. It is found in pemphigus, some forms of mucous membrane pemphigoid and other vesiculo-bullous dermatoses.
    b. **True.** The antigenic targets are located in and around the hemidesmosome/basement membrane complex.
    c. **False.** Sensitive detection systems are required to detect circulating autoantibodies in MMP. Mucosal biopsy is usually performed.
    d. **False.** Lichen planus is the most common cause of desquamative gingivitis. It may also be caused by mucous membrane pemphigoid, pemphigus, plasma cell mucositis and allergic reactions.
    e. **False.** Perilesional mucosa is required for direct immunofluorescence and the tissue must be snap-frozen or submitted to the laboratory in special transport medium.

2. a. **False.** Most estimates suggest that over 20% of the population are affected by RAU.
    b. **False.** Onset can be at any age but most commonly occurs at puberty.
    c. **False.** Haematinic deficiency may be found in up to 25% of RAU patients, in some populations.
    d. **True.** Herpetiform and major RAU may involve keratinised oral mucosa.
    e. **True.** Severe and atypical RAU has been reported in HIV sufferers.

3. a. **False.** Sawtooth rete ridges are characteristic of lichen planus in skin biopsies and are found in less than one-third of oral biopsies.
    b. **True.** Striae may be conspicuous or evident on close examination of gingival lesions in desquamative gingivitis caused by lichen planus.
    c. **True.** Solitary patches of lichenoid mucositis may be a reaction to dental materials.
    d. **False.** The subepithelial infiltrate typically comprises mostly T lymphocytes and histiocytes. A few B lymphocytes may be present.
    e. **True.** Topical corticosteroids are often used to treat symptomatic erosive lichen planus.

4. a. **True.** Most candidal infection is caused by *C. albicans*; other species such as *C. glabrata*, *C. krusei*, *C. tropicalis* and *C. parapsilosis* may cause oral infection. All are dimorphic.
    b. **False.** In chronic hyperplastic candidiasis (candidal leukoplakia), pseudohyphae invade the parakeratin layer.
    c. **True.** Autoimmune polyendocrinopathy syndrome is a rare autosomal recessive disorder; it is one form of diffuse mucocutaneous candidiasis.
    d. **True.** Significant systemic absorption of miconazole may occur and has been reported to potentiate the action of warfarin, resulting in severe purpura.

    e. **True.** Carriage rates are also increased in pregnancy and in denture wearers.

5. a. **False.** Initial HIV infection may be asymptomatic or may be associated with a 'flu-like illness, diarrhoea and a generalised stomatitis.
    b. **False.** Hairy leukoplakia is a warty plaque caused by Epstein–Barr virus overgrowth and occurs in CD4-cell lymphopenia related to HIV and non-HIV disorders.
    c. **False.** Kaposi's sarcoma is caused by human herpesvirus 8 (HHV-8), endemic in Mediterranean regions.
    d. **True.** HIV infection is associated with lymphoepithelial salivary cysts, dry mouth and malignant lymphoma.
    e. **True.**

6. a. **False.** Drug-induced gingival overgrowth (DIGO) is associated with phenytoin, ciclosporin and calcium-channel-blocking drugs such as nifedipine.
    b. **False.** An epulis is a localised swelling of the gingivae.
    c. **False.** Acute leukaemia more typically results in enlargement of the gingivae, through infiltration by leukaemic cells.
    d. **True.** Hereditary gingival fibromatosis is known to be caused by mutation of the SOS-1 gene on chromosome 2p.
    e. **False.** Excessive bleeding has been reported and such cases are best referred for specialist care.

7. a. **False.** Testing for α-gliadin antibody has been replaced by testing for endomysial or tissue transglutaminase antibody. A positive result should trigger referral to a gastroenterologist for further investigation.
    b. **False.** These features may be seen in orofacial granulomatosis.
    c. **True.** This is important particularly in the Plummer–Vinson syndrome.
    d. **True.**
    e. **True.**

8. a. **True.** However, herpes simplex type I is the more common cause.
    b. **False.** Acyclovir cream is not suitable for intra-oral use; systemic acyclovir may be prescribed if necessary.
    c. **False.** Herpes simplex is a DNA virus.
    d. **False.** It may rarely cause encephalitis.
    e. **False.** Herpangina is caused by coxsackievirus A.

9. a. **False.** White sponge naevus is an autosomal dominant disorder.
    b. **False.** It may also involve the anogenital region, nose and oesophagus.
    c. **True.** Biopsy is only made if there is doubt about the diagnosis.

d. **False.** It is caused by mutations in the genes for keratin 4 and 13.

e. **False.** Other very rare forms of hereditary white patch, such as those associated with tylosis and dyskeratosis congenita, are associated with malignancy.

10. a. **True.**
b. **False.** Migratory glossitis (geographic tongue) is not linked to systemic disease.
c. **True.** This is termed median rhomboid glossitis.
d. **False.** A red, beefy tongue is seen in haematinic deficiency.
e. **False.** Black hairy tongue is not a manifestation of a syndrome. Peutz–Jeghers is a syndrome of mucocutaneous melanotic pigmentation and gastrointestinal polyposis.

Extended matching items answers

EMI 1

1. **B.** Mucous membrane pemphigoid can affect the oral cavity, conjunctive and genital mucosa. Testing by indirect and direct immunofluorescence can be helpful in establishing the diagnosis.

2. **C.** Dysplasia and even invasive oral cancer can present clinically as a red patch. All such suspicious oral lesions should be biopsied or referred for consultant opinion.

3. **I.** Strawberry gingival papillae are a classical sign of a vasculitic disease, Wegener's granulomatosis. Ulceration may be present and prompt referral to a specialist unit is indicated.

4. **A.** Desquamative gingivitis is a clinical term describing red atrophic-looking gums. The most common underlying disease process is lichen planus, but vesiculo-bullous disorders can have similar clinical appearances.

5. **D.** Plasma-cell mucositis is a rare condition that affects the oral mucosa and that can extend into the supraglottic larynx. Mature plasma cells expand connective tissue papillae and this can result in a spongy appearance. Allergy to herbal and leaf products may be the cause in some patients.

6. **H.** Dentists may see children with primary herpetic gingivo stomatitis. Small grey vesicles are typical but quickly break down into small ulcers.

7. **G.** Linear gingival erythema is a recognised oral manifestation of HIV infection and is variant or erythematous candidiasis.

8. **F.** Leukaemia may present with gingival swelling or bleeding and may be confused with chronic periodontitis.

9. **E.** Over half of patients suffering from pemphigus present first with oral disease. Autoantibodies against desmoglein 3 occur and cause suprabasal oral keratinocytes to separate, resulting in intra-epithelial blisters. Testing by direct and indirect immunofluorescence may be helpful to establish the diagnosis.

10. **J.** These histological features are typical of giant-cell granuloma. The differential diagnosis should include central giant-cell granuloma and hyperparathyroidism.

EMI 2

1. **E.** Nicorandil is a drug given for intractable angina. Some individuals develop deep painful and persistent oral ulcers, often at fixed sites.

2. **A.** Hairy leukoplakia is caused by proliferation of Epstein–Barr virus (HHV4) in the upper layers of the oral epithelium in immunosuppressed patients. HIV infection or drugs given to prevent transplant rejection can predispose to HL.

3. **B.** Minor aphthae (recurrent oral ulceration) occurs on lining oral mucosa. Ulcers tend to last for less than 2 weeks and rarely exceed 5 mm in size. They are common in children and teenagers. Sudden onset in adult life may indicate an underlying systemic disorder.

4. **C.** White sponge naevus is caused by a mutation in keratin genes (often K4) and is autosomal dominant. No treatment is needed.

5. **J.** Traumatic ulcerative granuloma with stromal eosinophils (TUGSE) is caused by crush injury to tongue muscle. A thick fibrinous crust is present and the deeper muscle fibres are separated by histiocytic cells and eosinophils. Clinically the disorder can mimic carcinoma. Spontaneous resolution with conservative measures is observed.

6. **H.** Fordyce spots are normal sebaceous glands that occur in oral mucosa and oesophagus. In older patients or where atrophy is present they can be quite prominent.

7. **I.** When dental amalgam enters mucosal tissue it can form a pigmented lesion. Corrosion leads to spread of the particles with time and clinically the lesion appears to enlarge. Other causes of discrete pigmented lesions are melanotic macules, naevi and malignant melanoma.

8. **F.** Stomatitis nicotina or smoker's keratosis is a distinctive lesion of the soft palate. The red spots represent salivary duct openings. The lesion is not premalignant. Patients often give an unreliable smoking history.

9. **D.** Haemangiomas are blood-filled developmental lesions and are common in the tongue. Blood can be displaced by pressure or a fine needle can be used to sample contents to confirm the diagnosis.

10. **G.** Chronic hyperplastic candidosis is seen most often in denture wearers and smokers. *Candida* pseudohyphae extend into the keratin and provoke active chronic inflammation. Predisposing factors should be eliminated and systemic antifungal drugs can be prescribed if not contraindicated clinically.

Case history answers

Case history 1

1. Severe oral ulceration has been linked to nicorandil therapy. This is prescribed for uncontrollable angina and often cannot be substituted.

2. A full history should be obtained; full blood count and haematinics would be requested and other investigations may be needed.

3. Benzydamine hydrochloride (Difflam oral rinse or spray) may relieve pain and carmellose sodium (Orabase or Orahesive) may be used as a protective barrier. Topical steroids may be of benefit.

Case history 2

1. The features suggest frictional keratosis.
2. Marked wear facets are often seen in bruxism (habitual teeth grinding); a thickened band is often seen on the lateral tongue and buccal mucosa at the level of the occlusal plane owing to chronic trauma.
3. Provision of a protective splint may reverse frictional keratosis by eliminating mechanical trauma to the mucosa and correcting uncontrolled jaw movements or habitual chewing.
4. Classical histopathological features of frictional keratosis are acanthosis, hyperparakeratosis and maceration of the parakeratin layer with formation of bacterial plaque on its surface. Epithelial maturation is regular.

Case history 3

1. The features strongly suggest angina bullosa haemorrhagica.
2. Full blood count and coagulation screen to exclude a bleeding disorder.
3. A link between inhaled steroids and angina bullosa haemorrhagica has been suggested.
4. Reassure the patient and advise use a nebuliser, rinse out mouth after using inhaler, avoid excessively hot drinks and hard or rough foods.

Case history 4

1. Miconazole nitrate (Daktarin cream) has antifungal and antistaphylococcal activity. It is also available in a combined preparation with hydrocortisone (Daktacort). Nystatin cream may also be used.
2. Lip swelling, cobblestone mucosa, ulceration and granular gingivitis suggest a diagnosis of oral Crohn's disease (orofacial granulomatosis).
3. Mucosal biopsy would show non-caseating granulomas, scattered chronic inflammatory infiltration and dilated lymphatic vessels with lymphoedema.
4. It is important to investigate for Crohn's disease in the gastrointestinal tract.

Case history 5

1. Reticulated lesions of lichen planus are shown. The white lines are often referred to as Wickham's striae.
2. A band-like subepithelial lymphohistiocytic infiltrate, basal-cell liquefaction degeneration, Civatte bodies and sometimes sawtooth rete processes.
3. Hepatitis C infection has been linked with oral lichen planus.

Viva answers

1. Normal racial pigmentation; extrinsic causes such as paan chewing, smoking, chlorhexidine rinses and drugs; intrinsic causes such as melanin incontinence in Addison's disease, haemochromatosis and jaundice.
2. Triamcinolone as Adcortyl in Orabase, hydrocortisone as Corlan pellets, applied as directed in the British National Formulary, and betamethasone as Betnosol mouthwash.
3. A representative area should be selected and the biopsy should be of adequate size and depth. Crushing should be avoided and local anaesthetic solution must not be injected directly into the biopsy site. Normally biopsies are fixed in 10% neutral buffered formalin; at least 10 times the volume of the biopsy must be used. The specimen pot must be labelled and the request card should be completed carefully, providing full clinical details.
4. Swabs are taken to estimate growth, perform speciation and other microbiological tests. Smears are employed for rapid detection of pseudohyphae by periodic acid-Schiff base or Gram staining; this indicates candidal proliferation and is a good indicator of candidal infection.
5. Submucous fibrosis is related to paan chewing. Advice should be given to discontinue this habit and avoid other risk factors for oral cancer. Regular checking of the oral cavity is advised.
6. Fibrous, vascular and giant-cell types. Other disorders, including primary and secondary cancers, can present as a localised gingival swelling.
7. Erythematous candidiasis, hairy leukoplakia, HIV gingivitis, Kaposi's sarcoma.
8. Gingival and mucosal bleeding and purpura from thrombocytopenia; gingival enlargement caused by infiltration by leukaemic cells (especially in acute myeloid types); dry mouth; mucosal atrophy; and ulceration.

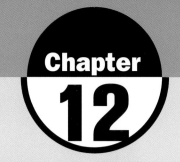
Premalignancy and malignancy

Overview

Cancer manifests in various ways in the oral cavity. It is essential that dentists are able to recognise malignancy and deal with it in a professional way. Premalignant disorders are also important and the terminology used to describe them can be confusing. A rather arbitrary distinction is made between premalignant conditions and premalignant lesions.

12.1 Premalignant conditions and lesions

Learning objectives

You should:
- understand the distinction between premalignant conditions and lesions
- know the oral premalignant conditions
- know the oral premalignant lesions
- be able to advise patients on protective measures and follow-up.

Premalignant conditions

Premalignant conditions are a group of disorders associated with a small increased risk of developing oral carcinoma. The common link is thought to be epithelial atrophy, which may confer greater susceptibility to carcinogens. Atrophic epithelium has altered cell turnover rates and is likely to be more permeable. Patients with premalignant conditions should be advised to eliminate tobacco or paan use and to limit alcohol intake, as these are risk factors for developing oral cancer.

Submucous fibrosis

Oral submucous fibrosis is related to using paan, which is a leaf quid containing areca nut. Many types exist, including fresh products consumed in the Indian subcontinent and southeast Asia as well as packed proprietary products. Tobacco, slaked lime, spices and other ingredients may be added; in southeast Asia, areca nuts are often chewed fresh. The mucosa and teeth become stained orange–brown because paan is held in the mouth for long periods. The affected mucosa becomes pale in colour and feels firm on palpation (Fig. 158). Fibrous bands may develop in the buccal mucosa and a pale, constricting fibrosis typically involves the palate. Mouth opening becomes restricted and swallowing may be difficult. The risk of developing oral carcinoma has been estimated at around 5%, although the risk of submucous fibrosis itself cannot be separated from the risks posed by carcinogenic substances in paan. In biopsy material, a subepithelial band of fine fibrillary collagen is seen in the lamina propria and the oral epithelium can be reduced to only a few cell layers in thickness. Keratinisation and chronic inflammation may be present in some cases. Where areas of erythroplasia and leukoplakia are present, biopsies may show epithelial dysplasia or even carcinoma.

Atrophic lichen planus

Links between lichen planus and oral cancer have been debated. Some evidence links atrophic variants of oral lichen planus, characterised by red areas of mucosal thinning and erosions, with an increased tendency to develop oral cancer. There are no proven associations between oral non-erosive lichen planus or cutaneous lichen planus and malignant transformation. Also a type of epithelial dysplasia known as **lichenoid dysplasia**, in which there is resemblance both clinically and microscopically to lichen planus, has been described. Other forms of **lichenoid mucositis**, such as lichenoid reaction and discoid lupus erythematosus, may additionally be confused with lichen planus. Tobacco or paan use should be discouraged in lichen planus sufferers.

Sideropenic dysphagia

A number of conditions can result in difficulty in swallowing. The association of primary iron-deficiency anaemia and difficulty in swallowing because of formation of a postcricoid fold (oesophageal web) is known as the Patterson–Kelly–Brown or Plummer–Vinson syndrome. Chronic iron deficiency results in generalised mucosal atrophy as iron is an essential growth requirement for the oral epithelium. Carcinoma may develop in the oesophagus and less commonly in the oral cavity.

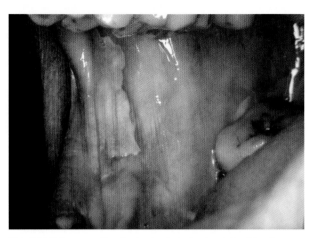

Fig. 158 Submucous fibrosis showing tethering bands involving the buccal mucosa.

Genetic disorders

The rare disorders **tylosis** and **dyskeratosis congenita** predispose to the development of leukoplakia and oral cancer.

Premalignant (precursor) lesions

Precursor oral lesions are areas of morphologically altered tissue in which cancer can arise. Various terms have been used to describe these lesions and diagnosis is often made by exclusion. Many lesions do not progress to cancer and some even regress. It is probable that a proportion of lesions diagnosed as premalignant are actually reactive, and for this reason the term 'potentially premalignant' is often used when considering leukoplakia and erythroplakia. Proliferative verrucous leukoplakia (PVL) is a clinically and histologically distinctive high-risk oral lesion.

Leukoplakia

Various definitions of leukoplakia have been proposed but it is essentially a predominantly white lesion that cannot be characterised as any other definable lesion. Leukoplakia is a clinical diagnosis and has a variable histology.

- Homogeneous leukoplakias are plaque-like lesions with a uniform smooth or wrinkled surface; there is less risk of malignant transformation.
- Non-homogeneous leukoplakias tend to be less circumscribed and show a greater range of appearances. Verrucous leukoplakia has a warty appearance and speckled leukoplakia has interspersed red areas. Heaping up of keratin, nodularity and ulceration may be present. The risk of malignant transformation is greater in non-homogeneous leukoplakia.

The diagnosis can only be made after careful clinical examination with representative mucosal biopsy, as these procedures are essential for exclusion of other defined disorders. A semantic problem exists in that diagnosis by exclusion may 'lump' more than one disease together and depends on which diseases are recognised as 'definable'. The prevalence of leukoplakia varies from 0.2 to 4% and the risk

factors are tobacco, paan, alcohol and possibly candidal infection.

The risk of malignant transformation is difficult to estimate in any individual case. Lesions in the floor of mouth and ventral tongue, and those showing evidence of epithelial dysplasia or carcinoma in situ, are at high risk (Fig. 159). Paradoxically, the risk of malignant transformation is greater in non-smokers than in smokers. Leukoplakia is very rare in non-smokers. The regression of leukoplakia in smokers following cessation suggests that a proportion of lesions are reactive, whereas leukoplakia in non-smokers more often represents a local cellular genetic change that tends to be progressive. However, there is evidence to suggest that smoking cessation in leukoplakia reduces risk, and an appropriate intervention is advised. Multifocal leukoplakia appears to be more risky than solitary lesions.

Other terms for leukoplakia

A variety of terms have been employed to describe precursor oral lesions.

Sublingual keratosis. This term is applied to leukoplakia affecting the floor of mouth and ventral tongue. One reported series described a malignant transformation in over 30% but this has not been confirmed by later studies. The term is not generally favoured because of lack of evidence supporting it as a distinct entity.

Candidal leukoplakia. It is possible for *Candida* pseudohyphae to invade the keratin on the surface of leukoplakia and it may cause a subepithelial chronic inflammatory response. The presence of microscopic dysplasia in this lesion causes concern. Candidal leukoplakia must be distinguished from chronic hyperplastic candidiasis which results in a firm warty or specked plaque that cannot be scraped off. It occurs most commonly on the dorsal tongue and buccal mucosa behind the angle of the mouth. Staining with periodic acid-Schiff's base (PAS) shows pseudohyphae of *Candida* species growing into the keratin layer, where they are typically associated with a neutrophil inflammatory infiltrate. There is marked epithelial hyperplasia with formation of elongated and blunted rete processes. Elimination of predisposing factors such as smoking, poor denture hygiene and haematinic deficiency, combined with systemic antifungal therapy, may cause

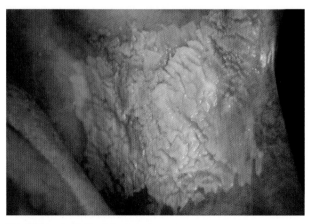

Fig. 159 Leukoplakia of the buccal mucosa.

resolution of the white plaque. Reactive cellular atypia may be seen but if dysplasia is present then the lesion must be considered to be Candidal leukoplakia.

Syphilitic leukoplakia. This is not relevant to contemporary practice but carried a high risk of malignant transformation when it was prevalent. It was a complication of tertiary syphilis and tended to affect the dorsum of the tongue.

Proliferative verrucous leukoplakia. The World Health Organization classification recognises this lesion as a high-risk precursor oral lesion. Minimal cellular atypia is present and greater emphasis is placed on the architecture when making the diagnosis.

Erythroplakia

Erythroplakia has been defined as a bright-red velvety change on the oral mucosa that cannot be characterised as any other definable lesion. There is a high risk of transformation. Histopathologically, erythroplakia tends to show dysplasia, often in a distinctive pattern with drop-shaped rete processes, marked nuclear and cellular pleomorphism and minimal keratinisation. Carcinoma in situ is often seen also.

12.2 Pathology and genetics

Learning objectives

You should:
- know the features of epithelial dysplasia
- understand what is meant by SIN
- know the management of precursor lesions.

Epithelial dysplasia and carcinoma in situ

The term **dysplasia** is used in a variety of contexts in pathology and means literally 'abnormal growth'. In the context of oral precursor lesions, it refers to a combination of cytological changes and disturbances of cellular arrangements seen during the process of malignant transformation. Epithelial dysplasia is graded by oral and maxillofacial pathologists into mild, moderate and severe grades. An alternative scheme uses the term 'squamous intraepithelial neoplasia (SIN 1, 2 and 3 respectively)'. The term **carcinoma in situ** is applied when abnormalities involve the entire thickness of the epithelium; in the SIN system severe dysplasia and carcinoma in situ are combined as SIN 3. The histopathological features recognised in dysplasia are given in Table 14.

Grading of dysplasia

Studies on histopathological grading show poor kappa agreement between even specialist pathologists. This problem arises because of lack of scientific evidence for weighting the various features of dysplasia. For example drop-shaped rete processes are generally accepted as a sinister feature, whereas increased mitotic rate may be seen in reactive processes. Both inter- and intra-observer variabilities between pathologists are high and the biological behaviour of the lesion does not always correlate with its

Table 14 Histopathological features of epithelial dysplasia

Feature	Comment
Nuclear and cellular pleomorphism	Variation in the sizes and shapes of cells and nuclei
Increased nuclear/cytoplasmic ratio	Can be quantified using cytophotometry
Nuclear hyperchromatism	Intense staining of nuclei
Prominent nucleoli	May be larger than normal and/or increased in number
Abnormal mitotic activity	Increased mitotic rate, mitotic figures present above the suprabasal layer, abnormal forms
Basal-cell hyperplasia	Several layers of basal cells may be seen; may result in drop-shaped rete processes
Disturbance of basal-cell polarity	Basal cells lose their orientation; nuclei lose their polarity
Abnormal maturation	Loss of normal stratification pattern; maturation present at inappropriate levels
Aberrant keratinization	May involve individual cells and may result in the formation of intraepithelial keratin pearls

grading. Problems may also arise because of non-representative sampling at the time of biopsy. Although histopathological grading is intrinsically unreliable, the presence of dysplasia in a suspicious lesion remains the best predictive indicator of malignant change.

Tumour suppressor genes and oncogenes

The process of malignant transformation is the result of accumulation of genetic damage. There may be genomic instability or stepwise accumulation of genetic events (Fig. 160). The latter process is thought to operate in most oral cancers and studies have demonstrated mutations, methylation, or loss of various tumour suppressor genes (e.g. p53, p16, p21, retinoblastoma, FHIT) in oral cancers. Loss of function of a tumour suppressor gene confers a selective growth advantage on the cell, resulting in an expanded population in which further genetic abnormalities are thought to arise. Abnormal oncogene activity may increase cell proliferation rates and drive malignant

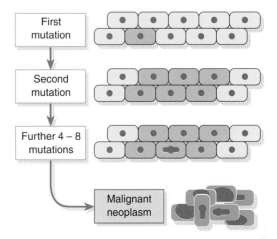

Fig. 160 The multistage hypothesis related to oral cancer.

progression. Dysplasia is likely to represent a histopathological change resulting from genetic alterations. Aneuploidy is a change in the number of chromosomes and is being investigated as a marker of malignant change using cytology methods.

Management of precursor oral lesions

Clinical risk factors for malignant change include tobacco habit, high alcohol intake and possibly poor diet. Clinical factors that must also be taken into account are:

- female gender
- extensive or spreading lesions
- lesions in the floor of mouth/ventral tongue, retromolar area or pillar of fauces
- red, speckled, verrucous or nodular appearance.

Most important is the presence of dysplasia or carcinoma in situ (SIN 3). Management should include:

- clear information and explanation of the significance of the lesion to the patient
- intervention to stop tobacco habit and limit alcohol intake
- treat anaemia and candidal infection if present
- surgical or laser excision or drug treatment may be considered
- regular review and observation: investigation if signs of cancer present.

Referral to a specialist centre is usually advisable for patients presenting with white or red mucosal patches, or other suspicious lesions. Biopsy is normally required for diagnosis and to determine whether epithelial dysplasia is present. Some patients may be followed up in primary care settings.

12.3 Oral cancers

● ●

Learning objectives

You should:
- know the epidemiology and types of oral cancers
- know the clinical and pathological features of squamous-cell carcinoma
- understand the management of squamous-cell carcinoma including its grading.

Most oral cancers do not arise in a clinically recognised premalignant lesion and are diagnosed as primary cancerous lesions. They are typically painless, unless infected or advanced, and often cause no symptoms. For this reason, the need to conduct a careful systematic examination for every patient cannot be stressed too much. Extra-oral examination should include both visual inspection of the face and neck and palpation of the neck (see Ch. 2). The patient's head should be tilted forwards and the lymph nodes in the neck palpated in relaxed tissue. A routine technique should be adopted, perhaps starting with the submental nodes and then moving to more posterior node groups. The oral mucosa and oropharynx should be examined carefully. The tongue should be protruded to detect lateral deviation and then relaxed and lifted to allow examination of its ventral surface and the floor of mouth. Correct positioning and the use of good illumination and mirrors are important factors. When oral cancer is detected, prompt referral is essential. The importance of attending at the hospital should be stressed, without provoking undue anxiety. Until a biopsy result is available, definitive diagnosis should be avoided. Any ulcer that fails to heal within a 3-week period should be regarded as suspicious and the patient should be referred to a specialist.

Epidemiology

Global incidence and trends

The global incidence of oral and oropharyngeal cancer has been estimated at over 405 000 new cases per year. Of these over 30 000 occur in the USA and around 4600 occur in the UK. There is marked geographical variation in distribution, with the highest incidence in the Indian subcontinent and southeast Asia, because of the particular use of paan and tobacco. Oral and oropharyngeal cancer ranks in the top ten in prevalence tables. The incidence of oral cancer is rising and more cases are seen in younger age groups. The male to female ratio of around 2.5:1 is also changing, with an increasing oral cancer incidence in women, particularly involving the tongue.

Morbidity and mortality

Overall 5-year survival for oral cancer is just over 50% but depends very much on the stage at initial diagnosis and clinical factors. Squamous-cell carcinoma of the lip has a better prognosis than intra-oral carcinoma. In general, prognosis is worse when tumours arise in the more posterior parts of the oral cavity and oropharynx than in the anterior area. Midline carcinomas in the floor of mouth and ventral tongue may, however, spread to both sides of the neck. Staging is a system used to describe the degree of spread or tumour 'load' and the most widely used TNM (tumour, lymph node, metastases) system is described in Tables 15 and 16. Survival at 5 years for TNM stage I oral carcinoma is around 80%, whereas survival is reduced to 15% for stage IV. Morbidity refers to the reduction in function, both physical and psychological. Again, morbidity tends to relate to stage, as large tumours may require removal of a large amount of tissue or radical radiotherapy. Hospital re-admission is frequent during treatment and in many cases tumours prove refractory to all forms of therapy. Quality of life can be assessed and is an important measure of morbidity. Good dental health is a significant factor.

Types of oral cancer

Squamous-cell carcinoma accounts for around 95% of all oral cancers. It arises from the epithelial lining of the oral cavity. It is described in detail in the next section. A number of other forms of malignant disease also arise in the oral cavity.

Minor salivary gland cancers. These tend to occur in the palate and upper lip and they present as rubbery nodules, sometimes ulcerated and painful. They are described in Chapter 13.

Malignant melanoma. This typically occurs in the palatal and gingival mucosa. A spreading brown-pigmented

Table 15 The TNM (tumour, lymph nodes, metastases) system used for determination of clinical and pathological stage of carcinoma. The system now includes an assessment of clinical risk

Component	Features
Primary tumour (T)	
TX	Primary tumour cannot be assessed
T0	No evidence of primary tumour
Tis	Carcinoma in situ
T1	Tumour ≤ 2 cm in greatest dimension
T2	Tumour 2–4 cm in greatest dimension
T3	Tumour > 4 cm in greatest dimension
T4	Tumour invades adjacent structures (bone, skin or deep muscle)
Lymph nodes (N)	
NX	Regional nodes cannot be assessed
N0	No regional lymph node metastasis
N1	Metastasis in a single ipsilateral lymph node, ≤ 3 cm in greatest dimension
N2	Metastasis in (a) a single ipsilateral lymph node 3–6 cm in greatest dimension, or (b) multiple ipsilateral lymph nodes, none > 6 cm in greatest dimension, or (c) bilateral or contralateral lymph nodes, none > 6 cm in greatest dimension
N3	Metastasis in a lymph node > 6 cm in greatest dimension
Distant metastasis (M)	
MX	Presence of distant metastasis cannot be assessed
M0	No distant metastasis
M1	Distant metastasis

patch or a raised ulcerated nodule, surrounded by pigmented mucosa, may be seen (Fig. 161). Prognosis is grave in nodular malignant melanoma.

Malignant lymphoma. Extranodal lymphoma arises principally in the oropharynx in the area of Waldeyer's ring. Nodular infiltration of the mucosa is seen and lymph nodes in the neck may become involved.

Table 16 Stage determination from TNM data

Stage	T level	N level	M level
0	Tis	N0	M0
I	T1	N0	M0
II	T2	N0	M0
III	T3	N0	M0
	or T1/2	N1	M0
IV	T4	N0/1	M0
	or any T	N2/3	M0
	or any T	any N	M1

Staging can also be based on pathological specimens and imaging.

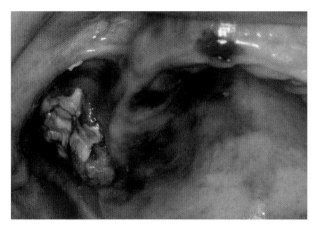

Fig. 161 A malignant melanoma involving the palate.

Leukaemia. Leukaemia may present with oral signs such as persistent gingival haemorrhage and oral ulceration. Acute myeloid leukaemia and childhood leukaemia may cause gingival enlargement because of direct infiltration of leukaemic cells (Fig. 162).

Metastatic deposits. Metastasis from primary cancers in the kidney, gastrointestinal tract, lung, breast, prostate and other sites occur in the oral cavity. Often they present as gingival nodules or as destructive bone lesions. Metastatic lesions in bone are usually radiolucent, but prostate and some breast metastases appear as radio-opacities in bone.

Rare neoplasms. Soft-tissue and bone tumours can arise in the oral cavity. Odontogenic malignant tumours are known but are very rare.

Squamous-cell carcinoma

Aetiology

Smoking

Cigarette smoking is the most important aetiological factor for intra-oral cancer in the Western world. Risk increases with cumulative dose, which is measured in 'pack-years'. There are no safe levels. The risk is greatest when combined with high alcohol intake. It is believed that carcinogens in tobacco smoke accumulate in the floor of mouth, accounting for the increased risk of squamous carcinoma at that site.

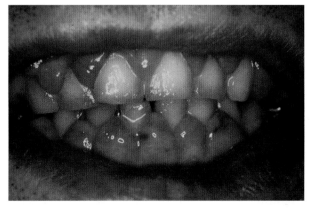

Fig. 162 Generalised gingival enlargement caused by acute leukaemia.

Paan and other tobacco use

Paan, also known as betel quid, is used throughout the Indian subcontinent. Leaf of the betel piper vine is used to form a rolled-up quid, into which areca nut is placed. Areca is thought to contain alkaloid carcinogenic precursors. In addition, tobacco, spices and slaked lime may be added. The quid is held in the oral cavity for a considerable time and is habit forming. Buccal and labial cancers are commonly associated with paan use. Other tobacco habits exist, including smearing tobacco paste into the mouth and reverse bidi smoking, which has been linked to palatal cancer. In recent times, areca nut has become popular in southeast Asia.

Alcohol

Alcohol is an important cofactor when combined with smoking but may not be a risk factor in its own right. It may increase epithelial permeability, allowing greater access of carcinogenic substances to the basal cells.

Ultraviolet light

Ultraviolet B is an important factor in lip cancer. Fair-skinned races in tropical latitudes are particularly at risk from sunlight. Protection, using measures such as sun block and wearing a wide-brimmed hat, is advocated where there is high risk.

Diet

Evidence is accumulating that a poor diet with low anti-oxidant action (deficient in fresh vegetable content) is an important contributory factor.

Viruses

Human papilloma virus (HPV) is an important cause. Studies have shown that HPV type 16 (and sometimes type 18) is an important factor. HPV is found in up to 70% of tonsillar (pharyngeal) carcinomas but is less frequently found in oral cancers. HPV positive tumours appear to have a better prognosis than non-HPV carcinomas, probably due to a better response to chemotherapy and radiotherapy.

Clinical features

The lip

Although the lip is the most common site for oral cancer, intra-oral cases are detected more often by dentists. The lower lip is almost exclusively affected, often to one side of the midline (Fig. 163). Shallow ulceration, crusting or thickening are typical presentations. Spread to the submental nodes tends to be slow; if detected early, this cancer has the best prognosis.

Intra-oral surfaces

The floor of the mouth, ventral tongue and lateral anterior tongue are most commonly involved. All too frequently, the tumour is symptomless and reaches an advanced stage before detection. The classical description is of a hard, fixed ulcer, with raised rolled margins and a necrotic base (Fig. 164). It is vital to remember that squamous carcinomas may also present as white or red mucosal patches, fleshy polyps, punched-out ulcers, indurated plaques or by

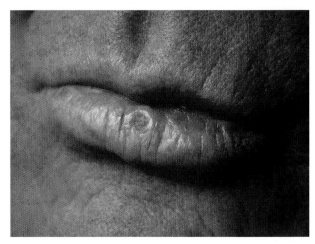

Fig. 163 A squamous-cell carcinoma of the lower lip.

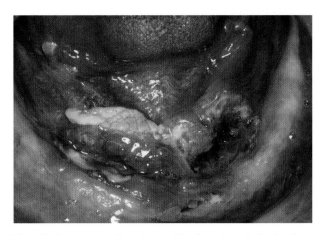

Fig. 164 A squamous-cell carcinoma of the floor of mouth showing the raised rolled borders. The lesion was painless and the patient presented requesting new dentures.

tethering mucosa. The tongue may become fixed to the floor of the mouth, making it difficult for the patient to raise it. Alternatively, the tongue may deviate to the side of an oropharyngeal tumour on protrusion (Fig. 165). Sometimes patients present with nodal metastasis from an occult primary lesion in the oropharynx.

Squamous-cell carcinoma also arises on the gingivae, alveolar ridge, buccal mucosa and palate, albeit less commonly. Bone invasion is an early feature of carcinoma arising in mucoperiosteum.

Head and neck

Dentists should also be aware of extra-oral cancers. Basal-cell carcinoma is not uncommon on the facial skin. Squamous-cell carcinoma arises in the maxillary sinus (Ch. 6), nasopharynx and larynx. Persistent hoarse voice can be a presenting sign of laryngeal cancer and should trigger referral to an otolaryngologist.

Pathology

Histopathological features

Microscopically, squamous-cell carcinoma comprises sheets of squamous epithelial cells supported by a fibrous

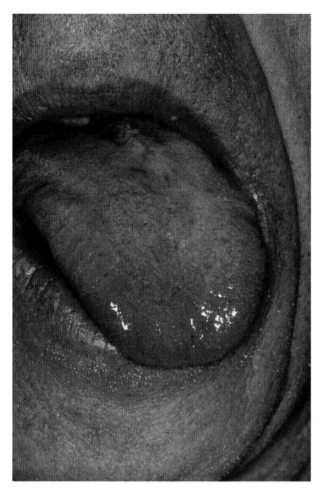

Fig. 165 Tongue deviation on thrusting the tongue outwards. The patient had a large carcinoma in the oropharynx, which had tethered the tongue on the left side.

stroma containing the tumour vasculature. The squamous cells can be recognised by their tendency to form flattened layers held together by prominent intracellular bridges (desmosomes). Often, individual cells undergo keratinisation and the most conspicuous feature is the formation of keratin pearls or whorls (Fig. 166). The vast majority of tumours are moderately differentiated, though examples of well-differentiated and poorly differentiated carcinomas occur. Increased mitotic activity is seen and bizarre mitotic figures are often present. Nuclear and cellular pleomorphism and nuclear hyperchromatism are typical features. Necrosis is present in some cases and is usually associated with poor prognosis. A key feature is invasion of the adjacent tissues by detachment and movement of the carcinoma cells. Invasion may be on a cohesive front or a diffuse non-cohesive front. Carcinoma spreads along anatomical planes. It may spread along nerves, vascular channels or into the sarcolemmal sheaths of muscle fibres. A chronic inflammatory response is usually seen at the invasive front. Many carcinomas are thought to arise in a wide field of mucosal change. Second primary cancers can arise at the same time (synchronous) or later than the presenting cancer (metachronous) and are a significant cause of poor outcome.

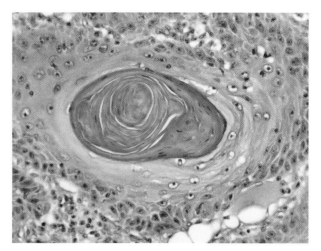

Fig. 166 A squamous-cell carcinoma showing a keratin pearl and cellular pleomorphism.

When an incisional biopsy is undertaken on clinically suspicious mucosal lesions, it is important to include the margin of the ulcer. The biopsy must be of sufficient depth and crush damage must be avoided. Failure to sample appropriately may lead to misdiagnosis.

Bone invasion

In addition to local spread into soft tissues, oral squamous-cell carcinoma can spread into adjacent bone. At first the periosteum acts as a barrier but cortical resorption can lead to entry of the carcinoma cells to marrow spaces and bone destruction. Radiographs show irregular bone destruction and teeth may be displaced or resorbed. Computed tomography (CT), magnetic resonance imaging (MRI) and particularly positron emission tomography (PET) scanning can help to determine the extent of bone and soft tissue spread (Fig. 167).

Metastasis

Carcinoma spreads to regional lymph nodes via the lymphatics. The primary site is important: lip cancers spread to the submental nodes, whereas intra-oral tumours are

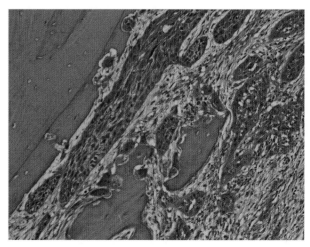

Fig. 167 Bone invasion by oral squamous-cell carcinoma.

more likely to spread to the cervical nodes (see Fig. 5, p. 12). Involved lymph nodes become first palpable and then fixed and hard. With increasing tumour deposition, nodes may become matted together or even cystic as a result of central necrosis. Tumours in the anterior floor of the mouth and tongue may metastasise to both sides of the neck. Imaging can also identify suspicious nodal metastasis to help treatment planning. Fine-needle aspiration can be used to detect cancer in equivocal nodes.

Distant metastasis is a relatively late event but spread may occur to the lungs, brain, viscera and bone. Chest radiography, isotopic bone scans and CT, MR or PET may be used to detect distant metastasis.

Grading and staging

Histological grading: prognostic features

Histological grading refers to those features seen in the microscope that can be related to the biological behaviour of the tumour. The degree of differentiation is not a particularly good indicator of prognosis. Pattern of invasion is more important; tumours that invade tissue on a non-cohesive front (single cells or narrow strands) have a worse prognosis than those that invade on a broad front. Anaplastic (undifferentiated) tumours have a very poor prognosis. Perineural and lymphovascular invasion are also indicators of poor prognosis. As yet, no molecular markers are in routine use.

Staging: TNM classification

Clinical and pathological staging refers to determination of the extent of tumour size and spread. The patient is examined carefully and imaging is used to aid in the detection of involved neck nodes. The TNM (Tables 15 and 16) system is widely used. Pathological staging (pTNM) is undertaken on surgically resectioned specimens and is more accurate than clinical staging.

Imaging of oral squamous-cell carcinoma

The role of imaging in oral cancer management includes:

- identifying tumour size and anatomical extent
- detection of regional nodes (staging)
- post-treatment follow-up.

Plain radiographs have a very limited role to play in assessment and management of oral squamous-cell carcinoma. Advanced lesions on the floor of the mouth may cause gross bone destruction in the adjacent mandible, but detection of early bony involvement has poor sensitivity. Radioisotope bone scans are used to detect such early bone destruction. These bone scans, particularly in combination with CT, lead to good diagnostic sensitivity in detection of bone involvement.

Imaging of oral squamous-cell carcinoma relies upon cross-sectional techniques (i.e. CT or MRI). Thin-slice (3–5 mm) CT sections are usually performed through the oral region and neck. Intravenous iodinated contrast is given and the scans are repeated, because neoplastic lesions of the floor of mouth and tongue base tend to enhance, which improves the delineation between normal and abnormal tissues. Contrast also highlights vessels, allowing them to

be more easily distinguished from nodes. PET can be used to detect small deposits of metastatic carcinoma and can often localise 'unknown' primary sites.

When examining images of submandibular and jugulo-digastric nodes of the internal jugular chain, those nodes with a diameter exceeding 1.5 cm are abnormal; in other parts of the neck 1 cm is the maximum size of normal nodes. A low-density centre may be seen in nodes containing tumour, although this finding may also be seen in inflammation. Neoplastic (and inflammatory) nodes frequently show ring enhancement following contrast injection. Imaging contributes to the clinical staging process not least because it shows nodes (retropharyngeal) beyond the scope of clinical examination.

Treatment

Surgery

Radical surgery is used to remove biopsy-proven primary oral cancers. It is first necessary to undertake a full hospital examination. This often includes examination of the upper aerodigestive tract under general anaesthesia to exclude second primary lesions. Other tests are used to exclude distant metastases. Informed patient consent and support are vital.

The surgical operation aims to remove the carcinoma, with a 2 cm margin of normal tissue beyond the clinical edge of the tumour where possible. When the carcinoma involves bone then part of the mandible or maxilla must also be removed. Reconstruction is required to maintain function after excision of all but the smallest lesions. This may be accomplished using local flaps or distant pedicled or microvascular free flaps. The latter may include bone as well as soft tissues. A large variety of flaps are available and this simultaneous resection and reconstruction has revolutionised the surgical management of patients with oral cancer. The emphasis is now on improving the quality of the functional and aesthetic result. The reconstruction may also involve the use of osseointegrated implants (Ch. 6).

Donor sites for flaps used in head and neck surgery include the lower limb, the upper limb and girdle, the anterior or posterior chest wall, the abdominal wall, the scalp and forehead. The radial free forearm flap is one of the most commonly used with the radial artery anastomosed to the linguo-facial trunk or superior thyroid artery. The flap is soft and pliable and good for intra-oral reconstruction and radial bone can be manipulated to provide a curved mandibular raplacement if required. However, there is risk of radial fracture and the quality of the bone is not ideal. Microvascular techniques are usually carried out with the aid of loupes or an operating microscope with care to avoid kinking or twisting of vessels.

A selective (removing lymph nodes at certain levels) or radical (removing nodes at all levels) neck dissection may be needed because of possible lymph node involvement. Neck dissection results in some morbidity and modern surgical techniques aim to minimise loss of function. Complications include haemorrhage, haematoma, oedema, Chyle leak, Horner's sydrome and infection. Decisions regarding the patient's need for postoperative radiotherapy are guided by histological evidence of tumour spread to the nodes and in particular to the extracapsular tissues. The issue of neck dissection where there is no clinical, radiological or cytological evidence of cervical nodal disease is contentious. Many centres routinely perform neck dissection in the clinically negative neck because occult metastatic disease may be present. Alternatively dye and radioactive tracers can be used to identify sentinel node basins in the direct drainage pathway of the tumour and individual nodes can then be removed and sampled thoroughly by the pathologist.

Radiotherapy

External beam (teletherapy) and implanted radioactive seeds or needles (plesiotherapy) can be used to treat oral cancer. Radiotherapy can also be used as an adjuvant therapy, combined with surgery. Acute mucositis occurs during treatment. Later complications include:

- osteoradionecrosis
- pathological fracture
- dry mouth
- radiation scar
- chronic ulceration.

A very rare late complication is the induction of neoplasms such as osteosarcoma.

Chemotherapy

Many oral and pharygeal cancer patients receive targeted drug therapy and modern chemotherapy as part of their management. Combinations of surgery, chemotherapy and radiotherapy are increasingly employed.

12.4 Role of the dentist in prevention, detection and treatment

Learning objectives

You should:
- understand how the general dental practitioner can educate patients in prevention of oral cancer
- be aware of the need to look for and follow-up suspicious lesions
- understand postoperative dental care for patients with oral cancer.

Prevention

Spending a few moments with a patient discussing giving up smoking is known as an anti-smoking intervention. It has been shown that such interventions are most effective when undertaken by health-care professionals and are a cost-effective method of prevention.

Early diagnosis and screening

Careful history taking and examination are essential for identification of suspicious oral mucosal lesions. Palpation of neck nodes and systematic examination of the oral mucosa should be routine practice. Use of tolonium blue as a screening test in primary care is not supported by robust evidence and it may generate false-positive results.

Referral

Delay should be avoided when a suspicious mucosal lesion is detected. Telephone referral to hospital with a confidential, detailed, follow-up letter to the specialist is a good option when cancer is suspected. It is important to avoid undue alarm to the patient and use of the word 'cancer' should be avoided. Many hospitals have schemes for 'fast-track referral' that can be employed effectively when cancer is suspected.

Dental care prior to radiotherapy

The dentist is an important clinician in the multidisciplinary team managing oral cancer. Preventive advice and completion of treatment to render the patient dentally fit are vital. Teeth with a poor prognosis may be extracted to avoid later problems with osteoradionecrosis and dental sepsis when radiotherapy is to be given to the jaws.

Post-treatment care

Once the acute mucositis associated with radiotherapy has subsided, patients may experience dry mouth, bone pain and increased caries rates. Surgical patients may require specialised restorative care and reconstruction. Recurrence or a second primary lesion is always possible and it is important to undertake regular review both to reassure and to detect any mucosal changes at the earliest opportunity. Maintenance of dental health is also important; radiotherapy is a high risk factor for caries and 6-monthly bitewing radiographs are recommended.

Self-assessment: questions

Multiple choice questions

1. Carcinoma of the lip:
   a. Is equally common on the upper and lower vermilion borders
   b. Is principally caused by smoking
   c. Usually arises in angular cheilitis
   d. Has a generally better prognosis than intra-oral cancers
   e. Often arises in a field of dysplastic change

2. Submucous fibrosis:
   a. Typically produces thickening of the buccal mucosa and soft palate, resulting in limited mouth opening and difficulty in swallowing
   b. Is caused by chewing betel nuts
   c. Is a hereditary disorder
   d. Has oral epithelium that usually shows atrophy
   e. Results in the presence of a fine fibrillary collagen layer in the lamina propria

3. Squamous-cell carcinoma of the floor of the mouth:
   a. Can be caused by irritation from calculus on the lingual aspect of the teeth
   b. May be related to pooling of carcinogens in the floor of mouth
   c. Can present clinically as a white patch
   d. Infiltration of the submandibular duct can cause symptoms of obstructive sialadenitis
   e. Can metastasise to both sides of the neck

4. The classification based on TNM (tumour, nodes, metastasis) findings:
   a. Is a system used for recording histopathological grading
   b. Primary carcinoma in the floor of mouth/ventral tongue can spread directly to level IV nodes
   c. Infiltration of adjacent structures by primary carcinoma without spread into the neck indicates stage IV disease
   d. Extracapsular spread of metastatic deposits in lymph nodes is an indicator of poor prognosis
   e. Stage I squamous-cell carcinomas have an 80% 5-year and 50% 10-year survival rate overall.

5. Histopathological features of oral epithelial dysplasia:
   a. Interobserver agreement of oral epithelial dysplasia grade amongst specialist pathologists is excellent
   b. Includes all of the following: acanthosis, acantholysis, drop-shaped rete processes, atypical mitotic activity and increased nuclear/cytoplasmic ratio.
   c. Indicate carcinoma in situ when the dysplasia involves the entire thickness of the epithelium
   d. Mild dysplasia progresses through moderate to severe dysplasia
   e. Dysplastic oral epithelium may be found in non-smokers and non-drinkers

6. Of the cancers in the orofacial region:
   a. The relative proportion of salivary cancers to adenomas is the same in minor and major salivary glands
   b. Malignant melanoma occurs only in the sun-exposed parts of the skin in the orofacial region
   c. Malignant lymphoma can arise as an extranodal tumour in the tissues of Waldeyer's ring
   d. Intra-oral basal-cell carcinoma most commonly arises in the floor of mouth and ventral tongue
   e. Kaposi's sarcoma is caused by HIV (human immunodeficiency virus) infection

Extended matching items

EMI 1. Theme: Histopathology of oral cancer and precursor lesions

Options:

A Carcinoma in situ
B Basaloid squamous-cell carcinoma
C Squamous-cell carcinoma
D Malignant melanoma
E Proliferative verrucous leukoplakia
F Spindle-cell carcinoma
G Oro-pharyngeal carcinoma
H Naso-pharyngeal carcinoma
I Submucous fibrosis
J Erosive lichen planus

Lead in: Match the histopathology report from the list below that is most appropriate for each diagnosis above.

1. Histological examination shows sheets of squamous cells supported by fibrous stroma. Keratin pearls are present and there is focal necrosis. The squamous cells are pleomorphic and possess hyperchromatic nuclei. Numerous atypical mitotic figures are present. The invasive front is non-cohesive and there is a moderate chronic inflammatory infiltrate at the invasive front.

2. Sections show oral mucosa. In the oral epithelium there is basal-cell crowding and hyperplasia. Atypical mitotic figures are present throughout the thickness of the oral epithelium. The squamous cells show nuclear and cellular pleomorphism, and keratin whorls are present. The rete ridges are drop shaped and individual cell keratinisation is present in some areas.

3. Sections show buccal mucosa in which there is mild epithelial atrophy with parakeratosis. The pattern of epithelial maturation is regular and the overall architecture is preserved. The rete processes are flattened and bands of hyaline collagen best seen in Van Geison stained sections are present in the lamina propria. A mild chronic inflammatory infiltrate is present in the subepithelial tissue.

4. Histopathological examination shows sheets of polygonal cells with large nuclei possessing prominent eosinophilic nucleoli and abundant basophilic cytoplasm. Nests of tumour cells are seen at the interface between the oral epithelium and lamina propria. Some individual atypical cells extend by Pagetoid spread into the oral

epithelium. The tumour cells are positive by immunoperoxidase for S 100, Melan-A and HMB 45 antibody staining.

5. Sections of this lesion from the base of the tongue show islands of submucosal squamous cells with rounded cytoplasmic outlines and basophilic cytoplasm. Microfocal keratinisation is present and comedo necrosis is seen. At the periphery of the islands the cells are often columnar and show palisading. The tumour cells exhibit marked nuclear and cellular pleomorphism in some areas and there is a high mitotic rate of > 15 figures per high power field.

6. Sections show oral mucosa in which there is acanthosis and marked hyperparakeratosis forming 'church spires'. The basal-cell layer is crowded and there is mild cellular atypia, with occasional hyperchromatic nuclei. Overall the degree of dysplasia can be graded as mild. Multiple levels have been examined and no invasive activity is seen.

7. Examination of this biopsy of an ulcerated polypoid swelling of buccal mucosa shows sheets of loosely arranged cigar- and kite-shaped cells. There is nuclear and cellular pleomorphism and the mitotic rate is < 2 figures per high-power field. The tumour cells stain with the cytokeratin markers AE1/AE3 and MNF 116. At the base of biopsy there are small islands of squamous-cell carcinoma and the adjacent mucosa shows severe epithelial dysplasia.

8. This tumour is formed by sheets of squamous cells supported by fibrous stroma. Keratin pearls are present and there is focal necrosis. The squamous cells are pleomorphic and possess hyperchromatic nuclei. Numerous atypical mitotic figures are present. Testing by FISH shows the presence of human papilloma virus type 16 and antibody staining shows overexpression of tumour p16 (CDKN2A).

9. Sections show a tumour composed of sheets of large poorly differentiated squamous cells admixed with a large number of lymphocytes. The tumour cells stained with cytokeratin antibodies AE1/AE3 and MNF 116. The cells also stained positively for Epstein–Barr virus (HHV4) using in situ hybridisation.

10. Sections show oral mucosa in which there is atrophy of the oral epithelium with mild parakeratosis. The basement membrane is thickened and a band of subepithelial lympho-histiocytic infiltrate is present. Basal-cell keratinocyte apoptosis is present and reactive cytological atypia is seen.

EMI 2. Theme: Oral cancer and precursor lesions

Options:

A Plummer–Vinson syndrome (Patterson–Kelly–Brown syndrome)
B Fanconi anaemia
C pStage IV Oral cancer (pT2, pN2b, pMx)
D pStage IV Oral cancer (pT4, pN1, pMx)
E Metastatic carcinoma from the breast
F Adenoid cystic carcinoma
G Leukaemia
H Extranodal non-Hodgkin malignant lymphoma
I Basal-cell carcinoma
J Carcinoma of the maxillary antrum

Lead in: Match the case from the list below that is most appropriate for each diagnosis above.

1. An 11-year-old child was found to have a painless ulcer on the lateral border of the tongue at routine dental check-up. On biopsy this was found to be a moderately differentiated invasive squamous-cell carcinoma. The child was small in stature and had learning difficulties. Café au lait spots were present on the skin.

2. A 32-year-old woman presented to her dentist with a sore tongue. On examination the tongue was smooth and glossy, with loss of papillae. On questioning it became clear that she had also been experiencing difficulty swallowing for some months. A blood test revealed a haemoglobin level of 8.5 G/L.

3. A 65-year-old man had a mandibular rim resection and neck dissection for squamous-cell carcinoma of the floor of mouth and ventral tongue. The pathologist described a tumour located mainly in the floor of mouth that was 28 mm in maximum width and 11 mm in depth. Five lymph nodes out of 48 recovered from the ipsilateral neck dissection contained metastatic squamous-cell carcinoma, two with extra-capsular spread.

4. A 58-year-old woman had a hemimandibulectomy and neck dissection for a squamous-cell carcinoma of alveolus and floor of mouth. The pathologist found the tumour to be 12 mm maximum diameter, invading the bone to a depth of 9 mm. One lymph node in the ipsilateral neck contained a deposit of metastatic squamous-cell carcinoma.

5. A 66-year-old woman presented to the dentist for a check-up. The dentist noticed a small nodular and ulcerated lesion on the cheek skin around the alar of the nose. The lesion had been growing slowly for 18 months.

6. An 80-year-old man presented to his dentist with bleeding gums. On examination there was gingival recession and the oral hygiene was only fair. The gingivae were discoloured and there was steady oozing of blood on gentle probing of the crevice.

7. A 52-year-old woman presented with left-sided facial palsy. A needle core biopsy of the left parotid gland was reported as showing small to medium-sized cells with hyperchromatic angular nuclei in a tubular and cribriform arrangement.

8. A 52-year-old woman presented with left-sided facial discomfort and a sensation of stuffiness. Two carious molars in the upper left quadrant were extracted and at review exuberant tissue was present in the tooth sockets.

9. A 54-year-old man presented with a nodular tumour involving the right side of the soft palate. On biopsy there were sheets of large malignant cells that were positive for CD20 and CD79a and negative for cytokeratin markers.

10. A 53-year-old woman presented with a gingival polyp in the left mandibular premolar area of 2 months' duration. The lower left side of the lip had become numb during the last week. Radiographs revealed destruction of the underlying bone and a needle core biopsy showed a malignant neoplasm composed of ductal cells in an abundant fibrous stroma.

Case history questions

Case history 1

A 68-year-old man attended his general medical practitioner with pain in his chest. He was referred to a cardiologist who diagnosed angina and advised him to stop smoking and to reduce his alcohol intake. The patient mentioned that he had mouth ulcers and he was advised to see his dentist as soon as possible. This advice was not followed and the patient did not make an appointment to see the dentist until 3 months later when the ulceration under his tongue was making it difficult to eat (Fig. 168).

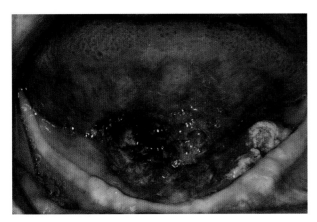

Fig. 168 Ulceration in the patient in Case history 1.

1. Which factors contributed to delay in diagnosis and providing treatment for this patient?
2. Assuming a provisional diagnosis of oral carcinoma, how should a biopsy be performed in this case?

The oral and maxillofacial surgeon advised surgical treatment, but the patient was deemed unsuitable for sentinel node biopsy.
3. Why was this?

Case history 2

An 85-year-old man presented with a 2-month history of a numb lip on the left side. His dentist had suggested that he leave his lower denture out for 2 weeks but this made no difference. A radiograph revealed a diffuse radiolucent lesion in the region of the left mental foramen. He was referred to the hospital where, on taking a full history, the patient admitted to haematuria and weight loss over the last 3 months. A lateral skull radiograph reveals multiple radiolucent lesions in the calvarium and jaws. The radiologist suggests multiple myeloma as a possible diagnosis.

1. Which tests could be used to investigate this?

A biopsy from the swelling over the mental foramen reveals carcinoma composed of clear cells and the pathologist suggests that this lesion might be a metastatic deposit.

2. Which primary sites are likely?
3. How should the patient be managed?

Case history 3

A 37-year-old woman presents for routine dental examination. Diffuse, red, velvety lesions are present on the buccal mucosa and retromolar areas in a bilateral distribution. The patient smokes 30 cigarettes per day and does not drink alcohol. A provisional diagnosis of erosive lichen planus is made and the patient is referred to the local oral medicine unit, where a biopsy is performed.

1. The oral medicine consultant made a clinical diagnosis of erythroplakia following biopsy. Which features are likely to have been seen in the biopsy specimen?
2. How might the patient be managed?
3. What is the risk of malignant transformation in this case?

Case history 4

A 38-year-old Swedish woman developed soreness of the tongue and was referred to a local otolaryngology unit. She is found to have iron-deficiency anaemia and she says she has been experiencing difficulty in swallowing. Endoscopy and barium swallow reveal an oesophageal web.

1. What syndrome does this patient have?
2. What changes may be seen in the oral epithelium in chronic iron-deficiency anaemia?
3. The patient used oral snuff (a tobacco product) and was advised to discontinue its use. She was surprised as snuff had been advised in a health promotion leaflet in Sweden. What is the basis for advising her to discontinue snuff use and why is its use advocated in Sweden?

Viva questions

1. What ingredients are found in paan?
2. A patient presents with cancer in the oropharynx. On protruding the tongue, it deviates to the left side. What is the significance of this sign?
3. What factor is common to the oral premalignant conditions?
4. What is meant by induration?
5. What are the clinical features of a cervical lymph node involved by metastatic carcinoma?
6. What is a blind biopsy?

Self-assessment: answers

Multiple choice answers

1. a. **False.** Cancer of the vermilion border affects mainly the lower lip.
   b. **False.** The principal aetiological factor is ultraviolet (ultraviolet B) exposure from sunlight.
   c. **False.** Angular cheilitis is most often caused by infection with *Candida* species or staphylococci and is not a precancerous lesion.
   d. **True.** Overall lip cancer has a better prognosis than intra-oral cancer. Early detection is a factor.
   e. **True.** Ultraviolet exposure is linked to solar keratosis, which is a dysplastic premalignant lesion often affecting the lower vermilion border.

2. a. **True.** Fibrous bands are often visible in the buccal mucosa and the affected areas appear pale and thickened on examination.
   b. **False.** There is no such thing as betel nuts. Paan is basically betel vine leaf into which areca nut is rolled. Paan quid is held in the mouth for prolonged periods.
   c. **False.** There is good epidemiological evidence linking submucous fibrosis to paan use.
   d. **True.** It can be reduced to only a few cell layers in thickness.
   e. **True.** Submucous fibrosis is characterised by deposition of fine collagen fibres beneath the oral epithelium. The papillary lamina propria is reduced and the abnormal collagen fibres tend to be orientated parallel to the surface of the mucosa.

3. a. **False.** Poor oral hygiene has been associated with oral cancer but is not considered a causative factor.
   b. **True.** Particularly from tobacco smoke.
   c. **True.** It also can appear as red patches.
   d. **True.** Squamous-cell carcinoma is often painless. In the floor of the mouth, direct infiltration of the submandibular salivary duct by the carcinoma may cause obstruction of the salivary flow. Obstructive symptoms may be the clinical feature leading to presentation.
   e. **True.** Particularly if the primary site is in the anterior floor of the mouth.

4. a. **False.** The TNM classification is used for tumour staging; grading is based on histological features.
   b. **True.** Although the neck is divided into anatomical compartments referred to as 'levels', primary oral carcinoma does not necessarily spread to the first level and then onwards in sequence from one level to the next, as was once thought. It has now been established that lymphatic channels communicate directly between the floor of mouth/ventral tongue and level IV in the neck. For example, a carcinoma arising in the floor of the mouth can spread directly to level IV without involving levels I–III.
   c. **True.** Infiltration of deep/intrinsic tongue muscle, bone and anatomical structures indicates stage IV disease.

   d. **True.** When squamous-cell carcinoma spreads to lymph nodes in the neck, the carcinoma cells travel via the lymphatic vessels to the lymph nodes. The metastatic cancer cells are seen first in the subcapsular sinus within the node and further proliferation may be restricted to the node interior. If the cancer cells are then seen to grow through the lymph node capsule and out into the surrounding tissue, this is described as 'extracapsular spread' by the pathologist. It is an important pathological feature because extracapsular spread is a powerful predictor of poor prognosis.
   e. **True.**

5. a. **False.** Grading of oral epithelial dysplasia is difficult and poor agreement even amongst specialist pathologists is recorded.
   b. **True.** Acanthosis is diffuse hyperplasia; acantholysis is disruption of the connections between keratinocytes.
   c. **True.** Often severe epithelial dysplasia involving almost the entire thickness is said to amount to carcinoma in situ.
   d. **False.** Histological progression of dysplasia is not always seen and regression of dysplasia is thought to occur.
   e. **True.** Oral epithelial dysplasia in non-smokers and non-drinkers causes concern clinically as transformation rates are reportedly higher.

6. a. **False.** Although minor gland salivary tumours account for only ~10% of all salivary gland tumours, the proportion of benign to malignant is approximately 55% to 45% in minor glands and 85% to 15% in the parotid.
   b. **False.** Malignant melanoma can occur in the oral mucosa, particularly in the palate and gingivae.
   c. **True.**
   d. **False.** Basal-cell carcinoma does not arise in the oral mucosa. Basaloid squamous-cell carcinoma is a variant of squamous-cell carcinoma with a poor prognosis.
   e. **False.** Kaposi's sarcoma is linked to human herpesvirus 8 infection and is associated with immunodeficiency.

Extended matching items answers

EMI 1

1. **C.** These features are typical of squamous-cell carcinoma.
2. **A.** Carcinoma in situ is defined by cellular atypia and disturbed maturation involving the whole thickness of the oral epithelium. For clinical management severe epithelial dysplasia often amounts to carcinoma in situ and in some classifications they are combined as squamous intraepithelial neoplasia grade 3 (SIN 3).

3. **I.** Submucous fibrosis is linked to paan (betel) chewing. Dense collagenous bands form in the oral mucosa and there may be limitation of mouth opening and difficulty in swallowing. Dysplasia and oral cancer may arise.

4. **D.** Malignant melanoma is an important tumour for dentists to be aware of. Melanoma may arise in the oral mucosa or facial skin.

5. **B.** Basaloid squamous carcinoma is a histological variant that is found most often in the base of the tongue and oro-pharynx. It tends to be submucosal and ulceration may not be seen.

6. **E.** The World Health Organisation classification recognises that proliferative verrucous leukoplakia (PVL) is a high-risk lesion that often transforms into cancer despite having minimal dysplasia.

7. **F.** Spindle-cell carcinoma is another recognised variant of squamous-cell carcinoma that sometimes arises after radiation therapy. The cells are lozenge or kite shaped and staining with cytokeratin antibodies is often needed to identify their epithelial character.

8. **G.** Some squamous carcinomas of the head and neck are linked to human papilloma virus, particularly type 16. HPV may account for up to 75% of oro-pharyngeal carcinomas.

9. **H.** Nasopharyngeal carcinoma is more common in the Chinese population and is linked to Epstein–Barr (HHV4) infection. This type of cancer is very radiosensitive and has a good response to treatment unless bone metastasis is present at diagnosis.

10. **J.** These features are typical of erosive lichen planus. Submucous fibrosis and erosive lichen planus are regarded as premalignant conditions because oral epithelial atrophy predisposes to the development of dysplasia and oral cancer.

EMI 2

1. **B.** There is a well-established link between Fanconi's anaemia and oral cancer in young patients.

2. **A.** Plummer–Vinson syndrome is characterised by formation of an oesophageal web and chronic iron deficiency anaemia. It is a premalignant oral condition.

3. **C.** In the UICC classification pT2 refers to a primary tumour between 2 and 4 cm in maximum dimension. pN2b denotes multiple ipsilateral involved nodes none greater than 6 cm in maximum dimension.

4. **D.** Invasion of adjacent structures including bone automatically upstages oral cancer to pT4 in the UICC system.

5. **I.** The alar of the nose is a likely site for basal-cell carcinoma. Dentists should be alert to these common destructive tumours when performing extra-oral examination.

6. **G.** Leukaemia may manifest as gingival swelling or chronic oozing of blood from the gingivae with bruising. It may be confused with chronic periodontal disease.

7. **F.** Adenoid cystic carcinoma typically shows perineural spread and may cause facial palsy, pain or paraesthesia. The Swiss cheese (cribriform) appearance is typical on biopsy.

8. **J.** Proliferation of tissue from tooth sockets can be a reactive healing response but the possibility of carcinoma should always be considered, especially in the maxilla. Imaging may be helpful in diagnosing carcinoma of the maxillary sinus.

9. **H.** Extranodal malignant non-Hodgkin lymphoma may involve the palate. The malignant cells will not stain with cytokeratin antibodies because these label epithelium. The antibody markers CD20 and CD 79a indicate that the tumour is a B-cell lymphoma.

10. **E.** Epulides should always be submitted for histological examination to exclude metastatic deposits. Breast and other cancers may metastasise to the gingival margin.

Case history answers

Case history 1

1. Oral cancer tends to be painless until advanced and many patients delay seeking advice until there is pain or oral dysfunction. Lack of awareness of oral cancer is common in the general public and in some health-care professionals. When patients complain of ulceration in the mouth, oral examination should be undertaken.

2. Incisional biopsy is normally performed by taking representative tissue of adequate size and depth from the margin of the lesion to include normal tissue. Many oral cancer centres prefer to see any suspected lesions and to undertake biopsy themselves. Sometimes imaging is undertaken first and biopsy may be done at the time of examination under general anaesthesia to exclude second primary lesions.

3. Sentinel node biopsy is a technique in which the lymph node or nodes draining the tumour site are identified by tracing techniques. The sentinel nodes are sampled and if no metastatic neoplasm is found, neck dissection is avoided. The technique is used only for T1 and T2 tumours and N0 nodes, judged clinically.

Case history 2

1. Examination of plasma proteins for monoclonal gammopathy, urine for Bence Jones protein, bone marrow aspiration or biopsy may be undertaken.

2. Renal clear-cell carcinoma, bladder or prostate are possible primary sites.

3. The patient should be referred to an oncologist.

Case history 3

1. Oral epithelial dysplasia is likely to have been seen. Erythroplakia tends to show drop-shaped rete processes and marked cellular atypia.

2. Erythroplakia is associated with high malignant transformation rates. The patient should be advised to give up smoking and to attend for regular follow-up. Consideration might be given to removing discrete areas by laser excision.
3. Malignant transformation rates of up to 50% (over many years of follow-up) are recorded in the literature. Rates are hard to estimate because of the poor quality of data in the literature.

Case history 4

1. Sideropenic dysphagia (Plummer–Vinson or Patterson–Kelly–Brown syndrome).
2. Oral epithelial atrophy and cellular atypia have been recorded.
3. Sideropenic dysphagia is a premalignant condition and the use of oral tobacco should be discontinued as it may result in malignant transformation. In some countries, washed oral tobacco (snuff) is promoted as an alternative to cigarette smoking to avoid the major health risks of smoking such as lung cancer and vascular disease.

Viva answers

1. Paan contains areca nut wrapped in piper betel vine leaf. Tobacco, slaked lime, spices and other ingredients may be added. Fresh, freeze-dried and other proprietary forms are available.

2. The tumour is on the left side; fixation of the tongue by oral cancer tends to cause the tongue to deviate to the ipsilateral side on protrusion.
3. Epithelial atrophy.
4. Induration is a clinical term referring to the thickening and fibrous texture of the tissues invaded by carcinoma cells. It is an important sign to detect when palpating a suspicious ulcer.
5. The neck node will be enlarged and fixed. It will typically be non-tender unless infection is present. Malignant nodes may be matted together to form a craggy mass. Central necrosis may lead to cystic change.
6. Blind biopsy is the term used to describe a procedure in which multiple biopsies are taken (usually of the nasopharynx or tonsil) to detect carcinoma where the primary site is not apparent on clinical examination. It is used when patients present with metastatic squamous-cell carcinoma in the neck with no obvious primary lesion.

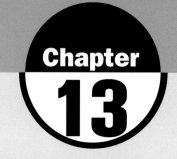
Salivary gland disease

Overview

The salivary gland can be affected by any condition that blocks the duct, whether extra- or intraductal blockage or duct wall thickening. Sjögren's syndrome is a chronic inflammatory disease of salivary and lacrimal glands. A number of tumours can also affect the glands themselves. The surgical management of salivary glands is described.

13.1 Anatomy

Learning objectives

You should:
- know the position of the salivary glands and the associated structures.

Minor salivary glands

The minor salivary glands are located in the submucosa and include the labial, buccal, palatal and lingual glands.

Submandibular gland

The submandibular gland is intermediate in size between the sublingual and parotid glands. It has a superficial part in the neck, a deep part in the floor of the mouth and it wraps around the posterior edge of the mylohyoid muscle. The superficial part is related to the facial artery, the facial vein, the cervical branch of the facial nerve, the mylohyoid nerve and the submandibular lymph nodes. The deep part is related to the lingual and hypoglossal nerves. Wharton's duct emerges from the deep part of the gland and continues forward to empty at the sublingual papilla in the floor of mouth. The sublingual gland empties into the floor of mouth directly or through Wharton's duct.

Parotid gland

The parotid gland is the largest of the paired salivary glands. It occupies the region between the ramus of the mandible and the mastoid process, extending upwards to the external acoustic meatus and is essentially pyramidal in shape. The external carotid artery (deep), the retromandibular vein (intermediate) and the facial nerve (superficial) pass through the gland. The majority of the gland lies superficial to the facial nerve. Stenson's duct runs through the cheek and drains into the mouth opposite the maxillary second permanent molar tooth.

13.2 Investigations

Learning objectives

You should:
- know the clinical features of salivary gland disease
- know which investigations are suitable for which symptoms.

History and clinical examination

As always, symptoms are often indicative of the abnormality present. These can include:

- slowly developing swelling or mass, suggesting a tumour
- swelling (at the site of a major gland) associated with sight/taste/smell of food, slowly subsiding subsequently, suggesting obstruction.
- pain and swelling (of a major gland) perhaps with a bad taste, suggesting infection
- dry mouth, suggesting a wide range of causes, including Sjögren's syndrome.

Look for asymmetry and obvious extra- or intra-oral swelling. In the case of the major salivary glands, establish if one or both glands are affected. Always palpate salivary glands bimanually. Is a swelling firm or soft? Larger calculi may be palpable as hard masses. In suspected inflammatory disease, see if clear saliva can be expressed from the duct orifice or, alternatively, whether turbid, mucopurulent secretion indicative of infection is present.

Malignant tumours in the salivary glands may present as fixed, firm, rapidly growing masses with pain and sometimes skin involvement. Facial nerve palsy is a sinister sign when a parotid mass is detected. Lymph node metastasis in the regional nodes may be present. It should be remembered that some salivary malignancies (e.g. adenoid cystic carcinoma) may be insidious. They may cause unilateral facial pain and remain undetected for a considerable period.

Hypersalivation may be a feature of certain neurological disorders. Sometimes it is confused with dribbling from the angle of the mouth caused by loss of neuromuscular control. Most often, hypersalivation is linked to a psychological disorder, when it is difficult to treat. It is sometimes seen in sialosis, which most commonly presents as painless bilateral parotid gland swelling.

Dry mouth is a frequent complaint and there may be a sensation of dry mouth with no objective reduction in flow. Sialometry is a simple first-line investigation that can help to identify reduced salivary flow (xerostomia). The most common cause of true xerostomia is the unwanted effects of drugs with sympathomimetic or antimuscarinic effect (e.g. tricyclic antidepressants and antihistamines). Treatment of xerostomia is discussed below with Sjögren's syndrome.

Sialometry

Normal whole unstimulated salivary flow rates can be assessed by asking the patient to gently dribble any saliva produced over a 5-minute period into a container. The normal flow rate is 0.3–0.4 ml/min; a flow rate of less than 0.1 ml/min indicates a clinically significant xerostomia.

Radiology

Selection of imaging methods in suspected or known salivary gland disease is determined for each patient on the basis of the question which the imaging investigation is expected to answer.

Is there a calculus present?

Plain radiographs. These are first choice for all glands.

Parotid glands. Intra-oral plain radiographs of the cheek (dental film placed in the buccal sulcus over the parotid orifice) and an antero-posterior radiograph of the face, with the patient requested to inflate the cheek, are required. Additional, lateral views are often taken, but any calculus may be superimposed upon bone or teeth and obscured.

Submandibular gland. The plain radiographic examination consists of a true occlusal radiograph of the floor of mouth (Fig. 169) and a 'special' (oblique occlusal) radiograph with the beam angled antero-superiorly while centred on the gland itself. Lateral views may be useful, although again a calculus may be superimposed upon bone and be difficult to identify.

Ultrasound. Alternatively, ultrasound examination may be used to identify calculi in either gland.

Is there an obstruction in the duct system? What is the condition of the duct system?

Sialography. Both these questions are best answered with sialography. Sialography is the introduction of a radio-opaque contrast medium into the orifice of one of the major salivary glands via a cannula. The media used are all iodine-containing solutions (usually low-osmolality aqueous solutions of iodine salts). The contrast is introduced slowly until discomfort is felt by the patient. Alternatively, the procedure is performed under fluoroscopic screening, allowing 'real-time' imaging. Usually two images are made at different angles (e.g. lateral and antero-posterior views).

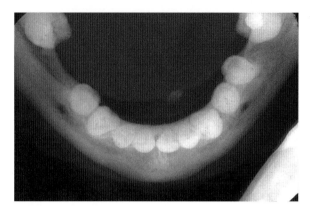

Fig. 169 True occlusal radiograph of the floor of mouth showing a small, well-calcified calculus close to the orifice of the left submandibular duct.

After this, the cannula is removed and a 'drainage' image obtained, usually after stimulation using a sialogogue (e.g. citric acid solution, lemon juice). Digital subtraction may be used to remove bone and tooth images, leaving the contrast image in isolation (Fig. 170).

Is there a mass present?

Ultrasound. This is the 'first line' investigation for a mass (Fig. 171). A high-frequency transducer is used to obtain images in several planes of the gland. Bony superimposition may prevent complete imaging of the deep lobe of the parotid and that part of the submandibular gland immediately adjacent to the mandible. Where a lesion is completely visualised on ultrasound and where there is no suggestion of malignancy an ultrasound examination is often sufficient for surgical planning.

Computed tomography (CT) or magnetic resonance imaging (MRI). Where the above criteria are not met (incomplete visualisation and/or evidence of malignancy), either CT or MRI is recommended.

Is there an abnormality of gland function?

Radioisotope imaging. This is a question usually asked in relation to Sjögren's syndrome. The only radiological

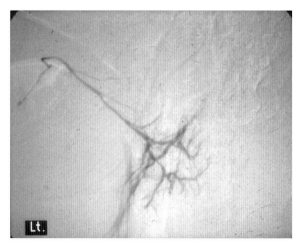

Fig. 170 Digital subtraction sialogram of a normal parotid gland. Digital subtraction removes the image of superimposed bone, allowing a clear image of the typically fine ducts of the normal gland.

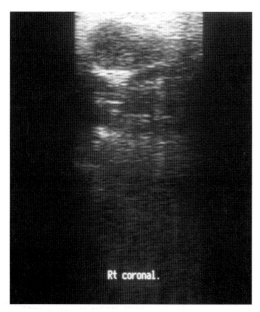

Fig. 171 Axial ultrasound image of a parotid gland containing a pleomorphic adenoma. The skin surface is at the top. The lesion is mainly hypoechoic with some areas of relatively higher echogenicity within. There is posterior enhancement.

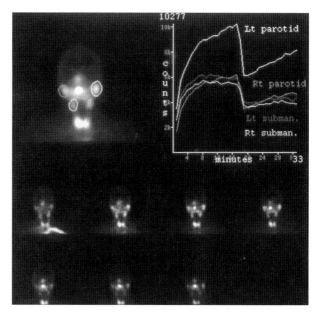

Fig. 172 Radioisotope scan of the salivary glands. Each image is taken with the patient facing the gamma camera, giving a 'face-on' image. The highly active bilobed area of activity at the bottom of each image is the thyroid gland. In this particular patient, the problem illustrated by the quantitative study was underactivity of the right parotid. Lt, left; Rt, right; subman., submandibular.

technique that can assess function is radioisotope imaging (nuclear medicine). This uses a radiopharmaceutical injected intravenously. The radiopharmaceutical is a molecule containing the isotope ^{99m}technetium as the pertechnate (a gamma ray emitter). Once in the bloodstream, this is handled by the body in the same way as iodine and is taken up by the salivary glands and then secreted in saliva. The gamma rays are detected by a gamma camera to produce an image representing the functional activity of the glands (Fig. 172). It is possible to quantify activity in addition to subjective assessment of images. This technique is also employed in rare cases where aplasia of one or more major glands is suspected.

Biopsy

Biopsy of labial minor salivary lobules is sometimes used to assess overall salivary function. Incisional biopsies of intra-oral salivary masses are undertaken through mucosa that will be later removed as a planned surgical procedure.

On no account should a discrete salivary gland mass in a major gland be subjected to incisional biopsy as this may lead to recurrence and is usually unnecessary. For example, there is a 9 in 10 chance that a single parotid mass is a pleomorphic adenoma and so the only acceptable biopsy is a superficial parotidectomy. This will ensure removal of the tumour together with a surrounding margin of normal tissue. Fine-needle aspiration or needle core biopsy is acceptable and is without the risk of implantation of malignant cells in the needle tract. Frozen section may be useful at surgery for tumours in parotid gland that are thought likely to be malignant, to establish whether the facial nerve may be preserved.

13.3 Salivary gland disorders

Learning objectives

You should:
* know the features, investigations and management of salivary gland disorders.

Obstructive salivary disorders

Obstructive salivary disease can be acute or chronic. The clinical features are characteristically pain and swelling of the affected gland just before meals. Astringent stimuli produce severe symptoms. Sometimes the swelling slowly subsides as saliva leaks past the obstruction, and a bad taste is suggestive of associated sialadenitis (Fig. 173).

Extraductal obstruction

Extraductal obstruction is caused by disease outside the duct wall. The most important cause is neoplasia, particularly squamous carcinoma in the floor of mouth or salivary neoplasms. Trauma may also lead to displacement of soft or hard tissue, resulting in duct obstruction.

Duct wall thickening

Duct wall obstruction may be related to fibrosis, leading to stricture. The orifices can become stenosed through trauma from dentures or teeth. Rarely, intraduct papillomas arise from the duct wall and obstruct the lumen.

Intraductal obstruction

Salivary calculus is the most common type of obstructive disorder (Fig. 174). The submandibular gland is most

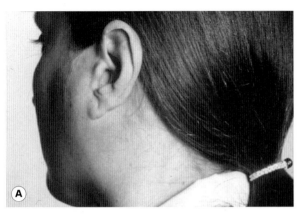

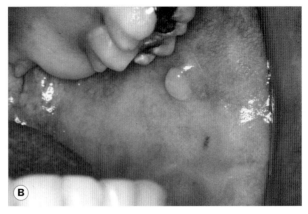

Fig. 173 An obstructive swelling of a parotid gland. **A,** extra-oral view; **B,** intra-oral view.

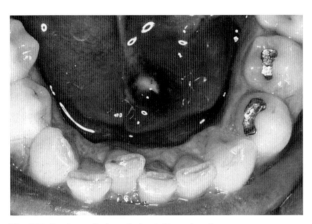

Fig. 174 A submandibular calculus in the oral cavity.

frequently involved (around 80% of cases), followed by parotid and, rarely, minor glands. The calculi (sialoliths) tend to be hard, yellowish and often have a lamellated, concentric-ring structure. They are composed of calcium phosphates, thought to be nucleated on microcalculi, which are commonly found in the major and minor glands. Salivary calculi may form in ducts within the gland substance.

Acute sialadenitis

Viral sialadenitis

Viral sialadenitis (mumps) is an acute contagious infection caused by a paramyxovirus. Spread is by direct contact with infected saliva and by droplets. There is a 2–3 week incubation period, and fever and malaise are followed by sudden, painful swelling of one or both parotid glands. In adults, viraemia results in involvement of internal organs such as the central nervous system and gonads. **Orchitis** (gonadal swelling) occurs in around 20% of affected adult males. Diagnosis is made on clinical grounds and bedrest is advised. As the disease occurs in minor epidemics, infected persons should avoid contact with those at risk. Virus is present in the saliva when symptoms commence and remains for approximately 6 weeks. One episode usually confers lifelong immunity.

Bacterial sialadenitis

Acute bacterial sialadenitis principally involves the parotid glands and is caused by bacteria entering the ductal system against the salivary flow. Reduced flow is a common predisposing factor and is a feature of many conditions, including chronic sialadenitis, Sjögren's syndrome and unwanted effects of drugs. *Streptococcus pyogenes, Staphylococcus aureus, Haemophilus* species, black-pigmented bacteroides and other oral bacteria may be detected in mucopurulent discharge from the duct opening, which is an important clinical sign. It is accompanied by swelling, pain, fever and erythema of the overlying skin. Treatment is by antibiotic therapy and gentle massage to encourage flow. Warm, salty mouthrinses may be helpful, and patients should be advised against placing a hot-water bottle over the gland as this may lead to a pointing abscess.

Chronic sialadenitis

Bacterial sialadenitis

Chronic bacterial sialadenitis is related to low-grade bacterial invasion through the duct system and often follows chronic obstructive disease. The submandibular salivary gland is most commonly affected. Typically, there is recurrent, painful swelling associated with eating or drinking. The duct orifice appears inflamed and a mucopurulent discharge may be seen on examination. Patients may complain of a salty or foul taste in the mouth. The gland may become firm and fibrotic at the end stage. Pathologically there may be duct ectasia, mucous metaplasia of duct epithelium, periductal fibrosis and elastosis, acinar atrophy and a chronic inflammatory infiltration. Interlobular fibrosis results in fusion of the lobules. Surgical removal is indicated in intractable disease. On sialograms, there are combinations of sialectasis (ductal dilatation), strictures, filling defects with calculi or stagnant secretions, and atrophy of minor salivary ducts (Fig. 175). In advanced disease, large abscess cavities may form.

Relapsing parotitis

Relapsing (recurrent) parotitis is an uncommon disorder affecting children and sometimes adults. Typically, sialography shows normal main ducts but punctate sialectasis

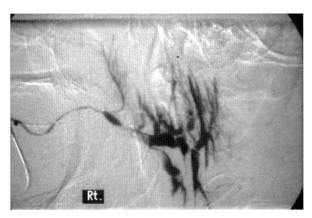

Fig. 175 Chronic sialadenitis of the parotid gland. The main duct has a reasonably normal diameter and course, but beyond the point of junction with an accessory gland (seen passing vertically upwards from the main duct) the gland is abnormal. The ducts are dilated and there is some atrophy of the peripheral ducts (compare with Fig. 169). A filling defect is visible centrally, indicating the presence of a substantial mucus plug or calculus.

peripherally. Some cases are bilateral, suggesting a congenital duct abnormality or tendency to reduced flow.

Radiation sialadenitis

Radiation sialadenitis occurs mostly after radiotherapy, particularly when given for head and neck cancers. There is acinar damage and progressive fibrous replacement. Depending on dose, some recovery may be seen. The glands are shielded where possible to avoid this unwanted effect (Fig. 176). See Sjögren's syndrome for treatment of xerostomia.

Sjögren's syndrome

Sjögren's syndrome is an autoimmune chronic inflammatory disease involving the salivary and lacrimal glands. It is characterised by polyclonal B-cell proliferation, probably as a result of loss of T-cell regulation. There is lymphocytic infiltration and destruction of glandular parenchyma (Fig. 177). Sjögren's syndrome can have widespread manifestations and is classified into:

- primary Sjögren's syndrome: association of xerostomia (dry mouth) and xerophthalmia (dry eyes)

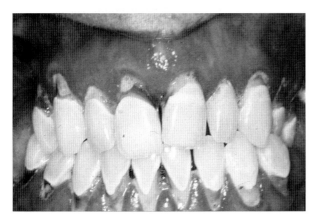

Fig. 176 A patient with radiation-related dry mouth, showing carious lesions.

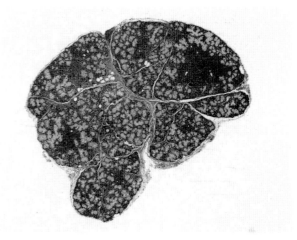

Fig. 177 Histopathological section of a labial gland biopsy in a patient with Sjögren's syndrome.

- secondary Sjögren's syndrome: association of either xerostomia or xerophthalmia and an autoimmune connective tissue disease.

There is some overlap between the two forms, though in general oral and ocular dryness is more severe in primary Sjögren's syndrome. Widespread symptoms may be experienced in both types, including nasal and vaginal dryness, dysphagia and dry skin. Fatigue syndrome is commonly present. Autoimmune connective tissue diseases that may be associated with secondary Sjögren's syndrome are given in Box 13. Rheumatoid disease (arthritis) is the most commonly associated disorder.

Clinically, middle-aged females are most commonly affected, though Sjögren's syndrome may occur in childhood. Sjögren-like features can be seen in other T-cell dysfunctions including HIV (human immunodeficiency virus) infection, therapeutic immunosuppression and graft-versus-host disease. Patients often complain of difficulty in eating dry foods and the tongue adhering to the palate. Symptoms are usually worst during the night and sleep may be disturbed. Difficulty in swallowing, speaking and wearing dentures may be experienced. The oral mucosa appears glazed and the tongue may become lobulated and beefy-red. Oral candidiasis is common and there may be patches of erythema or even ulceration. The major salivary glands may be enlarged. Sudden expansion may be a result of obstruction, acute infection or transformation to malignant lymphoma.

Box 13 Autoimmune diseases in secondary Sjögren's syndrome

- Rheumatoid disease (arthritis)
- Systemic lupus erythematosus
- Progressive systemic sclerosis
- Primary biliary cirrhosis
- Renal tubular acidois
- Mixed connective tissue disorder

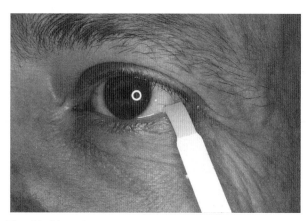

Fig. 178 Schirmer's test.

Diagnosis

Sjögren's syndrome is a clinical diagnosis and a number of investigations may aid in diagnosis. The ethics and costs of laboratory and clinical tests should be considered, particularly if results do not affect management.

Estimation of salivary flow (sialometry test) and lacrimal flow (Schirmer test; Fig. 178) are inexpensive simple tests. Often, detection of autoantibodies against SS-A(Ro) and SS-B(La) extractable nuclear antigens can be used as reasonably sensitive and specific tests. Other autoantibodies may be detected by arranging a panel of tests, as determined by evidence-based laboratory medicine. Tests that may be utilised for the diagnosis of Sjögren's syndrome are shown in Box 14. Sialographically, the classic features are varying degrees of punctate and globular sialectasis with fairly normal main ducts. However, secondary obstruction and infection means that changes often become similar to chronic sialadenitis (Fig. 179).

Labial gland biopsy is used sometimes to provide a histopathological diagnosis of Sjögren's syndrome. Infiltration of lymphocytes around intralobular ducts may be present resulting in focal lymphocytic sialadenitis. In major glands progressive lymphocytic infiltration is accompanied by acinar destruction and proliferation of residual ducts resulting in epimyoepithelial islands. Extensive change of this type results in a salivary lymphoepithelial lesion (SLEL) which in some cases progress to lymphoma.

Management

Sjögren's syndrome is generally managed by a multidisciplinary team. Dry mouth can be treated by:

- salivary stimulants if there is residual salivary function, such as chewing sugar-free gum, sucking specially formulated sugar-free pastilles (e.g. Salivix) or tablets (e.g. SST); sweets must be avoided because of the high caries risk
- saliva substitutes: these fall into three main groups
- carboxymethylcellulose based, e.g. luborant
- mucin based, e.g. Saliva Orthana
- gels containing enzymes normally present in saliva, e.g. BioXtra
- preventive advice relating to the high risk of caries and periodontal disease; in dentate individuals the use of a fluoride mouthwash may be recommended

---

Box 14 Diagnosis of Sjögren's syndrome

Diagnostic criteria

I. Ocular symptoms

A positive patient response to at least one of the three selected questions:

1. Have you had daily, persistent, troublesome dry eyes for more than 3 months?
2. Do you have a recurrent sensation of sand or gravel in the eyes?
3. Do you use tear substitutes more than three times a day?

II. Oral symptoms

A positive result to at least one of the three selected questions:

1. Have you had a daily feeling of dry mouth for more than 3 months?
2. Have you had recurrently or persistently swollen salivary glands as an adult?
3. Do you frequently drink liquids to aid swallowing dry food?

III. Ocular signs

Objective evidence of ocular involvement defined as a positive result in at least one of the following two tests:

1. Schirmer's test ($\leq$ 5 mm in 5 minutes)*
2. Rose Bengal score ($\geq$ 4 according to van Bijsterveld's scoring system).

IV. Histopathology

A focus score $\geq$ 1 in a minor salivary gland biopsy. A focus is defined as an agglomerate of at least 50 mononuclear cells; the focus score is defined by the number of foci in 4 mm^2 glandular tissue.

V. Salivary gland involvement

Objective evidence of salivary involvement defined by a positive result in at least one of the following three diagnostic tests:

1. Salivary scintigraphy
2. Parotid sialography
3. Unstimulated salivary flow ($\leq$ 1.5 ml in 15 minutes)*

VI. Autoantibodies

Presence in the serum of the following antibodies:

1. Antibodies to Ro (SS-A) or La (SS-B) antigens, or both.

Classification criteria

In patients without any potentially associated disease, the presence of any four of the six items is indicative of primary Sjögren's syndrome.

In patients with a potentially associated disease (for instance another connective tissue disease) item I or item II plus any two from among items III–V is indicative of secondary Sjögren's syndrome.

Exclusion criteria

Pre-existing lymphoma, acquired immunodeficiency disease (AIDS), sarcoidosis, graft-versus-host disease, sialoadenosis; use of antidepressant and antihypertensive drugs, neuroleptics or parasympatholytic drugs.

---

* As it has been demonstrated that this test may be reduced in normal subjects older than 60 years of age, it should be excluded from the criteria or not considered indicative for a diagnosis of Sjögren's syndrome in elderly subjects.

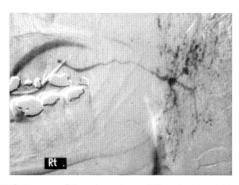

Fig. 179 Sialogram in Sjögren's syndrome. This patient has fairly classic radiological appearances in the parotid gland. The main ducts are fairly normal (although the main duct anteriorly is slightly dilated), but a striking feature is the presence of numerous small collections of contrast medium ('snow storm') overlying the gland.

- where xerostomia is severe but residual salivary gland function is present on stimulation, pilocarpine may be of benefit in radiation-induced xerostomia and Sjögren's syndrome.

Salivary gland tumours

Salivary tumours account for around 3% of human tumours but malignancy is comparatively rare. Most arise in the parotid gland, where around 90% of tumours are benign adenomas and only 10% are malignant. There is a higher relative proportion of malignant tumours in the submandibular and minor salivary glands; for example around 45% of salivary neoplasms arising in the palate (Fig. 180) prove to be malignant.

Many histopathological types have been classified and biological behaviour is variable. Only the most common types are described.

Benign tumours

Pleomorphic adenoma. Pleomorphic salivary adenoma is the most commonly encountered neoplasm, accounting for around 80–90% of all salivary tumours. In the major salivary glands, they present as slow-growing, painless nodules, often detected on routine extra-oral examination or palpation. The nodule can be soft or firm in texture and

is freely moveable. In the minor glands, pleomorphic adenoma typically presents as a rubbery nodule, principally in the palate and upper lip submucosa. Palatal lesions may be secondarily ulcerated.

Suspected pleomorphic adenomas are normally removed by excision biopsy with a margin of normal tissue. The adenomas are variable in appearance microscopically (Fig. 181) but are distinctive in having characteristic cellular and stromal elements. The cellular component is of ductal epithelial and myoepithelial cells, and these are arranged in sheets and strands. Ducts may form and sometimes squamous differentiation is present. The stromal component is rich in proteoglycans and can be organised as loose (myxoid) tissue or cartilage-like (chondroid) tissue; both types may be present. An important pathological feature to be aware of is that a capsule of compressed fibrous tissue forms around pleomorphic adenoma. Islands of tumour cells may extend beyond the capsule and 'shelling out' the adenoma in the past led to multifocal recurrence.

Warthin's tumour. Warthin's tumour (adenolymphoma) affects predominantly older men and arises almost exclusively in the parotid. Approximately 10% of cases are bilateral and the tumour presents as a discrete nodule, rarely exceeding 3cm in diameter. Microscopically, they have a papillary cystic structure comprising double layered, eosinophilic ductal cells supported by a lymphoid stroma. Smoking is thought to be an important aetiological factor.

Other adenomas. Other adenomas with varying patterns arise. These include basal cell, canalicular, trabecular and oncocytic types. Treatment is the same as for pleomorphic adenoma.

Malignant tumours

Outcome in malignant salivary gland tumours depends on histological type and grade as well as stage. Advanced malignant tumours with extensive spread or metastasis have a far worse prognosis than early stage tumours.

Adenoid cystic carcinoma. Adenoid cystic carcinoma affects middle-aged or elderly patients and accounts for

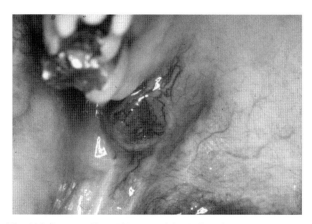

Fig. 180 A mucoepidermoid tumour arising in the palate.

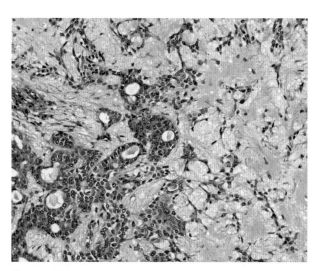

Fig. 181 Histopathological section of a pleomorphic adenoma.

around 30% of minor gland tumours. It is slow growing but may cause pain, palsy or paraesthesia because of its particular tendency to invade and spread along nerve pathways. Histopathologically, it shows a 'Swiss-cheese' appearance owing to microcysts filled by basement membrane material. Small darkly staining cells with indistinct outlines are typical (Fig. 182). It is infiltrative; metastasis develops as a late event and it has a poor long-term prognosis. It is treated by surgery, often with adjuvant radiotherapy.

Mucoepidermoid carcinoma. Mucoepidermoid carcinoma affects younger and middle-aged patients and it accounts for around 5% of minor gland tumours. Histopathologically, it shows mucous and squamous differentiation. Clinically, it shows a range of behaviour, from low-grade to highly malignant types.

Acinic-cell carcinoma. The acinic-cell carcinoma is uncommon. It shows differentiation towards salivary acinar cells; it is generally low grade but can be aggressive.

Polymorphous low-grade adenocarcinoma. Typically polymorphous adenocarcinoma occurs on the palate; it is a low-grade malignant tumour with a good prognosis despite its infiltrative growth pattern.

Other carcinomas. Carcinomas can arise in long-standing pleomorphic adenomas; when they invade adjacent tissues the prognosis is very poor.

Salivary duct carcinoma, basal-cell adenocarcinoma, sebaceous carcinoma and other rare types of carcinoma occur. Prognosis depends on both type and stage.

Other malignant tumours. Salivary glands can also develop malignant melanoma, lymphoma (sometimes arising in Sjögren's syndrome), metastases, myoepithelial tumours and rare types.

Salivary gland cysts

The most common salivary cysts occur in the minor salivary glands as a result of trauma. They present as blue, fluctuant swellings, which typically have a relapsing history. There are two types.

Mucous extravasation mucocoele. This is the most frequent type and it occurs in the lower labial mucosa (Fig. 183),

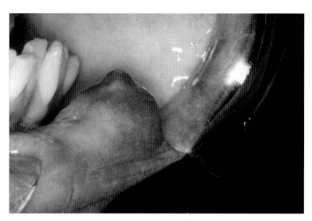

Fig. 183 A mucous extravasation mucocoele.

buccal mucosa and rarely at other sites. Trauma results in tearing of the duct, with leakage of saliva into the connective tissue. A granulation tissue capsule forms and mucin-filled, foamy macrophages are typically seen in the cyst fluid. Chronic inflammatory infiltration is usually seen also.

Mucous retention mucocoele. This type occurs less frequently and tends to be found in the upper labial mucosa. Trauma results in duct stricture and then expansion, forming a cyst lined by ductal epithelium. The cyst contains clear saliva, with minimal inflammatory or macrophage reaction.

Bilateral and multiple lymphoepithelial parotid cysts can be a feature of HIV infection. The cysts occur early in HIV disease and are not typically seen in advanced AIDS. Diagnosis is based on fine-needle aspiration and imaging. No intervention is normally required but if lymphomatous infiltration is suspected surgical excision may be performed.

13.4 Surgery

Learning objectives

You should:
* know the principles of surgery to remove salivary glands.

Surgical removal of minor salivary glands is the treatment of choice for mucous extravasation and retention cysts and tumours. Surgery of the major salivary glands is carried out when there is neoplastic disease, obstruction and sometimes in inflammatory disease.

Minor salivary glands

Excision of a cyst with associated glands and duct may be undertaken under local anaesthesia. Swellings thought to be tumours because of their history, site and appearance require wider excision. Ranulae (mucocoeles arising from the sublingual gland) should be excised together with the associated lingual gland. If large in size, then this may be more readily performed under general anaesthesia.

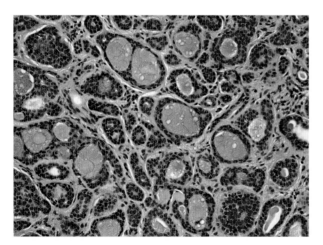

Fig. 182 Histopathological section of an adenoid cystic carcinoma.

Cryosurgery, in which subzero cooling is used to destroy tissues, may be used to remove small cysts. The probe of a liquid nitrogen apparatus is placed on the cyst for two to five cycles of about 30 seconds at −100 °C. The extreme cold results in an acute inflammatory response and tissue damage. The technique, which is very simple to use, results in significant postoperative swelling but excellent healing without a surgical scar. The disadvantage is that there is no histopathological examination. Cryosurgery may also be used for small vascular lesions such as haemangiomas.

Submandibular salivary gland

Surgical removal of a calculus from the anterior part of the duct of the submandibular salivary gland may be undertaken under local anaesthesia. A suture is placed about the duct behind the calculus to prevent it moving back into the gland and then the duct is dissected and opened via an intra-oral approach. The calculus is removed and the duct sutured open to prevent stricture. Should the calculus be sited more proximally, then removal of the gland may be necessary. In the case of surgical removal of the submandibular gland for this or another reason, the patient is advised of the following risks of the operation:

- possible facial nerve damage resulting in weakness of the lower lip
- possible lingual nerve damage resulting in lingual paraesthesia.

Surgical removal of the submandibular gland is undertaken under general anaesthesia with the patient supine and the head turned to the opposite side and extended. The skin is prepared and the submandibular incision made 2.5 cm below the mandible to avoid the facial nerve (Fig. 184). During dissection, vessels are identified and ligated before the gland is removed. A vacuum drain is placed to minimise haematoma formation and the wound is closed with sutures.

An alternative to surgery for calculus removal is radiologically guided retrieval of the calculus through the duct orifice using a basket retrieval catheter. This works best with small, freely moving calculi. Lithotripsy and balloon dilation may also be used and 70% of obstructed glands can be treated conservatively.

Parotid salivary gland

A calculus in the anterior part of the parotid salivary duct may be removed by an intra-oral approach under local anaesthesia, again with a suture placed behind to prevent the calculus slipping back into the gland. In the case of a calculus sited further back, or non-malignant disease in the superficial lobe, the glandular tissue superficial to the facial nerve may be removed (superficial parotidectomy), thus preserving the nerve. In the case of a malignant tumour, the whole gland may be removed (total parotidectomy) with sacrifice of the nerve. Non-malignant disease occurring in the deep lobe will require removal of the whole gland with preservation of the nerve. A patient undergoing parotidectomy is advised of the risks of the operation:

- possible facial weakness or expected facial paralysis depending on the type of surgery planned
- numbness of the ear on the side of surgery as the great auricular nerve has to be divided during surgery. Much less likely complications are:
- sweating around the ear when the patient eats because of regrowth of secretomotor parasympathetic nerve fibres (Frey's syndrome)
- salivary fistula.

Surgery is undertaken under general anaesthesia with the patient supine and the head turned to the opposite side. The skin is prepared and a preauricular incision made and extended behind the ear lobe over the mastoid process and down to the submandibular area (Fig. 185). A skin flap

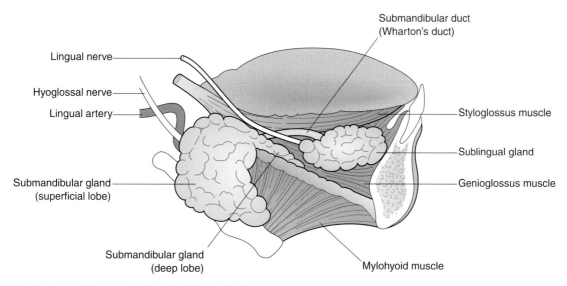

Fig. 184 Surgical approach for removal of a submandibular gland.

Lingual nerve

Hyoglossal nerve

Lingual artery

Submandibular gland (superficial lobe)

Submandibular gland (deep lobe)

Submandibular duct (Wharton's duct)

Styloglossus muscle

Sublingual gland

Genioglossus muscle

Mylohyoid muscle

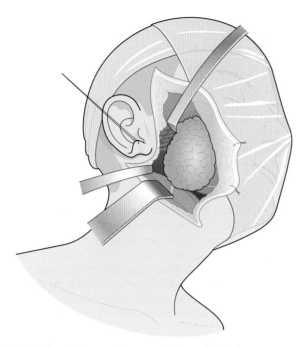

Fig. 185 Surgical approach for removal of a parotid gland.

is raised to expose the gland and the facial nerve trunk. An electric nerve stimulator may be used to help to identify the nerve if the patient has not been given a muscle relaxant drug as part of the anaesthetic technique at this stage. The gland may then be dissected above the nerve and removed. A vacuum drain is placed and the wound closed.

As with the submandibular gland, under certain circumstances calculi may be removed via the duct orifice by consevative methods (see above).

Self-assessment: questions

Multiple choice questions

1. Mumps (epidemic parotitis):
   a. Is caused by an adenovirus
   b. Is transmitted by droplets spread from infected saliva
   c. In adults may involve the central nervous system, pancreas, testes and ovaries
   d. Bilateral parotid involvement is more common than unilateral involvement
   e. Recurrent attacks are not uncommon

2. The following are likely causes of a localised swelling in the upper labial submucosa:
   a. Mucous extravasation mucocoele
   b. Mucous retention mucocoele
   c. Basal-cell adenoma
   d. Capillary haemangioma
   e. Warthin's tumour

3. Adenoid cystic carcinoma:
   a. May arise in the paranasal sinuses
   b. Arises from the adenoids
   c. Has a progressively worse survival at 5, 10 and 20 years, respectively
   d. Often exhibits perineural spread
   e. Has microcystic spaces containing basement membrane-like material

4. In Sjögren's syndrome:
   a. Secondary Sjögren's syndrome comprises dry eyes, dry mouth and a connective tissue (autoimmune) disorder
   b. Uptake of ^{99m}[Tc]-pertechnate by salivary glands is increased in Sjögren's syndrome
   c. Fatigue syndrome is associated with Sjögren's syndrome
   d. Salivary duct antibody is the most useful diagnostic immunotest for Sjögren's syndrome
   e. Polyclonal B-cell expansion is a feature of Sjögren's syndrome

5. Dry mouth:
   a. Caused by reduced salivary flow can be inferred when the resting rate falls below 5 ml/min
   b. Can be a feature of cystic fibrosis
   c. Typically is associated with cervical or root caries
   d. May be caused by anxiety
   e. Is an uncommon unwanted effect of drug therapy

6. Radiation effects on the salivary glands:
   a. Are more apparent in mucous acini than serous acini
   b. Some recovery is possible
   c. Include fibrosis after high exposure
   d. Can cause duct ectasia and squamous metaplasia
   e. Include endarteritis obliterans

7. Bilateral parotid swelling may be a feature of:
   a. Sarcoidosis
   b. Warthin's tumour
   c. Primary Sjögren's syndrome
   d. HIV (human immunodeficiency virus) infection
   e. Chronic lymphocytic leukaemia (CLL)

8. Salivary calculi (sialoliths):
   a. Of very small size (microliths) are commonly found in the major glands
   b. Form around nanobacteria that infect the ducts
   c. Can result in the submandibular saliva being supersaturated with respect to calcium and phosphate ions
   d. May be forced into the submandibular gland from the anterior duct during removal under local anaesthesia
   e. May not give rise to symptoms

9. Pleomorphic salivary adenoma:
   a. Carcinoma arising in pleomorphic salivary adenoma has a worse prognosis than mucoepidermoid carcinoma
   b. May contain myxoid and chondroid stroma
   c. May contain plasmacytoid or spindle-shaped myoepithelial cells
   d. May arise in the maxillary sinus and nasal septum
   e. Shows marked nuclear and cellular pleomorphism

10. Mucous extravasation mucocoele:
    a. Most commonly occurs in the buccal mucosa
    b. Has a granulation tissue capsule
    c. Often contains foamy macrophages
    d. May undergo spontaneous resolution
    e. Tends to have a relapsing clinical course

Extended matching items

EMI 1. Theme: Salivary gland disorders

Options:

A Mucous extravasation mucocoele
B Mucous retention mucocoele
C Heerfordt's syndrome
D Warthin's tumour
E Pleomorphic adenoma
F Facial nerve palsy due to perineural invasion
G Salivary lymphoepithelial lesion
H Sialosis
I Carcinoma in pleomorphic adenoma
J Mucoepidermoid carcinoma

Lead in: Match the case from the list below that is most appropriate for each diagnosis above.

1. A 55-year-old woman presented to her dentist with carious cavities that had occurred since her last check-up. The patient had noticed that her mouth was dry and on examination her parotid glands were enlarged. At the dental hospital her consultant performed a needle core biopsy, which was reported as containing confluent sheets of non-caseating granulomas. She was referred on to an ophthalamic specialist who found that she had uveitis on slit-lamp examination.

2. A long-standing tumour was removed from the parotid gland. The pathologist reported that the tumour was composed of sheets, strands and islands of ductal cells separated by myxochondroid tumour. Plasmacytoid myoepithelial cells were present in some areas and islands of squamous cells were also present. The tumour was enclosed by an intact pseudo-capsule formed by compressed fibrous tissue into which tumour pseudopodia extended.

3. A 15-year-old girl presented with a relapsing swelling on the lower labial mucosa. The pathologist reported that the lesion was a cyst that was lined internally by granulation tissue. The lumen contained foamy macrophages.

4. An elderly man presented with bilateral swellings of the parotid gland. On ultrasound the tumours were cystic and were up to 3 cm in diameter. A fine-needle aspirate showed lymphocytes and clusters of oncocytes. Following the aspiration the gland became painful but after 2 weeks the tumour had reduced in size considerably.

5. A 62-year-old woman developed a rapidly growing swelling of the left parotid gland which was fixed to skin. A biopsy was reported as showing multiple patterns of carcinoma, including salivary duct carcinoma. Hyaline and myxoid scar tissue was also present.

6. A 42-year-old woman presented with a parotid tumour. A needle core biopsy showed a tumour composed of cells with hyperchromatic, angular nuclei and scant basophilic cytoplasm. The features were those of adenoid cystic carcinoma. A worrying sign of salivary malignancy was present.

7. A 13-year-old boy presented with a swelling of the right parotid gland that had steadily enlarged and which had not improved after a course of antibiotics. Ultrasound showed a fairly well circumscribed cystic tumour which was removed. The pathologist reported that the tumour contained goblet cells, squamous cells, clear cells and 'intermediate' cells.

8. An overweight 56-year-old man developed type II diabetes. His parotid glands became enlarged over a 2-year period and he felt that his mouth was too full of saliva. The dentist noticed that he had acid erosion on the palatal surfaces of his upper anterior teeth.

9. A 70-year-old patient who suffered from Sjogren's syndrome for many years experienced enlargement of one of her parotid glands. A superficial parotidectomy was performed and the pathologist reported that the parotid parenchyma was expanded by a lymphoid infiltrate and epi-myoepithelial islands were present.

10. A 15-year-old girl presented with a relapsing swelling on the upper labial mucosa. The pathologist reported that the lesion was a cyst that was lined internally by ductal epithelium. The lumen was filled with mucoid fluid and a small lamellated calculus was present.

EMI 2. Theme: Salivary gland disorders

Options:

A Xerostomia
B Hypersalivation
C Cystic HIV salivary disease
D Canalicular adenoma
E Obstuctive sialadenitis
F Mumps
G Relapsing childhood parotitis
H Acute bacterial sialadenitis
I Ranula
J Sialoblastoma

Lead in: Match the case from the list below that is most appropriate for each diagnosis above.

1. A 21-week-old infant developed an enlarging mass in her right parotid gland that encroached onto the sternomastoid and elevated the ear.

2. A dentist noticed that one of his 60-year-old patients developed fresh carious lesions between each visit and had recently developed cervical cavities in the anterior incisor teeth.

3. A 7-year-old boy experienced facial swelling and a febrile illness. His mother described his face as 'being out like a box' and thought that he had a dental abscess.

4. A 57-year-old patient developed a fluctuant swelling in the floor of the mouth that was translucent on transillumination.

5. A 60-year-old man developed a cystic lump in the submucosa of the upper lip. Smaller lumps were found adjacent the main lesion and were removed.

6. A 32-year-old man presented with pain and swelling under the angle of the mandible at meal times. Afterwards there was an unpleasant taste in the mouth.

7. A 78-year-old man complained of producing too much saliva. It leaked onto his pillow and he was constantly swallowing.

8. A 28-year-old man developed gross bilateral parotid swelling. On imaging he had multiple cystic changes and a fine-needle aspirate showed lymphoid cells.

9. A 14-year-old girl presented with acute parotid swelling and pain. She had experienced two previous attacks, one on the other side.

10. A 37-year-old man experienced pain and swelling of his right parotid gland 2 days after blowing up a balloon.

Case history questions

Case history 1

A 24-year-old woman attended for dental care. She mentioned that she had found a small lump just in front of her left ear. On examination there was a freely moveable, rubbery nodule, 1 cm in diameter, just below and anterior to the tragus of the left ear. She was referred to an oral and maxillofacial surgeon who undertook some investigations and subsequently performed a superficial parotidectomy. The histopathologist reported the nodule as a pleomorphic salivary adenoma.

1. Which investigations are available to the oral and maxillofacial surgeon for preoperative diagnosis of a lump in the parotid gland?
2. What is the rationale of undertaking a superficial parotidectomy for this benign neoplasm?
3. What are the key histopathological features of pleomorphic salivary adenoma?
4. Why is it advantageous to remove this benign neoplasm as soon as practicable after diagnosis?

Case history 2

A 9-year-old boy presents with unilateral parotid swelling of a few days' duration. He had suffered a previous similar episode, which was thought to be mumps although not entirely typical. Antibiotic therapy was prescribed and the swelling subsided within a few days. The symptoms recurred a few weeks later and again after 3 months. His mother mentioned at that time that he occasionally made a 'funny face' by blowing out his cheeks.

1. What is the most likely diagnosis?
2. Sialography is avoided in children unless essential; what features would be expected in a patient with this disorder?
3. How should the condition be managed?

Case history 3

A 73-year-old woman with a long history of Sjögren's syndrome developed rapid enlargement of the left parotid gland. She suffered from rheumatoid arthritis. The swelling had been present for 5 weeks before she attended her dentist. On examination, the left parotid gland is enlarged and feels both thickened and firm on bimanual palpation. Ipsilateral non-tender cervical lymph nodes are also palpable.

1. Does the patient suffer from primary or secondary Sjögren's syndrome?
2. What is the most likely cause of the recent parotid swelling?
3. How may this diagnosis be confirmed?

Case history 4

A 38-year-old woman presents with swelling and pain for 3 days involving the left parotid gland. On examination, the overlying skin appears erythematous and the gland is tender on palpation. A mucopurulent discharge from the left parotid duct is seen. A diagnosis of acute bacterial sialadenitis is made and a swab of the discharge was sent to the microbiology department.

1. Which investigations on the swab should be requested?
2. Which bacterial agents are most likely to be involved?
3. Which predisposing factors may be present?
4. How should the case be managed?

Case history 5

A 34-year-old man working as a chef complains that his face is swollen at the angles of the jaw, making him look like a hamster! He is obese and has recently been found to be diabetic. On examination, there is bilateral, symmetrical enlargement of the parotid glands. They are not tender and a copious flow of clear saliva could be obtained from the ducts.

1. What diagnosis is most likely?
2. Which predisposing factors can be associated with this disorder?
3. What histopathological features are seen in this condition?

Case history 6

A 47-year-old man presents with intermittent pain and swelling in the left submandibular area for 4 months. Symptoms were worst just before eating and persisted throughout the meal. He noticed an unpleasant taste in the mouth for some time after eating, as the swelling subsided.

1. What is the most likely diagnosis?
2. Which features should be looked for particularly on examination?
3. How may imaging help to provide useful clinical information?
4. Which histopathological features might be expected in the submandibular salivary gland?

Viva questions

1. Suggest some common causes of dry mouth
2. What types of tumour commonly affect the salivary glands?
3. What are the possible causes of obstruction of the submandibular salivary gland?
4. What are the possible complications of the surgical removal of a parotid salivary gland?
5. What is a labial gland biopsy? How is it undertaken?

Self-assessment: answers

Multiple choice answers

1. a. **False.** Mumps is caused by a paramyxovirus. It is difficult to detect this directly but the virus can be grown from throat swabs or saliva. Serology will show a rise in antibody titre between acute and convalescent specimens.
    b. **True.** Direct contact and droplet spread from saliva are the principal routes of transmission. Virus is present in saliva during the prodromal phase and for about a week after resolution of the sialadenitis.
    c. **True.** Orchitis is the most common manifestation. It is thought to occur in about 20% of adult mumps in males and has been linked to infertility. Meningitis and meningoencephalitis are rare complications.
    d. **True.** Bilateral parotitis is seen in around 70% of cases. Submandibular glands are occasionally involved also, resulting in a 'box-like' facies.
    e. **False.** Long-lasting immunity is generally conferred and recurrent infection is extremely rare.

2. a. **False.** Mucous extravasation mucocoeles are common in the lower lip, especially in the occlusal plane, but are very rare in the upper lip.
    b. **True.** Mucous retention mucocoeles tend to occur in the upper lip and buccal mucosa, most commonly in older patients.
    c. **True.** Basal cell, trabecular and canalicular adenomas are found in the upper lip. Some may show cystic change and some are multifocal.
    d. **True.** The lips are richly vascular, and vascular malformations are not uncommon in the submucosa. They typically blanche on pressure and may be pulsatile.
    e. **False.** Warthin's tumour (adenolymphoma) is a parotid lesion, though ectopic examples have been described.

3. a. **True.** Adenoid cystic carcinoma can arise in the paranasal sinuses, including the maxillary sinus, lacrimal gland, trachea and in more distant glandular tissues.
    b. **False.** The word 'adenoids' is a lay term for nasopharyngeal tonsillar tissue or thickened nasal/antral mucosa.
    c. **True.** In a meta-analysis of survival data, survival rates were quoted at approximately 75% at 5 years, 40% at 10 years and 15% at 20 years.
    d. **True.** Perineural invasion often leads to palsy, pain or paraesthesia as presenting signs.
    e. **True.** The microcystic spaces impart the Swiss-cheese appearance. They contain 'connective tissue mucin', which stains with Alcian blue. It includes basement membrane constituents.

4. a. **False.** Some textbooks do give this definition, but most clinicians recognise that either dry mouth or dry eyes with a connective tissue disorder can be defined as secondary Sjögren's syndrome.
    b. **False.** Scintiscanning can be used but uptake is decreased.
    c. **True.** This is common.
    d. **False.** Antibodies against extractable nuclear antigens are the most sensitive and specific indicators, particularly SSA and SSB.
    e. **True.** Polyclonal B-cell expansion may result from loss of T-cell regulation.

5. a. **False.** The lower limit of normal resting salivary flow is approximately 0.1 ml/min.
    b. **True.** Cystic fibrosis is a genetic disorder where secretion is abnormal.
    c. **True.** Preventive advice should be given to those with xerostomia as increased caries rates are seen.
    d. **True.** It is a consequence of adrenergic hormone release.
    e. **False.** Unwanted effects of drug therapy are one of the most common causes of dry mouth. Patients must not be advised to discontinue their medication but the responsible physician may be contacted for advice.

6. a. **False.** Both mucous and serous acini are equally sensitive.
    b. **True.** Some recovery of function is possible after low-dose irradiation.
    c. **True.** This can cause stricture of the duct.
    d. **True.** Particularly when head and neck cancers are treated.
    e. **True.** This is proliferation of the intimal layer and results in narrowing or obliteration of the vascular lumen.

7. a. **True.** Sarcoidosis is a multisystem chronic granulomatous inflammatory disorder that can involve the salivary glands and cause swelling and dry mouth. Parotitis, facial palsy, uveitis in sarcoidosis is known as Heerfordt syndrome.
    b. **True.** Up to 10% of Warthin's tumour are bilateral cases.
    c. **True.**
    d. **True.** Bilateral lymphoepithelial cysts of the parotid gland, Sjögren-like syndrome and malignant lymphoma may occur.
    e. **True.** CLL may infiltrate any organ. Bilateral parotid enlargement and dry mouth are rare manifestations.

8. a. **True.** Microcalculi are commonly seen histologically.
    b. **False.** It has been claimed that renal calculi form around 'nanobacteria' but even the existence of these organisms is debatable.

c. **True.** The saliva will be in dynamic equilibrium with the calcium- and phosphate-containing calculi.

d. **True.** A suture may be placed to avoid this well-recognised hazard.

e. **True.** Sometimes calculi are found incidentally on routine examination. Treatment may not be necessary.

9. a. **True.** Carcinoma arising in pleomorphic adenoma is a very aggressive neoplasm; mucoepidermoid carcinoma has a range of clinical behaviour.

b. **True.** Both loose (myxoid) tissue and cartilage-like (chondroid) tissue can occur in the stroma.

c. **True.** Plasmacytoid (hyaline) myoepithelial cells are a key feature.

d. **True.**

e. **False.** 'Pleomorphic' in pleomorphic salivary adenoma refers to the variety of features which may be encountered; it is cytologically bland.

10. a. **False.** It is most common in the lower labial mucosa.

b. **True.** It occurs around saliva that leaks from a tear in a salivary duct into connective tissue.

c. **True.** They occur in cyst and fluid.

d. **True.** However, they can relapse.

e. **True.**

Extended matching items answers

EMI 1

1. **C.** Sarcoidosis is a chronic granulomatous condition that may affect the parotid and cause uveitis. Facial nerve palsy and fever may be present. This is Heerfordt's syndrome (uveo-parotid fever).

2. **E.** Pleomorphic adenoma is sometimes referred to as 'mixed tumour' because the neoplasms contain both epithelial ductal and myxochondroid stromal elements. The hyaline plasmacytoid myoepithelial cell is a characteristic feature.

3. **A.** Mucous extravasation mucocoele is most common on the lower lip. The duct of a minor salivary gland is ruptured by trauma. Saliva leaks out and granulation tissue walls this off forming a cyst. Foamy macrophages are commonly present.

4. **D.** Warthin's tumours are benign and typically present in the parotid gland. There is a strong link with smoking and 10% are bilateral.

5. **I.** Carcinoma can arise from pleomorphic adenoma, usually after several years. Multiple patterns of carcinoma are suggestive of this diagnosis. Often a 'ghost' or scarred remnant of the original pleomorphic adenoma can be found embedded in the tumour.

6. **F.** Facial nerve palsy is a sign of malignancy when a salivary tumour is present in the parotid gland.

7. **J.** Mucoepidermoid carcinoma tends to occur in a younger age group than other salivary cancers. The features in this case suggest a low-grade carcinoma. High-grade mucoepidermoid carcinoma is more infiltrative and tends to be solid.

8. **H.** Sialosis is caused by salivary acinar hyperplasia and is known to occur in a variety of disorders including diabetes, alcoholism, sympathomimetic drug use, obesity and endocrine disorders. The acid erosion of the palatal enamel suggests bulimia which is also a cause of sialosis.

9. **G.** Sjogren syndrome is an autoimmune condition in which B cells accumulate in the salivary tissue. As the condition advances the salivary acini are destroyed, the ducts form epimyoepithelial islands and lymphoid cells accumulate. This lesion is termed a salivary lymphoepithelial lesion (SLEL). It is known that SLEL can progress to malignant lymphoma.

10. **B.** Mucous retention mucocoele is less common that extravasation cyst and tends to occur in the upper lip. The duct is blocked, sometimes by calculus and the duct expands to produce an epithelial lined cyst.

EMI 2

1. **J.** Sialoblastoma is a rare salivary tumour that presents in the neonatal period.

2. **A.** Caries is a feature of xerostomia (dry mouth) due to loss of buffering power and the protective effect of saliva on enamel. Patients sometimes do not complain of dry mouth clinically even when it is severe. Xerostomia is a common unwanted effect of drugs, but may also be caused by underlying diseases such as Sjogren syndrome.

3. **F.** Mumps virus causes swelling of the parotid and submandibular glands. Unilateral disease can be confused with dental abscess when carious teeth are present.

4. **I.** The term ranula is used to describe a mucous extravasation mucocoele arising from the main submandibular duct.

5. **D.** Canalicular adenoma is a salivary neoplasm typically found in the upper lip. It shows a loose structure with beading of the tumour cell strands. Multiple tumours may be present.

6. **E.** Obstructive sialadenitis is most commonly seen in the submandibular gland but the parotid may also be affected. Calculus forms in the main duct and chronic infection may contribute to progressive fibrosis and loss of functional elements.

7. **B.** Hypersalivation (ptyalism) is a sensation of producing too much saliva. Many patients with this complaint have normal flow rates on testing. Sometimes the condition is due to drooling because of loss of muscle action and surgery can help.

8. **C.** Bilateral multicystic salivary disease is a recognised manifestation of HIV infection.

9. **G.** Relapsing childhood parotitis is an unusual condition characterised by duct ectasia. Acute episodes are managed by antibiotic therapy, warm mouthrinses and gentle massage. The condition often resolves after puberty.

10. **H.** Acute parotitis is caused by oral bacteria that ascend the parotid duct. The gland should be gently pressed and mucopurulent saliva from the parotid

papilla sampled for microbial analysis. Broad spectrum antibiotics may be useful in combination with gentle massage and mouthrinses.

Case history answers

Case history 1

1. History and clinical examination including palpation of the swelling are most informative. Ultrasound, sialography, computed tomography, magnetic resonance imaging and positron emission tomography are useful imaging modalities. Fine-needle aspiration biopsy (FNAB) or narrow-cutting core biopsy can be used for pathological diagnosis. Final tumour diagnosis is sometimes made after excision biopsy.
2. Pleomorphic salivary adenoma cells tend to extend into the capsule surrounding the tumour and enucleation may be followed by multifocal recurrence. Extracapsular dissection, superficial parotidectomy or other procedures aim to remove the adenoma with a margin of normal tissue to avoid this problem.
3. Key histopathological features are sheets, strands and islands of ductal epithelial and myoepithelial cells; myxoid or chondroid stroma; plasmacytoid (hyaline) myoepithelial cells; cytological blandness; extracapsular extension; and variability in appearance.
4. Early removal of pleomorphic adenoma is advised (a) to reduce morbidity; (b) to avoid the risk of malignant transformation; and (c) to allow thorough histopathological sampling for diagnosis.

Case history 2

1. The most likely diagnosis is recurrent childhood sialadenitis.
2. Childhood sialadenitis is characterised by main duct ectasia and strictures with destruction of secretory tissue.
3. Acute episodes of infection may necessitate antibiotic therapy; gentle external massage may help to encourage salivary flow. Habits such as inflating the cheeks should be discouraged, as infection arises from bacteria ascending the ducts.

Case history 3

1. Secondary Sjögren's syndrome; around 10% of patients with rheumatoid arthritis have been estimated to have Sjögren's syndrome.
2. Malignant lymphoma. There is a progression from B-cell infiltration, through lymphoepithelial lesion to malignant lymphoma in some cases. Low-grade B-cell lymphoma is the most common type. Acute infection or obstruction may also cause sudden swelling of the parotid gland.
3. Imaging studies may reveal a space-occupying mass but biopsy is needed if malignant lymphoma is suspected.

Case history 4

1. Culture and sensitivity.
2. *Streptococcus pyogenes, Staphylococcus aureus, Haemophilus* species and other normal oral flora may be isolated.

3. Reduced salivary flow such as in chronic sialadenitis, HIV infection, Sjögren's syndrome, obstructive disease, postirradiation changes and side effects of drugs.
4. Antibiotic therapy should follow current guidelines, such as those in the British National Formulary, taking into account the microbiology findings. Patients should be advised to avoid applying heat to the gland and should gently massage the gland by placing two fingers over the angle of the mandible and gently moving upwards and forwards. Warm salt mouthrinses may also help. Review should be arranged and proper assessment undertaken when the acute symptoms have subsided.

Case history 5

1. Sialosis (acinar hypertrophy).
2. Drugs, alcoholism, diabetes, liver cirrhosis, metabolic and hormonal disturbances, bulimia.
3. Enlargement of secretory acinar cells with cytoplasm packed with zymogen granules.

Case history 6

1. Obstructive sialadenitis owing to calculus formation. Other causes of obstruction should also be considered.
2. Calculus in the submandibular duct may be visible but is more often detected by bimanual palpation. The floor of mouth may be dried with gauze and salivary flow observed from the duct orifice. A sialogogue, such as chewing a citric acid tablet, may reproduce the signs and symptoms. Turbid saliva suggests infection and should be sampled for microbiological analysis.
3. Occlusal radiography with exposure adjustment for soft tissue may reveal radio-opaque calculus in the submandibular duct. The second imaging investigation is sialography, which sometimes dislodges the calculus.
4. Obstructed glands may recover following removal of calculus. In chronic obstructive sialadenitis, it may be necessary to remove the submandibular gland. Principal histopathological features are duct ectasia with mucous metaplasia, inter- and intralobular fibrosis, acinar atrophy, acinar loss and chronic inflammatory infiltration. Intraglandular calculus may form.

Viva answers

1. Unwanted effects of drugs, Sjögren's syndrome, anxiety, mouth breathing, dehydration, uncontrolled diabetes mellitus, and generalised chronic inflammatory or neoplastic disorders.
2. Pleomorphic adenoma is the most common tumour; other less-rare types are Warthin's tumour, adenoid cystic carcinoma, acinic-cell carcinoma and mucoepidermoid carcinoma.
3. These can be classified as extraductal (e.g. pressure from an adjacent tumour or displaced anatomical structure), ductal (e.g. fibrous stricture of the duct wall) and intraductal (e.g. calculus, mucous plug).

4. Facial nerve weakness or palsy, loss of sensation of the ear, Frey's syndrome (gustatory sweating), salivary fistula and cosmetic defect.

5. Labial gland biopsy is taken to provide a sample for histological assessment of salivary tissue, avoiding parotid biopsy. It is used most often as a diagnostic procedure in Sjögren's syndrome. Under local anaesthesia, a 1 cm vertical or horizontal incision is made in the lower labial mucosa, and 10–12 lobules removed. There must be no disease in the overlying mucosa. Care must be taken to avoid damage to the labial neurovascular bundles.

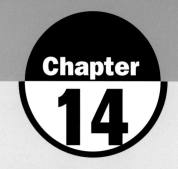

Facial pain

Overview

This chapter focuses on the common and significant causes of orofacial pain excluding those related to dental and periodontal pathology. For many patients orofacial pain is the stimulus to seek dental care, thus the treatment of patients in pain is, unfortunately, going to form a significant part of your practice. In terms of orofacial pain, the basis of accurate diagnosis and appropriate treatment is the information that is obtained from the patient. Consequently, history-taking skills need to be utilised to their best effect.

14.1 Assessment of a patient suffering from orofacial pain

Learning objectives

You should:
- know how to take an informative history
- know what examination to undertake.

Assessment of orofacial pain requires eliciting as much information from the patient as possible. The basic information you need must include:

- the nature of the pain: encourage the patient to describe the pain in their own words by the use of open questions rather than supplying them with a list of descriptors of pain from which to select; the latter can be useful if a patient is finding it particularly difficult to describe their pain
- when the pain first began
- the duration of each episode of pain
- the frequency of the painful episodes: how often do episodes of pain occur; what is the longest and shortest time the patient has been symptom free
- the site(s) affected: ask the patient to point to the source of the pain and/or outline the area affected by it; does the pain radiate to other areas? Is it confined

to the distribution of a particular nerve(s) or does it cross anatomical boundaries, for example the midline?
- initiating factors: anything that the patient remembers occurring immediately before or at the same time as the start of their symptoms
- precipitating factors: anything which now seems to induce the patient's symptoms
- exacerbating factors: anything which makes the patient's symptoms worse
- ameliorating factors: anything which relieves, either partially or totally, the patient's symptoms
- associated signs and symptoms
- previous investigations
- previous treatment
- relevant medical/dental/social/family history.

Much of this information will emerge naturally, in most cases, by simply asking the patient to tell you about their pain. Verbal and non-verbal communication skills should be used to encourage the patient to tell their story in a way that is mutually beneficial. At the end of the consultation, the patient should feel that they have been able to impart information that they felt was relevant and the dentist should have guided them through this process to yield up the information required to reach a differential diagnosis.

A thorough extra-oral (including the temporomandibular joint and muscles of mastication) and intra-oral examination (see Ch. 2) is obviously mandatory. Additional components of the examination procedure may be required depending on the differential diagnosis, for example assessment of cranial nerve function in patients presenting with symptoms of trigeminal neuralgia. The differential diagnosis will be based on a combination of the outcome of the examination and history. The special investigations that are carried out (these may not always be necessary) will be aimed at clarifying the differential diagnosis and should be carefully tailored to fulfil this purpose, not used as a general screening procedure.

While this chapter will not be considering those diseases of the teeth and their supporting structures that give rise to orofacial pain, it is important to stress that dentists need to be particularly skilled in excluding such structures as the source of the patient's pain. The principal causes of pain arising from the teeth and their supporting structures are listed below, with reference to the appropriate sections of this book and its companion volume (*Master Dentistry*, Vol. 2, *Restorative and Paediatric Dentistry*, edited by Heasman). You must know the signs of symptoms of these conditions and apply this knowledge when reaching a differential diagnosis in the case of a patient with orofacial pain.

- Dentine sensitivity (Vol. 2)
- Pulpitis (Ch. 5, this volume)
- Periapical periodontitis
- Periodontal abscess (Ch. 5, this volume).

14.2 The neuralgias

Learning objectives

You should:
- know the typical clinical presentations of the various neuralgias
- know any special investigations
- understand the management options.

Trigeminal neuralgia

The majority of cases (> 85%) of trigeminal neuralgia are of classic type (CTN). Compression of the trigeminal nerve in the region of the dorsal root entry zone (DREZ) by a blood vessel has emerged as the leading cause of CTN.

Clinical presentation

Sex. More common in females than males.

Age. Predominantly affects individuals over the age of 50 years. This is highly significant, as its presence in younger individuals is suggestive of multiple sclerosis.

Nature. A sharp, stabbing, episodic, electric shock-like pain. Often the pain is so intense that the patient has to stop what they are doing.

Duration. Usually of seconds duration. Occasionally a dull pain persists in the background after the sharp pain has resolved. In severe cases, the episodes of pain may be so close together that they seem continuous, but this is unusual. Spontaneous remission of symptoms can occur, but both this and their recurrence are unpredictable.

Site. The pain is localised to one or more divisions of the trigeminal nerve, most commonly the second and third division. The patient outlines the distribution of the appropriate division(s) when asked to indicate the area affected by the pain. The pain does not usually cross the midline.

Initiating factors. The pain is induced when a particular area of the skin or mucosa is stimulated, the so-called 'trigger zone'. For example, washing the face, shaving, putting on make-up, eating, speaking and exposure to cold may all induce pain.

Associated signs and symptoms. The absence of associated signs and symptoms of sensory or motor deficit is important. Neurological assessment is mandatory to ensure that the symptoms of trigeminal neuralgia are not the result of a lesion (neoplastic or non-neoplastic) within the posterior cranial fossa. The patient's medical history may already have revealed the existence of such a lesion or the presence of multiple sclerosis.

Special investigations

Magnetic resonance imaging (MRI) is now considered mandatory. In many cases it demonstrates the intimate, potentially causative, relationship between the trigeminal root and an adjacent blood vessel. MRI is of particular value in excluding posterior cranial fossa lesions and, to some extent, multiple sclerosis.

Medical management

The therapy of choice is carbamazepine. Reduction or complete resolution of symptoms following its use is considered to be virtually diagnostic of trigeminal neuralgia. However, it should be prescribed cautiously, starting at a dose of 100 mg twice or three times daily and increasing slowly until the patient's symptoms are controlled. This is usually achieved at between 200 and 400 mg three times daily. Gradual increase in dosage is important as elderly patients are particularly susceptible to carbamazepine's many side-effects. Some of these, for example nausea, ataxia and dizziness, make taking carbamazepine completely unpalatable to the patient or significantly limit its dose. Others, including leukopenia and skin reactions, necessitate its withdrawal; patients should be informed of the signs and symptoms of these conditions when the drug is prescribed. Full blood count, liver and renal function tests should ideally be carried out prior to its prescription and at regular intervals during at least the first months of treatment. If withdrawal of carbamazepine proves to be necessary, oxcarbazepine or gabapentin provide alternatives. Should the dose of carbamazepine be limited the skeletal muscle relaxant baclofen or the anti-epileptic lamotrigine may be added.

Surgical management

Although the evidence base for surgical interventions is weak, microvascular decompression (MVD) appears to have the best outcome and is emerging as the preferred option in those patients who are fit for open surgery. In this procedure the offending blood vessel is lifted away from the trigeminal root and permanently repositioned. In comparison to peripheral destructive procedures such as neurectomy or central destructive procedures such as percutaneous radiofrequency thermocoagulation, MVD has a low rate of complications. It is, however, important that MVD is performed sooner rather than later as success declines with duration of trigeminal neuralgia symptoms. This is leading to a change in approach with clinicians raising the awareness of patients to the possibility of surgical intervention much earlier in the medical treatment phase rather than as a last resort. Other central procedures include retrogasserian glycerol injection and gamma knife stereotactic surgery. These have largely replaced peripheral procedures although local anaesthetic injected into the trigger zone will provide temporary relief of symptoms (bupivacaine has a longer duration of action) and is useful in confirming the diagnosis.

Glossopharyngeal neuralgia

Glossopharyngeal neuralgia is an extremely uncommon condition.

Clinical presentation

Nature. There is sharp, stabbing, episodic, electric shock-like pain. Pain may be so severe that the patient tries to keep their tongue still and avoids swallowing.

Duration. Usually of seconds duration. Spontaneous remission of symptoms can occur but both this and their recurrence are unpredictable.

Site. The pain is localised to the postero-lateral tongue and fauces but felt within the ear on the affected side.

Initiating factors. The pain is induced by stimuli such as eating, drinking, swallowing, speaking and coughing.

Associated signs and symptoms. The absence of associated signs and symptoms of sensory or motor deficit is important. Neurological assessment is mandatory to ensure that the symptoms of glossopharyngeal neuralgia are not the result of a lesion (neoplastic or non-neoplastic) within the posterior cranial fossa or jugular foramen. The patient's medical history may already have revealed the existence of such a lesion.

Special investigations

Special investigations do not contribute directly to the diagnosis of glossopharyngeal neuralgia but are important in excluding posterior cranial fossa or jugular foramen lesions. MRI or CT are both appropriate.

Medical management

The therapy of choice is carbamazepine. The same considerations apply with respect to dose and side-effects as for trigeminal neuralgia.

Surgical management

The principles of surgical management are the same as those for trigeminal neuralgia: that is, chemical, thermal or physical damage to the appropriate nerve. However, it is usually not possible to use local injections or cryotherapy. Surgical section of the glossopharyngeal nerve can be effective as can other central surgical techniques but these are not without significant side effects.

Preherpetic neuralgia

Development of the classic vesicles of herpes zoster (Ch. 11; Fig. 186) is, in some cases, preceded by facial pain. This leads to the diagnosis being made retrospectively in many cases.

Clinical presentation

Nature. An aching or burning pain, which can mimic chronic pulpitis.

Duration. Continuous.

Site. The pain is limited to the distribution of the division(s) of the trigeminal nerve in which the lesions of herpes zoster subsequently develop. It may be localised by the patient to a particular tooth or teeth.

Associated signs and symptoms. The development of clinical signs of herpes zoster within a few days of the onset of the pain confirms the diagnosis.

Special investigations

Vitality testing, bitewing and periapical radiographs should be carried out when the pain is localised to the teeth to exclude dental pathology.

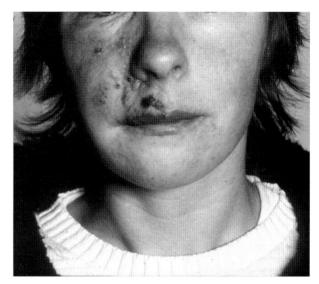

Fig. 186 Vesicles of herpes zoster.

Medical management

Appropriate treatment of herpes zoster (Ch. 11).

Postherpetic neuralgia

Postherpetic neuralgia occurs in about 10% of patients who have had herpes zoster infection and it persists in approximately 5%.

Clinical presentation

Sex. More common in females than males.

Age. Usually over 50 years.

Nature. An intense, unpleasant, burning pain.

Duration. May be present continually.

Site. The pain is localised to the area of the distribution of the division(s) of the trigeminal nerve involved in the preceding episode of herpes zoster.

Accompanying signs and symptoms. History and possibly scars of herpes zoster. The severity of the pain may lead to anxiety and depression.

Special investigations

Investigations may have been carried out previously to confirm the diagnosis of herpes zoster but infection is often diagnosed on clinical grounds alone.

Medical management

There is evidence that prevention or amelioration of postherpetic neuralgia can be achieved by the use of antiviral drugs such as famciclovir to treat the preceding herpes zoster infection. If postherpetic neuralgia develops, its medical management is difficult. Conventional non-steroidal anti-inflammatory agents are largely ineffective, as is carbamazepine. There is some evidence base for the use of tricyclic antidepressants and these along with gabapentin, pregabalin and opioid analgesics have been advised as first-line treatment. Topical therapies such as lidocaine patches and capsaicin may also be of benefit.

Surgical management

Local anaesthetic blockade of the stellate ganglion using bupivacaine may produce short-term relief in some patients.

14.3 Pain of vascular origin

Migraine

Clinical presentation

Sex. Migraine is more common in females than males.

Age. Wide age range from childhood onwards.

Nature. Intense, severe, persistent aching pain.

Duration. Usually of hours or days.

Site. The pain is usually unilateral but may not always affect the same side of the head. Certain variants are centred on the eye.

Initiating factors. A variety of stimuli may induce the headache, for example certain foodstuffs (e.g. chocolate, bananas), alcohol, stress, hormonal changes during the menstrual cycle, the contraceptive pill or noise.

Associated signs and symptoms. In classic migraine, the headache is preceded by an aura, which may include nausea, vomiting, visual disturbances (photophobia, flashing lights) and other disturbances of sensory and/or motor function.

Special investigations

CT and MRI do not contribute directly to the diagnosis of migraine but, where signs and symptoms are atypical, are important in excluding the presence of intracranial lesions.

Medical management

Analgesics such as paracetamol or aspirin are effective, particularly when used in combination with an antiemetic such as metoclopramide. If such drugs are ineffective the use of serotonin $5HT_1$ agonists, for example sumatriptan, is appropriate. In terms of prophylaxis, useful drugs include pizotifen, beta-blockers, tricyclic antidepressants or sodium valproate.

Cluster headaches

Clinical presentation

Sex. More common in males than females.

Age. Predominantly affects individuals under the age of 50 years.

Nature. An intense aching pain that disturbs sleep; attacks may occur at the same time each day.

Duration. Typically, there are intermittent episodes of pain of between 15 and 180 minutes' duration on a daily basis for several weeks, interspersed with pain-free periods of months rather than days in duration.

Site. The pain is localised to one side of the face, typically affecting the cheek, orbit, forehead and temple. The pain does not cross the midline.

Initiating factors. Alcohol, vasodilators, high altitude.

Associated signs and symptoms. Flushing of the cheeks, watering of the eyes and nasal congestion on the affected side.

Special investigations

CT and MRI do not contribute directly to the diagnosis of cluster headaches but are important in excluding intracranial lesions.

Medical management

The most widely used treatments once an attack commences is sumatriptan. Drugs effective in preventing attacks of cluster headaches such as calcium channel blockers (e.g. verapamil) may be taken as prophylaxis.

Giant-cell arteritis (cranial arteritis, temporal arteritis)

Giant-cell arteritis may occur alone or as a component of polymyalgia rheumatica.

Clinical presentation

Sex. More common in females than males.

Age. Usually over 50 years.

Nature. Severe, throbbing headache.

Duration. Usually of hours or days.

Site. The pain is unilateral and most frequently affects the temple.

Initiating factors. None.

Associated signs and symptoms. The temporal artery throbs and is prominent and tender to the touch. Eating may result in pain in the muscles of mastication. If the lingual artery is affected, pain may be experienced in the tongue; ultimately ulceration as a result of necrosis secondary to ischaemia can occur. More generalised signs and symptoms include fever, general malaise and weight loss. If pain and stiffness affecting the shoulders, upper arms and pelvis are present in addition to the characteristic unilateral headache, a diagnosis of **polymyalgia rheumatica** should be considered.

Special investigations

The eosinophil sedimentation rate (ESR) is normally grossly elevated as are serum interleukin 6 levels. Biopsy of the temporal artery reveals skip lesions interspersed with areas of apparently normal vessel wall. In affected areas, the media and intima are infiltrated by inflammatory cells, amongst which giant cells are prominent. The lumen of the vessel is narrowed secondary to thrombosis and fibrosis.

Medical management

Treatment with high-dose prednisolone (40–60 mg daily) should be commenced promptly to ensure that blindness secondary to ischaemia of the optic nerve does not occur. As the ESR falls, this dose can be reduced to 7.5–10 mg. Long-term therapy is required (3 to 6 years) to limit relapse.

14.4 Atypical orofacial pain

You should:
- understand that atypical facial pain is a diagnosis of a particular set of symptoms
- know the features of atypical odontalgia
- understand the relevance of a history of stress in some patients.

Atypical facial pain

The term atypical facial pain can foster the belief that this diagnosis is reached simply by excluding other causes of facial pain. However, atypical facial pain results in a particular constellation of symptoms, which form the basis of its diagnosis.

Clinical presentation

Sex. More common in females than males.

Age. Usually over 50 years.

Nature. A gripping, vice-like, aching pain. Patients sometimes describe a feeling of pressure.

Duration. Usually present continually and has often been so for months or years with intermittent increases in severity.

Site. The pain more commonly affects the maxilla than the mandible; it may be uni- or bilateral and crosses anatomical boundaries.

Initiating/ameliorating factors. There are no clear initiating, ameliorating or exacerbating factors. Analgesics are usually ineffective.

Duration. Many patients give a history of consulting several general dental and medical practitioners, specialist physicians and surgeons. Teeth may have been extracted in an attempt to alleviate the patient's symptoms to no benefit.

Clinical examination

A careful clinical examination is important to exclude other causes of facial pain.

Medical history. The medical history may reveal other conditions such as irritable bowel syndrome, back pain, pelvic pain and fibromyalgia. In some patients, there may be a history of depression and/or anxiety; patients may be reluctant to disclose these conditions directly, if at all, but the patient's drug history can be informative.

Social history. The patient's social history is a significant but difficult area. The fruitfulness of this area of inquiry depends very much on the quality of the dentist's communication skills: the ability to create the appropriate conditions for disclosure of such information. A patient may well expect to be asked about their smoking habits but be less willing to divulge details concerning their personal circumstances during a consultation with their dentist. Sources of stress and distress should be identified: for example bereavement, significant illness of, or anxiety about, family or friends, job loss, breakdown of relationships, an unhappy home and/or work life, fear of serious illness.

Special investigations

Special investigations are intended to exclude any causes of facial pain that remain following the history and examination phase of the consultation. An assessment of the patient's mental state may be made, where appropriate, using an instrument such as the Hospital Anxiety and Depression Scale.

Medical management

In a proportion of patients with atypical facial pain, resolution or reduction in symptoms occurs following confirmation and discussion of their diagnosis. This should include reassurance with respect to the non-neoplastic nature of the cause of their symptoms and, if relevant, exploration of their possible relationship to stress, anxiety and depression. In other cases, symptoms persist and pharmacotherapy may be of benefit. There is evidence to support the use of various antidepressant drugs drawn from the tricyclic antidepressant (e.g. dothiepin, amitriptyline) and selective serotonin reuptake inhibitor (e.g. fluoxetine) groups. However, the benefits of such drugs do not appear to be related to their antidepressant properties as they are of benefit in individuals free from depression. Encouraging results have also been obtained using psychotherapeutic approaches such as cognitive behavioural therapy. Therefore, for some patients, involvement of a psychologist and/or psychiatrist in their assessment and management may be appropriate.

Atypical odontalgia

Atypical odontalgia can be thought of as the dental equivalent of atypical facial pain. The characteristics of the pain and those patients who experience it are broadly identical; all that differs is the site of the pain. The patient localises the pain to a tooth or group of teeth that are clinically and radiographically normal. In some cases, the patient may have already insisted on the extraction of one or more teeth by another dental practitioner with no or only temporary relief of symptoms, which now affect the extraction site and/or adjacent teeth. It is clearly important to resist extracting healthy teeth in such patients.

14.5 Burning mouth syndrome

You should:
- know the clinical presentation of burning mouth syndrome
- know which conditions have similar symptoms and need to be excluded
- understand the link with stress and anxiety in some patients.

Burning mouth syndrome (BMS; glossodynia, glossopyrosis, oral dysaesthesia) is characterised by a burning sensation affecting the oral mucosa present in an individual in whom other local and systemic causes of such a sensation have been excluded as far as is possible (e.g. xerostomia, incorrectly designed dentures, diabetes, anaemia). The aetiology and pathogenesis of burning mouth syndrome

Fourteen

remain uncertain; changes in the oral environment, abnormalities of the peripheral (including neuropathy) and/or central nervous systems and psychosocial issues have all been implicated and are supported by varying degrees of evidence.

Clinical presentation

Sex. More common in females than males.

Age. Usually over 50 years.

Nature. A burning sensation. The patient may describe the mucosa as feeling as if it has been scalded or sprinkled with pepper.

Duration. Present on a daily basis often for a considerable period of time (months or years). Several different patterns have been described and a classification system suggested:

type 1: not present on waking, severity increases as the day goes on

type 2: present on waking and throughout the day

type 3: intermittent, unpredictable pattern of occurrence.

The patient's symptoms do not disturb their sleep.

Site. The burning sensation most commonly affects the tongue, lips and hard palate either singly or in combination. In terms of single sites, the tongue is most commonly affected. Type 3 BMS often affects unusual sites such as the throat or floor of mouth.

Initiating/ameliorating factors. There are no clear initiating, ameliorating or exacerbating factors. However, patients may report that the burning sensation is not present when they are eating or occupied and is noticed more when they are at rest. Analgesics are usually ineffective.

Associated symptoms. Alterations in taste sensation (dysgeusia), dry mouth.

Duration. Many patients give a history of consulting several general dental and medical practitioners, specialist physicians and surgeons.

Clinical examination

Significant findings in the patient's medical and social history might be similar to those discussed above under atypical facial pain.

A careful clinical examination is important to detect any local causes for the patient's symptoms, for example signs of conditions such as erythema migrans, glossitis, lichen planus and candidiasis; evidence of parafunctional habits such as bruxism, tooth clenching or tongue thrusting; assessment of the design of the patient's dentures, particularly with respect to adequacy of freeway space and positioning of the teeth with respect to the tongue space; and xerostomia.

Special investigations

Investigations are targeted at detecting any causes of burning sensations affecting the oral mucosa. A full blood count and haematinics to diagnose anaemia and/or deficiency of iron, folate or vitamin B_{12} should be carried out. The presence of candidal infection should be excluded by the use, at the very least, of swabs and smears but ideally by a more quantitative method such as oral rinse or saliva sample. The presence and degree of xerostomia should be assessed by sialometry. Blood glucose and glycosylated haemoglobin should be measured for possible diabetes. While patients may attribute their symptoms to allergic reactions, most commonly to dental materials, in the absence of a clear history or clinical signs current evidence does not justify the use of allergy testing, such as patch tests, in this group of patients.

Medical management

Any possible local and systemic causes of burning sensations affecting the mouth detected on examination or following special investigations should be treated. Where no such causes are detected or where their successful treatment does not bring about resolution of symptoms the diagnosis of burning mouth syndrome is confirmed. In a proportion of patients with BMS, resolution or reduction in symptoms occurs following confirmation and discussion of their diagnosis, including reassurance with respect to the non-neoplastic nature of the cause of their symptoms, exploration of their possible relationship to stress and anxiety, and exclusion of local and systemic causes. In other cases, symptoms persist but patients are able to come to terms with them once they are convinced of the absence of a serious underlying cause. Unfortunately many of the treatments currently in use for burning mouth syndrome have not been subjected to randomised controlled trials. For example, in terms of systemic therapies, antidepressants drawn from the tricyclic group (e.g. nortriptyline) are widely used to good effect but stronger evidence exists for the use of serotonin reuptake inhinbitors (e.g. paroxetine). In contrast, cognitive–behavioural therapy does provide an evidence-based alternative to systemic drug treatment.

Self-assessment: questions

Multiple choice questions

1. In irreversible pulpitis the pain normally
   a. Is exacerbated by biting down on the affected tooth
   b. Is poorly localised
   c. Is of short, less than 10 minutes, duration
   d. Does not respond to simple analgesics such as paracetamol

2. Trigeminal neuralgia
   a. Is normally treated with carbamazepine
   b. Can be a presenting symptom of multiple sclerosis
   c. Usually crosses the midline of the face
   d. Only occurs in response to touching a 'trigger point'
   e. Does not wake the affected individual from sleep

3. Giant-cell arteritis normally
   a. Occurs most commonly in men
   b. Affects only the temporal artery
   c. Results in a slightly elevated ESR
   d. Can be treated successfully with systemic steroids
   e. Causes blindness

4. Postherpetic neuralgia
   a. Is the only type of facial pain associated with herpes zoster infections
   b. Is well controlled by the use of carbamazepine
   c. Is an invariable consequence of herpes zoster infections
   d. Is never accompanied by facial palsy

5. Atypical facial pain
   a. Is more strongly associated with depression than anxiety
   b. May be alleviated by simple reassurance
   c. May be caused by anaemia
   d. Is a diagnosis of exclusion

Extended matching items

Options:
A. Trigeminal neuralgia (classical trigeminal neuralgia – CTN)
B. Atypical facial pain
C. Giant-cell arteritis
D. Post-herpetic neuralgia
E. Cluster headache
F. Short-lasting unilateral neuralgiform headache attacks with conjunctival injection and tearing (SUNCT)
G. Classical migraine without aura
H. Glossopharyngeal neuralgia
I. Trigeminal neuralgia (symptomatic trigeminal neuralgia – STN)
J. Burning mouth syndrome

Lead in: Match the case history from the list below that is most appropriate for each diagnosis above.

1. A 33-year-old man complains of an intense aching pain which occurs once a day and lasts for about an hour. He outlines the affected area which extends upwards from his right cheek to his forehead. The episodes of intense pain have been going on for about a week. His nose feels blocked and runs when the pain is present. He experienced similar symptoms about 3 months ago which lasted for a couple of weeks and resolved spontaneously.

2. A 36-year-old woman gives a 2-week history of a sharp pain lasting for a few seconds which comes on when she touches the left-hand side of her upper lip. One burst of pain can follow immediately after the preceding one. When you are taking her history she mentions that about a month ago she consulted her GMP about a deterioration in hearing affecting her left ear.

3. A 58-year-old man gave a history of a stabbing pain affecting his left temple. Each burst of pain lasts for about 4 minutes, he can experience three of these each waking hour. He is concerned that he may have developed an infection in his left eye, which looks red.

4. A 62-year-old woman gives a history of a sharp pain lasting for a few seconds whenever she touches the skin over her lower jaw. It is making it difficult for her to carry out daily activities like washing her face or eating. The pain is confined to the left-hand side. Once an episode of pain is complete she can be pain free for about an hour even if she touches her face in the area affected by the pain. She has been taking paracetamol at regular intervals but this has made no difference to the pain.

5. A 65-year-old woman complained of a deep-seated aching sensation affecting the right-hand side of her face from her top jaw up to her forehead. She has suffered from the pain on a more or less continuous basis for about 4 years. There are no exacerbating or ameliorating factors. Analgesics have proved ineffective. Her GMP referred her to an ENT consultant who carried out an MRI to check for sinus problems. She has also been seen by two other dentists and had root canal treatment on several teeth, two of which have subsequently been extracted. On examination you detect no abnormalities.

6. A 25-year-old woman complains of episodes of aching pain affecting her right or left forehead, temple and cheek. She experiences these a couple of times each month and gives a 6-month history. The pain is normally present for between 12 and 48 hours and makes it very difficult for her to concentrate on anything. She occasionally feels nauseous when the pain is present and tries to avoid situations that she knows will be noisy.

7. A 71-year-old woman attends your surgery complaining of a sharp pain which affects the back of her tongue and the area just beneath the angle of her

jaw always on the left-hand side alone. The pain lasts for about a minute and comes on when she swallows or chews. Her lower left first and second molar teeth are present and restored but they appear sound, are vital and are not tender to percussion.

8. A 65-year-old woman presents with a throbbing pain affecting her left temple. The headache began about a week ago and is accompanied by pain in the muscles around her jaw joint on eating. She has no previous history of facial pain or headache. Intra-oral examination is unremarkable. There is no evidence of dental pathology or parafunctional habits.

9. An 80-year-old woman who moved into residential care 3 months ago is brought to your surgery. The elderly lady is complaining of an intense burning sensation affecting the right-hand side of her face which has been present for at least the past 3 months. The lower part of her face is spared. Nothing seems to make it better or worse. The patient is a poor historian and the carer knows little of her history before she came to live at the care home. On examination you notice some scarring of the skin of her right cheek and forehead but nil else of note. The patient was recently prescribed a low dose of amitriptyline for anxiety by her GMP and this seems to have helped a little with the pain.

10. A 56-year-old woman complains of a burning sensation affecting her tongue. It is present on a more or less continuous basis and gets worse as the day goes on. Her GMP prescribed a mouthwash for her but this has not been of any benefit. She is edentulous but leaving her dentures out makes no difference to the pain. Her medical history is unremarkable and on examination her tongue appears completely normal.

Case history questions

Case history 1

A 50-year-old partially dentate male experiences a sharp pain from his teeth whenever he consumes cold foods and on exposure to cold air. The pain lasts only for as long as the stimulus is present. On examination, generalised gingival recession is present.

1. What is a likely diagnosis?
2. What elements in the patient's history indicate this diagnosis?
3. What would be the relevant findings on examination?
4. Are further investigations appropriate and if so what?
5. What would be a treatment plan?

Case history 2

A 25-year-old female attends the surgery complaining of pain on eating or clenching her teeth. She localises the pain to her upper right first permanent molar. On examination intra-orally, this tooth appears sound; however, the lower right first permanent molar has a large mesial-occlusal-distal (MOD) amalgam. The latter tooth is tender to percussion (TTP).

1. What is a likely diagnosis?
2. What elements in the patient's history indicate this diagnosis?
3. What would be the relevant findings on examination?
4. Are further investigations appropriate and if so what?
5. What would be a treatment plan?

Case history 3

A 65-year-old man complains of a sharp pain affecting his right cheek. The pain is of short duration but extremely severe, like being stabbed with a needle or an electric shock. When he was at rest, the pain rarely occurred. It was more likely to come on when he was speaking or eating. Washing his face and shaving were particularly problematical. The pain never crosses the midline. The patient is generally fit and well although he gave a history of a recent deep-vein thrombosis and now takes warfarin. On examination, the pain is induced when the patient's left cheek is touched. The patient is edentulous.

1. What is a likely diagnosis?
2. What elements in the patient's history indicate this diagnosis?
3. What would be the relevant findings on examination?
4. Are further investigations appropriate and if so what?
5. What would be a treatment plan?

Case history 4

A 70-year-old lady is referred to the dentist by her medical practitioner. She gives a 5-year history of facial pain affecting her maxilla. Various upper teeth had been extracted over this period with no sustained benefit but now the pain was not localised to a particular tooth. She describes a relentless dull ache that varies in severity but is always present. Overall it has not changed much since its onset. Nothing really made it better or worse; she has tried various analgesics but nothing was effective. She had recently been seen by an otolaryngologist to have her sinuses checked; no abnormalities had been detected. In addition, a previous dentist had referred her to a local oral and maxillofacial surgeon, who had not detected any abnormality but had arranged for her to be seen by a neurologist who had carried out a CT scan, which was normal. On extra-oral examination, there was no tenderness of the muscles of mastication and no abnormality intra-orally. The patient's remaining teeth appeared sound.

1. What is a likely diagnosis?
2. What elements in the patient's history indicate this diagnosis?
3. What would be the relevant findings on examination?
4. Are further investigations appropriate and if so what?
5. What would be a treatment plan?

Case history 5

A 36-year-old male complains of an aching pain affecting the right-hand side of his maxilla. The pain seems to arise from his teeth, particularly those towards the back of his mouth in his upper jaw. About 2 years previously he had experienced some discomfort in the same area but this had only come on after eating cold foods and had lasted for about 15 minutes. His current symptoms do not seem to be brought on by anything. Each episode of pain lasts for about an hour and is relieved by taking paracetamol. On examination intra-orally, the patient's upper and lower molars on the right-hand side are heavily restored but not tender to percussion. Electric pulp testing shows a reduced response from his upper right first permanent molar compared with the corresponding tooth on the left-hand side.

A 55-year-old woman visits your surgery complaining of a burning sensation affecting her palate that had started a couple of months ago. This is not present on waking but increases in severity as the day goes on. She suffers from non-insulin-dependent diabetes controlled by diet alone and hypertension for which she is taking lisinopril; she is otherwise fit and well. The patient is edentulous; her current dentures are 2 months old and replaced the previous set, which she had used for the past 20 years. She has recently taken early retirement and lives with her husband, who continues to work. She is a lifelong non-smoker. Since her diabetes was diagnosed 5 years ago, she has not drunk any alcohol; prior to this she had consumed between 4 and 5 units per week. There was a family history of non-insulin-dependent diabetes. She expresses concern that her symptoms might indicate that she was developing oral cancer.

1. What is a likely diagnosis?
2. What elements in the patient's history indicate this diagnosis?
3. What would be the relevant findings on examination?
4. Are further investigations appropriate and if so what?
5. What would be a treatment plan?

Essay question

You are given the following history. Using this case as a basis, discuss the aetiology of a burning sensation affecting the oral mucosa, demonstrating how you would reach a diagnosis of burning mouth syndrome (BMS).

Self-assessment: answers

Multiple choice answers

1. a. **False**. The pain associated with irreversible pulpitis normally arises spontaneously and is not induced or exacerbated by applying pressure to the affected tooth. However, lying down and hot stimuli may induce/exacerbate the pain.
    b. **True**. As with reversible pulpitis the pain of irreversible pulpitis is usually poorly localised by the affected individual but does not normally cross the midline unless upper or lower anterior teeth are affected.
    c. **False**. The pain of irreversible pulpitis is usually long lasting and present for hours rather than minutes.
    d. **False**. Non-opiate analgesics such as paracetamol are normally effective in controlling the pain associated with irreversible pulpitis.

2. a. **True**. Carbamazepine is the drug of choice for the medical management of trigeminal neuralgia but the role of surgery in the treatment of this condition should not be overlooked. The latter provides a valuable alternative in those patients where pharmacotherapy is precluded, ineffective or poorly tolerated.
    b. **True**. Trigeminal neuralgia predominantly affects individuals over the age of 50 years. Its occurrence in a younger individual raises the possibility of multiple sclerosis. Similarly this association should also be borne in mind when investigating the cause of facial pain in a person known to suffer from multiple sclerosis.
    c. **False**. One of the diagnostic features of trigeminal neuralgia is the anatomical distribution of the pain which is confined to the area innervated by the affected division(s) of the trigeminal nerve.
    d. **False**. Whilst pain triggered by touching a particular area of the face/oral mucosa is a classical feature of trigeminal neuralgia, episodes of pain may also occur spontaneously. The clinical presentation of trigeminal neuralgia does not always meet the typical diagnostic criteria.
    e. **False**. Patients suffering from trigeminal neuralgia may give a history of being woken from sleep by their pain.

3. a. **False**. Giant-cell arteritis affects females more commonly than males.
    b. **False**. Whilst the term temporal arteritis is often used, the vasculitis which it describes has the capacity to affect large, medium-sized and small arteries in the craniofacial region in general and is believed to form part of a spectrum of disease culminating in polymyalgia rheumatica.
    c. **False**. Giant-cell arteritis is normally characterised by the presence of an elevated ESR of the order of 40 mm h^{-1} or greater, although in 20% of cases the ESR may be within normal limits.

    d. **True**. Systemic steroids are initially prescribed at high dose, typically 40–60 mg prednisolone daily. Maintenance therapy at a lower dose, e.g. 7.5–10 mg may be continued for several years to prevent relapse.
    e. **True**. Ischaemia of the optic nerve secondary to involvement of the ciliary arteries may lead to blindness if treatment is not commenced promptly.

4. a. **False**. In some individuals pre-herpetic neuralgia, which may mimic dental pain, precedes the development of the vesiculo-bullous lesions which characterise herpes zoster.
    b. **False**. Post-herpetic neuralgia is a difficult condition to treat effectively. Carbamazepine is largely ineffective, however some benefit may be derived from the use of tricyclic antidepressants.
    c. **False**. Post-herpetic neuralgia has a variable incidence, the likelihood of its occurrence increases with age, and it is more likely to affect women than men. Approximately 50% of those affected will continue to experience symptoms for longer than three months.
    d. **False**. Ramsay Hunt syndrome is characterised by herpes zoster affecting the external auditory meatus and pharynx accompanied by an ipsilateral facial palsy.

5. a. **True**. Depression is more strongly associated with atypical facial pain than anxiety; the reverse appears to be the case in burning mouth syndrome.
    b. **True**. Just as in burning mouth syndrome simple reassurance accompanied by supportive listening plays a significant role in the management of atypical facial pain.
    c. **False**. There is no evidence to support an association between anaemia and atypical facial pain.
    d. **False**. Whilst the exclusion of other causes of facial pain is important when making a diagnosis of atypical facial pain, the latter does have characteristic features which contribute to its diagnosis, e.g. non-anatomical distribution; description of a gripping, vice-like relentless pain; maxilla affected more commonly then the mandible.

Extended matching items answers

1. **E**. Pain is unilateral, severe and has occurred previously but age and duration of pain make CTN unlikely, however could be atypical variant or STN. Associated nasal congestion and rhinorrhea is significant and not usually associated with TN. Therefore on balance E, but MRI scan indicated in view of suspicion atypical or STN.
2. **I**. The clinical features are strongly suggestive of TN. The patient's age is a cause for concern, CTN would be extremely unusual in someone of her age.

The absence of a refractory period after triggering of the pain is also somewhat atypical. Therefore STN should be seriously considered. The presence of ipsilateral hearing loss raises further concerns as to the possibility of a central lesion being present. Even if the patient were in the usual age group for CTN this would raise the possibility of STN.

3. **F.** On first reading this case has many of the features of trigeminal neuralgia. The 4-minute duration of the pain is possibly longer than one might normally expect for TN and the ophthalmic is the least commonly affected division of the trigeminal nerve. The presence of conjunctival injection shifts the balance in favour of SUNCT but an overlap is recognised between the two conditions. MRI indicated.

4. **A.** The patient gives a classic description including distribution of pain, trigger zone and a refractory period after stimulation. Whilst CTN is highly likely, MRI is obligatory to exclude STN and assess possibility of DREZ compression.

5. **B.** Although the pain is unilateral the patient's description of a continuous aching pain which is has been present and stable for several years; without exacerbating or ameliorating factors; unresponsive to analgesics is strongly suggestive of atypical facial pain. The absence of positive findings on examination and investigation is characteristic. MRI is often performed although rationale for this is unclear; its prime purpose is to provide reassurance to both clinician and patient of the absence of significant associated pathology. However, the history of this patient at this stage makes that extremely unlikely.

6. **G.** This pain is episodic but episodes have a long duration compared to all the other conditions and are not clustered. It has affected either side of the face/head. Accompanying nausea and phonophobia are indicative of migraine.

7. **H.** Whilst the tongue is commonly affected in burning mouth syndrome the pain is of too short a duration and is described as sharp. The involvement of the area just below the angle of the jaw and pain on chewing might suggest dental pathology but the teeth are sound and not TTP. Similarly, were it not for the involvement of the tongue, a diagnosis of TN might be considered. However, taking into account the sites affected, the nature of the pain and when it is experienced the diagnosis is glossopharyngeal neuralgia.

8. **C.** The recent onset of unilateral pain of this nature in this site without any previous history should immediately raise the possibility of giant-cell arteritis. The patient is in the right age group (usually = 50 y). The accompanying pain in the muscles of mastication on chewing could represent temporo-mandibular joint dysfunction but is entirely consistent with giant-cell arteritis.

9. **D.** Some elements of the history – continuous pain, no exacerbating or ameliorating factors, some benefit from amitriptyline – are compatible with a diagnosis of atypical facial pain. The pain does, however, have a reasonably well-defined anatomical distribution apparently sparing the area innervated by the mandibular division of the trigeminal nerve. The intense burning quality of the pain is also suggestive of post-herpetic neuralgia and the presence of scarring on the skin of the patient's face reinforces this by providing evidence of previous skin lesions possibly related to herpes zoster.

10. **J.** The duration and nature of the pain exclude H. The absence of mucosal abnormality and the fact that the symptoms persist even when the denture is not worn point to J. The lack of response to topical agents is not unusual. The patient's normal medical history seems to rule out systemic factors such as anaemia and diabetes but it would be prudent to carry out appropriate blood tests. Candidal infection can be excluded by performing appropriate microbiological investigations and xerostomia by sialometry, although the normal findings on examination make both of these unlikely.

Case history answers

Case history 1

1. Dentine sensitivity.
2. Sharp pain, tooth related, cold stimuli, lasts for as long as the stimulus is present.
3. Gingival recession.
4. No further investigations.
5. Advise use of a toothpaste for sensitive teeth. Apply a sealant to exposed cervical dentine. Check tooth-brushing technique.

Case history 2

1. Periapical periodontitis affecting the lower right first permanent molar.
2. Pain on eating and clenching teeth together. The pain is well localised but there may be confusion over whether the pain is coming from an upper or a lower tooth.
3. Suggested tooth is sound, but the opposing tooth is heavily restored and TTP.
4. Vitality testing and periapical radiograph of lower right first permanent molar.
5. Endodontic treatment or extraction.

Case history 3

1. Trigeminal neuralgia.
2. Severe pain, like being stabbed with a needle or an electric shock; provoked by movement of the face and touching the face; confined to the left cheek and never crosses the midline.
3. Pain is induced by touching the patient's left cheek; patient is edentulous.
4. No other investigations.
5. Consider prescription of carbamazepine but check for possible drug interactions. Metabolism of warfarin is accelerated by carbamazepine, reducing its anticoagulant effects. Contact the patient's medical

practitioner and inform of the diagnosis; liaise with respect to treatment and referral to a neurologist. Monitoring and adjustment of anticoagulant therapy will be necessary if carbamazepine is prescribed.

Case history 4

1. Atypical facial pain.
2. Long history but non-progressive; extraction of teeth in the affected area; relentless, some variation in severity but always present; no exacerbating or ameliorating factors; analgesics ineffective; extensively investigated (otolaryngology, oral and maxillofacial and neurology referrals).
3. No abnormality was detected at examination including the temporomandibular joint and the muscles of mastication.
4. Vitality testing of remaining teeth should be carried out, following up any significant findings with bitewing and periapical radiography.
5. The diagnosis should be discussed with the patient: cause uncertain 'medically unexplained symptoms'; further dental treatment of no benefit; suggest referral to oral medicine consultant for confirmation of diagnosis.

Treatment options: leave things as they are, pharmacotherapy (e.g. tricyclic antidepressants), psychotherapy (helping the patient to live with the pain).

Case history 5

1. Possible reversible (acute) pulpitis 2 years previously and now irreversible (chronic) pulpitis.
2. Initial symptoms induced by cold stimuli and of relatively short (15 minutes) duration; the onset of the current symptoms is spontaneous and they have a long duration (more than 1 hour).
3. Heavily restored teeth; reduced vitality but not tender to percussion.
4. Bitewing radiograph of right-hand side shows recurrent caries in the upper right first permanent molar.
5. Removal of the restoration in the upper right first permanent molar, excavation of caries and placement of temporary dressing.

Essay answer

Your essay should include the following information.

1. Definition of BMS. A burning sensation affecting the oral mucosa in the absence of clinically detectable lesions.

2. History of the complaint. The age and sex of the patient, the affected site and the pattern of pain are all appropriate to this diagnosis. Brief discussion of the usual sites affected in BMS and the different pain patterns experienced.
3. Clinical examination. No abnormality is detected extra- or intra-orally. Various oral mucosal disorders can give rise to a burning sensation; good examples would be lichen planus, erythema migrans, candidiasis, glossitis.
4. Medical history. Non-insulin-dependent diabetes controlled by diet alone? Is control adequate? Poorly controlled diabetes may result in xerostomia and an increased susceptibility to oral candidiasis. Both of these may give rise to a burning sensation. There is no suggestion of anaemia or nutritional deficiency in the medical history but it has been suggested that these may cause BMS-like symptoms.

Medication. The patient is taking lisinopril, an angiotensin-converting enzyme, the side-effects of which can include xerostomia and a burning sensation affecting the oral mucosa. Explore the temporal relationship between the onset of symptoms and the commencement of medication.

5. Further investigations. Suggest special investigations to exclude issues arising from the medical history: sialometry, isolation and quantification of *Candida* species, full blood count, haematinics, random blood sugar and glycosylated haemoglobin.
6. Dental history. Provision of a new full set of dentures coincides with the onset of symptoms. Do the symptoms resolve/improve if she leaves her dentures out? Allergy to dental materials has been suggested as a cause of BMS-like symptoms but evidence to support this is weak. It is accepted that denture design faults (e.g. adequacy of freeway) can result in such symptoms. There is no evidence of denture stomatitis on clinical examination.
7. Social history. Onset of BMS symptoms may be associated with 'stressful' events or changes of lifestyle. Patient has recently retired.
8. Additional information. The patient expresses anxiety concerning the possibility of oral cancer. Such anxieties may exacerbate or cause BMS.

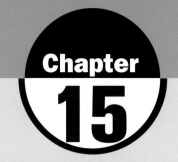

Disorders of the temporomandibular joint

Chapter 15

Overview

The temporomandibular joint occurs between the mandible and the temporal bone. The joint itself can show pain/dysfunction and internal displacement of the disc. It is also affected by trauma and by systemic diseases such as rheumatoid arthritis.

15.1 Anatomy and examination

Learning objectives

You should:
- understand the anatomy of the joint
- know the clinical examination and radiological appearance of the joint
- be aware of the technique of arthroscopy.

Anatomy

The temporomandibular joints (TMJs) are the two joints between the mandible and the temporal bone. They are unique in the body in that they contain two joint spaces separated by a fibrocartilage disc (Fig. 187).

Components

The mandibular condyle

The mandibular condyle is a bony ellipsoid structure attached to the mandibular ramus by an elongated neck. Its mediolateral dimension (around 20 mm) is larger than the antero-posterior dimension (8–10 mm). Its articulating surface is covered in a thin layer of fibrocartilage. There is usually a clearly demarcated ridge running mediolaterally along its anterior surface. This is the edge of the articulating surface. Below the ridge is a hollow, marking an attachment of the lateral pterygoid muscle.

The mandibular (glenoid) fossa

The mandibular fossa is a hollow on the inferior surface of the squamous temporal bone. The fossa is bounded anteriorly by a ridge of bone, the articular eminence, which forms the anterior margin of the joint. The fossa is covered in a thin layer of fibrocartilage. The mastoid air cells often extend into the bone of the articular eminence and the bone of the fossa.

Interarticular disc

The interarticular disc is a biconcave sheet of avascular fibrous connective tissue that divides the joint into a superior and inferior joint space. At its anterior margin, it blends with fibres of the lateral pterygoid muscle. Posteriorly, it attaches to looser connective tissue (bilaminar zone) containing nerves and lined with synovial membrane.

Capsule

The TMJ has a fibrous capsule attached to the rim of the mandibular fossa and the neck of the condyle. The disc attaches to it medially and laterally. The lateral aspects of the capsule are thickened by the lateral (temporomandibular) ligament.

Ligaments

The lateral ligament lies lateral to the TMJ and runs from the root of the zygoma to the posterior aspect of the condylar neck. It limits antero-posterior joint movement. The sphenomandibular and stylomandibular ligaments are also part of the joint complex and probably also serve to limit movement.

Joint movement

The joint has a combination of rotatory movement of the condyle in the lower joint space and anterior translation of the condyle, with sliding of the disc forwards along the articular eminence (Fig. 188).

Examination

Clinical examination

The dental examination should be systematic and include the TMJ and the masticatory muscles.

Joint examination

Movement. Face the patient and ask him/her to open slowly to maximum. Normal range (inter-incisal) is 35 to 40 mm. If opening is thought to be reduced, ask whether the limiting factor is pain or an obstruction. Note the path of opening and any lateral deviation.

    Pain on palpation. Palpate in front of the ear and within the external auditory meatus.

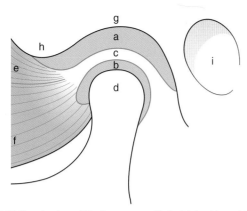

Fig. 187 The structure of the temporomandibular joint. a. Upper joint space; b. lower joint space; c. interarticular disc; d. condylar head; e. lateral pterygoid muscle superior head; f. lateral pterygoid muscle inferior head; g. mandibular fossa; h. articular eminence; i. external auditory canal.

Auscultation. This needs a stethoscope to be done properly. However, clicks may well be audible without a stethoscope. A click implies a disc displacement that reduces into a normal position on opening. Crepitus (cracking/grating noise) implies degenerative change or, sometimes, acute inflammation.

Muscle examination

Muscle tenderness suggests some abnormal function (clenching, bruxism). Masseter and temporalis muscles are assessed by direct palpation. The lateral pterygoid is indirectly examined by noting the response (in terms of any preauricular pain) to attempted opening against the restriction of the examiner's hand below the chin. The medial pterygoid cannot be examined.

Radiology

Most clinical problems related to the TMJ are caused by muscular parafunction (e.g. bruxism) or internal disc derangements. Neither is likely to be associated with any relevant bony abnormalities. Consequently, radiography is not normally indicated unless there is any suggestion of bony abnormality, such as might be the case in rheumatoid arthritis or osteoarthrosis. Many panoramic X-ray machines allow specific images of the condyles to be taken without unnecessary radiography of the rest of the jaws. The only radiographic projection to show the whole joint is the transcranial oblique lateral view.

A clinical diagnosis of suspected internal derangement might lead to a requirement for imaging of the disc. This is done by either magnetic resonance imaging (Fig. 189) or TMJ arthrography (Fig. 190).

Arthroscopy

Arthroscopy allows visual examination of the upper joint space and an opportunity for minor surgical treatment. A small arthroscope can be used to facilitate lavage and division of joint adhesions. The lower joint space is difficult to access without risk of damage to the articular disc. Arthroscopy is undertaken under local anaesthesia; however, if lengthy arthroscopic surgery is to be

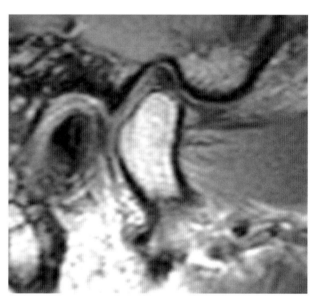

Fig. 189 Magnetic resonance image of a TMJ. The disc can be seen as the darker structure between the condylar head and the temporal bone.

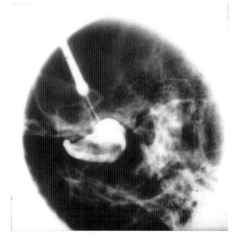

Fig. 190 TMJ arthrogram. Contrast is injected into the joint spaces below and, sometimes, above the disc. Consequently, the disc is outlined rather than directly seen.

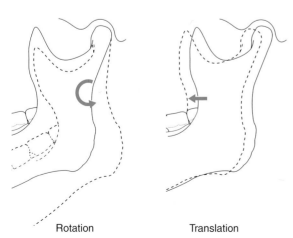

Rotation　　　　　Translation

Fig. 188 Movement of the temporomandibular joint.

undertaken, then a conscious sedation technique would be appropriate or even general anaesthesia.

15.2 Disorders of the joint

You should:
* know the symptoms of TMJ pain/dysfunction and its management
* know the features of disc displacement with and without reduction
* know the management of displaced discs.

Pain/dysfunction

The most common TMJ disorder is pain or dysfunction.

Clinical features

Symptoms are a combination of:

* headache
* limitation/deviation of jaw opening
* joint sounds
* pain on palpation of the TMJ
* pain on palpation of the associated muscles.

Joint sounds alone, or with headache, are not diagnostic of TMJ pain/dysfunction.

Radiology

There is no abnormality visible.

Management

* Reassurance and explanation to patients
* Jaw rest and soft diet
* Analgesics/anti-inflammatory drugs
* Occlusal splints to interfere with parafunction may offer some help
* Physiotherapy
* Muscle relaxants.

Internal derangement

The articular disc normally sits above the anterior aspect of the condylar head, with the disc posterior attachment lying within 10° of the vertical (Fig. 191). A disc may be anterior to this 'normal' position in asymptomatic individuals, suggesting that an anterior disc position is a normal variant. Thus an internal derangement is best thought of as an abnormality in position that interferes with function and that may be associated with other symptoms. An anterior disc 'displacement' is the most common internal derangement, but antero-medial, medial, and antero-lateral displacements are all seen.

Disc displacement with reduction

Reduction means that a displaced disc 'reduces' into a normal position on opening but reverts to an abnormal position on closing (reciprocal click) (Fig. 192A).

Clinical features

* Clicking on opening
* Clicking on closing
* Transient jaw deviation during opening/closing.

Radiology

No abnormalities are apparent on plain radiographs. Disc imaging shows the displaced disc in a closed/rest position (Fig. 192B).

Management

* Consider no treatment other than reassurance and explanation
* Occlusal splints to interfere with parafunction may offer some help
* Physiotherapy.

It should be emphasised that treatment should only be considered where the abnormality is affecting the patient's quality of life; a clicking joint may be considered as normal.

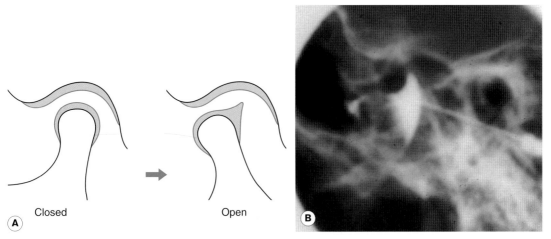

Fig. 191 The normal articular disc in the closed and open positions (**A**) and in an arthrogram showing the maximum opening (**B**).

Closed   Open

Ⓐ   Ⓑ

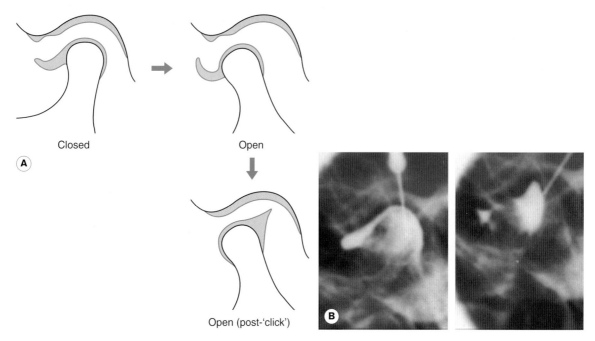

Fig. 192 A displaced disc with reduction showing the movement diagrammatically and arthrographically in open and closed positions.

Disc displacement without reduction

If there is no reduction, a displaced disc remains in a displaced position regardless of the stage of opening. This interferes with movement and may cause pain (Fig. 193A).

Clinical features
- Reduction in opening
- In unilateral cases, lasting deviation on opening
- No click
- Pain may be present in front of the ear.

Radiology

Plain films usually show nothing. In long-standing cases there may be signs of osteoarthrosis (see below).

Disc imaging shows an abnormal disc position in all movements (Fig. 193B). In long-standing cases, perfora-tion of the disc may be seen and joint space adhesions inferred.

Management
- Explanation of the condition and reassurance
- Muscle relaxants and physiotherapy
- Manipulation under anaesthetic
- TMJ surgery.

Surgical treatment of internal derangement

Surgery is only indicated where non-surgical methods have failed and symptoms are severe. Meniscoplasty is a proce-dure to reposition the disc. Access to the joint is gained via a vertical incision in front of the ear (preauricular incision) most commonly, although some favour an incision behind or within the ear. Various techniques have been devised to avoid damage to the facial nerve. The capsule is then

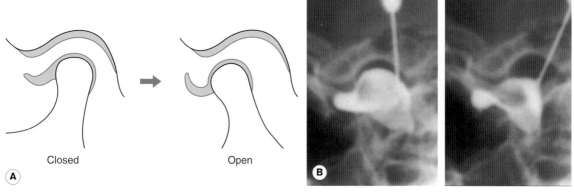

Fig. 193 A displaced disc without reduction showing the movement diagrammatically (**A**) and on arthrography (**B**).

opened, the disc visualised, repositioned and sutured in place. Studies suggest various success rates such as 90% of patients show improvement in symptoms, 5% no better and 5% worse.

The disc may be removed (menisectomy) if it cannot be repositioned because of deformity or degeneration. It may have been replaced with an alloplastic material in the past but is more likely to be replaced now with an autogenous tissue such as temporalis muscle or auricular cartilage.

15.3 Conditions affecting the joint

Learning objectives

You should:
- know the effects of trauma on the joint
- know what systemic diseases will also affect the TMJ.

Osteoarthrosis

Osteoarthrosis is a non-inflammatory disorder of joints in which there is joint deterioration with bony proliferation. The deterioration leads to loss of articular cartilage and bone erosions. The proliferation manifests as new bone formation at the joint periphery and subchondrally. It has an unknown aetiology, but previous trauma, parafunction and internal derangements are all suggested as aetiological factors.

Clinical features
- Pain localised to the TMJ region
- Limitation of opening, worse with prolonged function
- Crepitus
- Tender on palpation of TMJ.

Radiology

Plain films show erosions of the articular surfaces of the condyle and, less commonly seen, of the mandibular fossa. Sclerosis of the bone and marginal bony proliferation ('lipping' or osteophytes) are seen (Fig. 194) and narrowing of the radiographic joint space. Bony proliferations may break away and be seen as loose bodies in the joint space.

Management
- Explanation and reassurance
- Anti-inflammatory drugs
- Physiotherapy
- Restore deficiencies in the posterior occlusion to reduce loading on TMJs
- Intra-articular steroid injections (advanced disease)
- Surgery (advanced disease; final option) to smooth irregular condylar head where there are osteophytes or irregularities.

Rheumatoid arthritis

Rheumatoid arthritis is a disorder associated with synovial membrane inflammation in several joints. The TMJs are involved in approximately half of affected individuals.

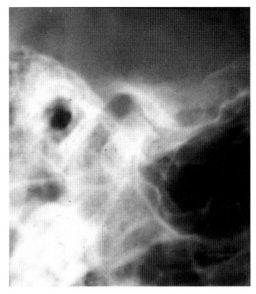

Fig. 194 Radiograph of osteoarthrosis showing marginal bony proliferation ('lipping').

Villous synovitis leads to the formation of synovial granulomatous tissue (pannus) that involves fibrocartilage and the underlying bone. The pannus releases enzymes that cause cartilage/bone destruction.

Clinical features
- Pain over TMJs
- Tenderness over TMJs
- Swelling over TMJs
- Stiffness and limitation of opening
- Crepitus
- Developing anterior open bite and retrusion of chin in advanced disease
- Joints of hands, wrists, knees and feet commonly involved.

Radiology

Radiology demonstrates reduction in bone density in the TMJ. There is marked erosion of the condylar head and articular fossa and narrowing of the joint space.

In long-standing disease, there is:
- destruction of entire condyle
- anterior open bite
- secondary osteoarthrosis
- ankylosis.

Management
- Analgesics/anti-inflammatory drugs
- Steroids
- Physiotherapy.

Juvenile chronic (rheumatoid) arthritis

Juvenile chronic rheumatoid arthritis differs from rheumatoid arthritis in the age of onset (mean age 5 years), the severe systemic involvement and the absence (in some cases) of rheumatoid factor.

While it shares clinical and radiological features with rheumatoid arthritis, the age of onset means that there is often a severe effect on mandibular growth, leading to a 'bird face' appearance owing to the mandibular retrusion, often accompanied by an anterior open bite. The disease often has periods of remission/quiescence, during which time the erosions of the joint may 'smooth over' with formation of a new cortex. Ankylosis may occur.

Trauma

Trauma may have a number of effects upon the TMJ. Fractures are discussed in Chapter 8.

Effusion

Effusion is influx of fluid into the joint, usually either bleeding following trauma or inflammatory exudate. It is important to differentiate this from septic (infective) arthritis.

Clinical features

- Pain over joint
- Swelling over joint
- Limitation of movement
- Sensation of a blocked ear
- Difficulty in occluding posterior teeth.

Radiology

There is a widened joint space.

Management

- Anti-inflammatory drugs
- Rarely, surgical drainage may be needed.

Dislocation

In dislocation of the TMJ, the condyle is abnormally positioned outside the mandibular fossa but within the joint capsule. Dislocation may occur during trauma or be caused by failure of muscular coordination.

Clinical features

- Inability to close the jaw
- Pain
- Muscle spasm.

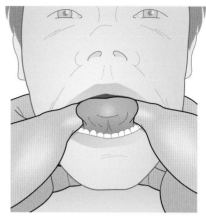

Fig. 195 Manual manipulation to reduce a dislocated jaw.

Radiology

Radiography confirms a clinical diagnosis. The condyle may translate beyond the articular eminence normally, without a dislocation, so clinical information is essential. The condyle will be anterior and superior to the 'summit' of the articular eminence.

Management

Manual manipulation to reduce the dislocation (Fig. 195). Intravenous sedation with midazolam provides muscle relaxation and greatly facilitates this manoeuvre. The patient should avoid wide mouth opening for some days and use the hand to prevent this when yawning.

Ankylosis

Fusion across a TMJ may occur as a result of trauma, mastoid infection or juvenile chronic arthritis. Surgical treatment is by joint replacement with a prosthetic joint unless the patient's facial development is not yet complete, when a costochondral (rib) graft is used in an attempt to provide a bony replacement that may grow.

Self-assessment: questions

Multiple choice questions

1. The following contribute to mouth opening:
   a. Medial pterygoid muscle
   b. Lateral pterygoid muscle
   c. Masseter muscle
   d. Temporalis muscle
   e. Stylomandibular ligament

2. The following radiographs/imaging methods can be used to measure joint space width:
   a. Panoramic radiograph
   b. Transpharyngeal radiograph
   c. Transcranial oblique lateral radiograph
   d. Transorbital (Zimmer) radiograph
   e. Computed tomography (CT)

3. Condylar hyperplasia:
   a. Is a developmental disorder
   b. Is an inflammatory disorder
   c. Is assessed using radioisotope imaging
   d. Is usually self-limiting
   e. Causes ankylosis

4. Erosion of the condyle may occur in:
   a. Pain/dysfunction
   b. Internal derangement
   c. Psoriasis
   d. Synovial chondromatosis (SC)
   e. Dislocation

5. Deviation to the left side on opening could be caused by:
   a. Right TMJ disc anterior displacement without reduction
   b. Left TMJ disc anterior displacement without reduction
   c. Right TMJ effusion
   d. Left TMJ effusion
   e. Bony ankylosis

Extended matching items

EMI 1

Options:
A Osteoarthrosis
B Pain/dysfunction syndrome
C Joint effusion
D Fracture of condylar neck
E Ankylosis
F Juvenile chronic arthritis
G Internal derangement: anterior displacement with reduction
H Internal derangement: anterior displacement without reduction
I Rheumatoid arthritis
J Joint dislocation

Lead in: Match the case history given below that is most appropriate for the diagnosis listed above.

1. An 11-year-old patient, following trauma to the jaw as an infant, developed a worsening facial asymmetry and now has extreme limitation of opening. He has no other joint problems in the body.

2. A 25-year-old male has just had a blow to the face playing rugby. He complains of pain over his right TMJ and limitation of jaw movement. On examination there is no gross facial asymmetry. There is a tender swelling over the affected joint and the ipsilateral posterior teeth don't seem to occlude completely.

3. A 25-year-old woman complains of an annoying 'click' in her left TMJ on opening and closing. On examination, there is no facial asymmetry when the jaw is closed, but a transient deviation of the jaw during opening and closing the mouth. Maximal opening is normal.

4. A 45-year-old woman with a long history of 'TMJ trouble' complains of dull pain and grating sounds over her right TMJ. The symptoms are sometimes worse after a meal, but her jaw is also stiff in the morning with some difficulty in opening.

5. A 35-year-old woman with a long history of clicking and occasional pain from her right TMJ presents with an acute event, consisting of limited opening, deviation of the jaw towards the affected side on attempted opening and pain localised to the joint region. These symptoms were present upon waking up in the morning and have been unchanged since. She mentions that the click that has always been there is no longer present.

6. An 18-year-old male student complains of aching jaw joints, headaches and limitation of mouth opening over the previous 2 weeks. There is no history of trauma or of previous TMJ-related symptoms. On examination, the reduced opening is confirmed, with a path of opening that is rather irregular. There is tenderness over the TMJ regions and of the muscles of mastication bilaterally. There are inconsistent jaw sounds but no predictable 'click' in either joint.

7. A 9-year-old boy has a 3-year history of right TMJ pain and tenderness. Recently, symptoms have developed bilaterally. On examination the mandible appears rather underdeveloped, there is an asymmetry with the right side appearing relatively small and there is an anterior open bite. Enquiry indicates that he has symptoms in other joints in the body.

8. A 50-year-old woman presents with an inability to bring her teeth together properly and pain over the TMJs bilaterally. This occurred suddenly after yawning widely. There is a history of this occurring once before, a few years ago. On examination there is an obvious anterior open bite, with an occlusion limited to her most posterior teeth. There is marked tenderness over the TMJ regions.

9. A 30-year-old man who has been assaulted complains of pain over his left TMJ and an inability both to open his mouth fully and to bring his teeth together properly. On examination, there is a deviation towards the affected side on attempted opening. Intra-orally there is a posterior open bite on the contralateral side. There is tenderness over the affected joint.

10. A 55-year-old woman presents with swelling, pain and tenderness over her TMJs. She says that her mouth opening is limited and there is a feeling of stiffness when she tries. This has been going on for some months, gradually getting worse, and she also has 'joint trouble' in her hands and feet. She also mentions that her 'bite' doesn't feel right. Enquiry reveals no history of joint clicking or trismus prior to the current problem.

EMI 2

Options:

A Panoramic radiograph (collimated to TMJ regions)
B Transpharyngeal radiograph
C Transcranial oblique lateral radiograph
D Reverse Towne's radiograph
E Lateral cephalometric radiograph
F No imaging needed
G Axial CT with parasagittal reconstruction
H Cone beam CT
I Arthrography
J Magnetic resonance imaging

Lead in: Select the appropriate imaging technique from the above list for the investigation of patients with the following provisional clinical diagnoses. Some conditions may require more than one kind of imaging investigation.

1. Osteoarthrosis
2. Pain/dysfunction syndrome
3. Joint effusion
4. Fracture of condylar neck
5. Ankylosis

6. Juvenile chronic arthritis
7. Internal derangement: anterior displacement with reduction
8. Internal derangement: anterior displacement without reduction
9. Rheumatoid arthritis
10. Joint dislocation

Case history questions

Case history 1

1. What diagnosis is suggested?
2. What would be the management?

Case history 2

1. What diagnosis is suggested?
2. What would be the management?

Case history 3

1. What diagnosis is suggested?
2. What would be the management?

Case history 4

1. What diagnosis is suggested?
2. What would be the management?

Viva questions

1. Is a clicking temporomandibular joint (TMJ) abnormal?
2. What clinical signs would suggest that a patient was a bruxist?
3. Are TMJ disorders a manifestation of mental illness?
4. Should you take a panoramic radiograph for patients with TMJ disorders?
5. What are the indications and contraindications for TMJ arthrography?
6. How would you examine the lateral pterygoid muscle when assessing a patient with a TMJ disorder?
7. What are the uses of arthroscopy in managing TMJ disorders?
8. When might you use a soft bite guard for a patient with TMJ problems?

Self-assessment: answers

Multiple choice answers

1. a. **False.** It helps in closing the mouth.
    b. **True.** Only the lateral pterygoid muscle is a 'mouth opener'. In fact it has two parts; its lower head is active in opening, protrusion and lateral movements, while its upper head has activity during mouth closing.
    c. **False.** It helps in closing the mouth.
    d. **False.** It helps in closing the mouth.
    e. **False.** The stylomandibular ligament extends from the styloid process on the skull base to the angle of the mandible; its role is probably to limit movement of the mandible but it has no active role to play.

2. a. **False.** Panoramic radiographs are taken with the jaw protruded and, therefore, cannot show any information about joint space width.
    b. **False.** The transpharyngeal radiograph is taken with the mouth open.
    c. **True.** A 'closed' transcranial oblique lateral radiograph is the only radiograph that shows joint space width. However, the angulation used means that it is the joint space width in the lateral part of the joint that is demonstrated.
    d. **False.** This rarely used antero-posterior radiograph is taken with the mouth open. The X-ray source has to be positioned close to the eye and consequently gives a high dose to the lens.
    e. **True.** CT can give measurements of joint space width. However, conventional axial scans must be reassembled in a two-dimensional reconstruction to make measurement easier, so fine sections are best. Direct sagittal scanning is preferable.

    Joint space narrowing is a sign of osteoarthrosis. However, it is important to remember that imaging should not be carried out just to ensure that all pathological findings have been demonstrated. The purpose of imaging is to aid in diagnosis and to make a contribution to management. If you have established the diagnosis clinically and know what treatment you are going to do, then the presence/absence of joint space narrowing is irrelevant!

3. a. **True.** Condylar hyperplasia is a developmental anomaly causing excessive growth of the condyle, leading to a developing facial asymmetry, enlargement of the condyle and sometimes deformity of the condylar head. It usually arises before age 20 years and is commoner in males.
    b. **False.**
    c. **True.** Radioisotope bone scanning (using ^{99m}Tc-labelled methylene bisphosphonate as the radiopharmaceutical) is used to assess activity in the condyle; ideally surgery is carried out when the activity is reduced to background level.
    d. **True.** The jaw on the affected side often shows an increase in height of the ramus and body. There may be a posterior open bite on the affected side but often there is compensatory maxillary alveolar overgrowth. Treatment is ideally by orthognathic surgery, but this should be delayed until the condition has stopped developing.
    e. **False.** Ankylosis is not associated with the condition.

4. a. **False.** Erosion of the condylar head is a fairly non-specific feature. It is most commonly seen in osteoarthrosis.
    b. **True.** Erosion in internal derangements represents advanced disease with progression to osteoarthrosis.
    c. **True.** Psoriasis is a seronegative systemic arthritis. Radiologically and clinically it is similar to rheumatoid arthritis.
    d. **True.** SC is a rare disorder where there is formation of multiple cartilagenous and osseocartilagenous nodules in the synovial membrane of joints. These nodules can detach and become loose in the joint spaces. Patients with SC have variable symptoms ranging from none to pain, swelling, joint noises and trismus. Treatment is by surgery to remove the nodules and resect the abnormal synovial membrane.
    e. **False.** There is no association with erosions.

5. a. **False.** Deviation occurs towards the affected side.
    b. **True.** Any limitation on TMJ movement will lead to deviation of the jaw towards the affected side.
    c. **False.** This would cause deviation to the right.
    d. **True.** Effusion will limit movement, causing deviation to the left.
    e. **False.** Bony ankylosis would not show this sign because true ankylosis will prevent all but a tiny degree of jaw movement.

Extended matching items answers

EMI 1

1. **E.** The problem is localised to a single joint in the body and has a clear relationship to trauma when an infant, so ankylosis seems a likely diagnosis and juvenile chronic arthritis seems unlikely. Bony ankylosis means that mandibular movement is essentially non-existent, although a few millimetres of movement may be observed through flexing of the bone. Sometimes, however, the ankylosis is due to fibrous union of the joint components, and a little greater movement may be possible. Radiography should be able to differentiate the two types.

2. **C.** Trauma has precipitated this problem, so the differential diagnosis is essentially between C, D and J. In this case the occlusion is a helpful clue. If there

247

was a unilateral fracture of the condylar neck, then there would probably be a posterior open bite on the contralateral side. Dislocation is usually bilateral and gives an anterior open bite. Effusion, apart from other local signs of inflammation, tends to produce difficulty in bringing the posterior teeth together, but no dramatic change in the occlusion. Of course, if there is any doubt, radiography should be used as a help.

3. **G.** Reciprocal clicking is the essential sign of anterior disc displacement with reduction. In the absence of other symptoms, such as pain, difficulty in eating etc., this can be seen as normal variation rather than disease.

4. **A.** This condition is more common in older patients and in women. It may follow on from an internal derangement or after trauma. The condition comes and goes and may gradually burn out. Management should, therefore, be aimed at symptomatic relief. In some respects, the symptoms in this patient could be consistent with rheumatoid arthritis, but the absence of other joints with disease makes this most unlikely.

5. **H.** Patients with a reducing disc (disc displacement with reduction) sometimes present with a sudden event of inability to open their mouth (disc displacement without reduction). The event usually arises suddenly, during eating, yawning or, as here, appears on waking from sleep.

6. **B.** The muscle tenderness, the headaches and jaw limitation all fit with this diagnosis. The absence of any 'click', either current or historical, goes against a diagnosis of internal derangement.

7. **F.** The age of the patient tends to give this one away, as does the evidence of multiple joint involvement. Almost half of patients with this condition will have TMJ involvement and most will ultimately have bilateral disease. Retrognathia and anterior open bite are prominent features because of destruction of the normal condylar growth centre. Asymmetry is also fairly common, reflecting differential degrees of involvement of the joints.

8. **J.** The features are certain to be dislocation, because of the sudden onset during yawning and the occlusal effects. Patients who dislocate their jaw in this way may suffer recurrent events, as in this case. The anterior open bite, with 'gagging' on the posterior teeth, is also seen in bilateral condylar fractures, but in the absence of trauma this would not be in the differential diagnosis here. The only other possible diagnosis would be an acute internal derangement problem, where the condylar head had passed anterior to a lax interarticular disc and could not reduce back to allow closure; such an event would be unlikely to occur bilaterally.

9. **D.** This scenario fits well with a fractured neck of condyle. The key factor that helps differentiate this case from other trauma-associated TMJ problems is the occlusion. As discussed in Chapter 8, a fracture at this site will lead to an altered occlusion due to the likely displacement of the condylar fragment and the consequent upward movement of the ipsilateral ramus.

10. **I.** The symptoms might suggest pain/dysfunction or anterior disc displacement without reduction. The absence of a previous click, however, would tend to exclude the latter diagnosis. The clues here are the problems with other joints and the complaint about the 'bite'. In rheumatoid arthritis, destruction of the articulating surface of the condyles may occur, leading to a superior position of the condyles in the fossae. This may lead to an altered occlusion and anterior open bite.

EMI 2

1. **A** is the simplest choice. Radiological findings in osteoarthrosis include sclerosis, joint space narrowing, flattening of the articulating surfaces and osteophyte formation. B is of historical interest, while C needs special equipment that dentists would not have.

2. **F.** As there is nothing to image in this condition, and as the provisional diagnosis is reached on clinical evidence, no imaging is required.

3. **F** or **A.** This diagnosis is often reached on clinical evidence and radiology can do nothing to improve the treatment. In reality, however, some imaging may be needed to confirm that there is no fracture and, in such cases, a panoramic radiograph may be sufficient.

4. **A** and **D.** When evaluating fractures, it is *de rigueur* to have two images at different angulations, and this pair offers a 90° difference. It is becoming increasingly common for G or H to be used in this situation; while either provide excellent images of the TMJ, they also deliver higher radiation doses than A and D, and relative cost/benefit has not been evaluated.

5. **A** followed by **G** or **H.** Once the diagnosis has been made using clinical information and A, cross-sectional imaging is appropriate to aid the surgeon in planning intervention.

6. **A** and **E.** The lateral cephalometric radiograph will be important as a means of recording objectively the facial changes associated with this condition.

7. **F.** So long as no treatment is needed and the clinical features so clear, imaging is not going to change management.

8. **I** or **J.** Here, intervention is likely, so imaging if the meniscus position is required. Magnetic resonance imaging is the preferred method for this, although a few centres will still perform arthrography.

9. **A** and possibly **E.** A may show the characteristic erosion of the condylar heads and assist in confirming diagnosis. E would be appropriate if there is evidence of a changing occlusion, as was the case with juvenile chronic arthritis.

10. **A.** The radiograph is used to confirm that the condylar heads lie anterior to the articular eminences.

Case history answers

Case history 1

Amanda is a 22-year-old dental receptionist who complains of sharp pain in the right preauricular region that increases when trying to move her jaw, with an associated headache. This has been present for 3 months. There are no joint noises when she opens her mouth and there is very limited opening. There is a deviation of the jaw to the right that occurs only in the final stages of opening. She says that she used to have a clicking jaw but no longer does so.

1. The previous history of clicking suggests that there was, in the past, a displaced disc in the right TMJ that could reduce when opening. The change in symptoms, with loss of the click and limitation of opening with late deviation, is typical of a non-reducing disc displacement. A displaced disc without reduction is usually preceded by a reducing disc.
2. Describe the problem to Amanda and try to reassure her. Treatment should be carried out in conjunction with her doctor, unless you are a hospital practitioner. A referral for physiotherapy would be appropriate and a muscle relaxant drug could be prescribed. Benzodiazepine drugs are used for their muscle relaxant effects. The form may be diazepam 5 mg at night, or temazepam elixir (10 mg in 5 ml) at night. Review the patient after 1 month. Longer review might be useful, particularly if there has been some improvement, as spontaneous resolution can occur. In the absence of any improvement, it may be appropriate to consider disc imaging and manipulation of the jaw under general anaesthesia.

Case history 2

Mrs Johnson is a 50-year-old woman who attends the surgery complaining of a chronic localised pain over her left TMJ and limited opening. The masticatory muscles are not particularly tender. She finds opening her mouth wide for dental treatment painful. She says that the pain gets worse as the day goes on. You notice crepitus on examining the TMJ.

1. The symptoms and signs suggest that the diagnosis is osteoarthrosis.
2. First, take a radiograph of the affected TMJ to confirm the diagnosis by identification of the radiological signs of the disease. A transpharyngeal view or a panoramic (TMJ programme) radiograph would be reasonable. Alternatively a transcranial film might be useful to examine the joint space. Mrs Johnson is concerned about the effect this condition is having on her life. Therefore, it is worth attempting treatment. Reassure the patient and describe the nature of the condition. Examine the mouth and assess whether there is a satisfactory posterior occlusion. Prescribe a non-steroidal anti-inflammatory drug. An appropriate prescription would be 400 mg ibuprofen three times a day *after* food for 1 month. This should not be prescribed for patients with any history of peptic ulceration or asthma, during pregnancy or for patients with kidney or liver disorders. A course of physiotherapy would be valuable. Review after 1 month. In the absence of improvement, refer to a specialist clinic. The specialist may consider intra-articular steroid injection or, as a last resort, surgery.

Case history 3

David is a 19-year-old man who was struck on the left side of his chin during a game of Saturday football. He arrives at the surgery on Monday morning in pain from the right TMJ. He cannot open his mouth as wide as he could. His right TMJ/preauricular region is very tender and swollen and he deviates towards the right side on opening.

1. There is a clear link to the traumatic incident and the differential diagnosis is a joint effusion or a fracture of the right condylar neck.
2. Check the occlusion. An effusion would either have no effect on the occlusion or cause a difficulty in approximating the posterior teeth on the affected side. A fractured condylar neck is often associated with premature contact between the posterior teeth on the ipsilateral side and a posterior open bite on the contralateral side. Take a radiograph. A panoramic film is a valuable imaging method for suspected mandibular fractures. This might be supplemented by other views (e.g. a reverse Towne's view) if the panoramic suggests a fracture. An effusion would probably not give any radiological signs on a panoramic view. If the diagnosis is joint effusion, then reassurance, resting the joint and use of anti-inflammatory drugs on a short-term basis would probably suffice. If a fracture is confirmed, then the patient should be referred to a hospital oral and maxillofacial surgeon. If the occlusion is normal, then management would be conservative, that is, the same as for an effusion. If the occlusion is abnormal, this would indicate a 2-week period of intermaxillary fixation (IMF) or, on occasion, open reduction and fixation.

Case history 4

Mr Jones is a busy bank manager and your regular patient. At a check-up, he mentions that he has pain when opening his mouth, associated with intermittent clicking from the left TMJ. There is pain when you palpate the muscles of mastication and when you palpate the left preauricular region. There is a slight reduction in mouth opening and the jaw deviates towards the left side on opening.

1. The symptoms and signs are consistent with pain/dysfunction syndrome.
2. Reassure the patient and explain that this is a common condition. Point out that pain/dysfunction may spontaneously subside but may recur. Advise jaw rest, soft diet, the use of anti-inflammatory drugs and construct a soft bite guard. Consider referral for a course of physiotherapy. Review.

Viva answers

1. 'Clicking' of the jaw is a result of an atypical disc position, usually an anterior displacement. Magnetic resonance imaging studies of normal individuals show that a substantial proportion have an anterior disc position. Therefore, the presence of a jaw click is not

in itself abnormal and there should be no attempt to 'treat' it unless there are other symptoms or signs.

2. Bruxism is associated with the following:
   - tooth attrition with unusual wear facets
   - tooth sensitivity, particularly of anterior teeth
   - frequent fracture/replacement of restorations
   - scalloping of the lateral border of the tongue
   - ridging of the cheek mucosa along the occlusal plane.

3. No. However, 30–40% of patients attending for a TMJ disorder will also have a mental disorder. The most common disorder is a depressive illness. It is possible that when people become depressed they become more aware of physical symptoms.

4. No. The majority of patients with TMJ disorders have pain/dysfunction or an internal derangement. Neither have radiological signs. A panoramic radiograph is often taken as a 'check' for other pathology. This is unsupportable as radiographic screening using panoramic radiographs has no scientific basis. A radiograph (a panoramic may be the best choice) is indicated where the suspected diagnosis is osteoarthrosis and after trauma when a fracture is a possible diagnosis.

5. The main indication for arthrography would be an internal disc derangement that has not resolved following conservative treatment and where either manipulation under general anaesthesia or surgery is being contemplated. Generally magnetic resonance imaging is preferred to arthrography but is often less readily accessed. Contraindications include local infection and iodine allergy. Very anxious patients and needle phobics may not be appropriate candidates for arthrography.

6. Lateral pterygoid muscle is not accessible for direct examination. Some authorities suggest palpation behind the maxillary tuberosity as a method of direct examination but it is of dubious value, particularly as anyone would find palpation here uncomfortable. The muscle is best assessed by measuring the response to opening the jaw against the resistance of the operator's hand. Place your hand under the patient's chin and ask them to open against it. If there is muscle spasm, there will be preauricular pain on attempted opening. This procedure can be repeated with lateral movements.

7. Arthroscopy is a minimally invasive surgical technique in which an instrument is passed into the upper joint space, permitting direct imaging via a camera and surgical procedures to be performed. Lavage, biopsy and sectioning of adhesions can be performed.

8. A soft bite guard is a useful first-line treatment for patients with pain/dysfunction syndrome. Its method of action is not understood, but it may work as a habit breaker in parafunction or simply as an absorber of occlusal forces. It is usually worn at night for 6 weeks.

Radiation protection

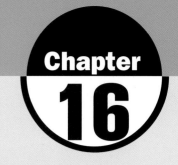

Chapter

16

Overview

Ionising radiation is used in medicine and dentistry to visualise dense internal structures. In dentistry, the potential problems are stochastic tumour-inducing effects. This chapter discusses the doses and risks in different types of dental radiography and the indications for the use of different views. Methods to protect both the patient and the dentist are discussed, together with the components of a quality assurance programme.

16.1 Ionising radiation and its effects

Learning objectives

You should:
- know what ionising radiation is
- know how it interacts with matter
- know what its somatic and genetic effects are
- know the doses and risks in dental radiography.

The use of ionising radiation in medicine and dentistry is governed by the statutory requirements laid down in the Ionising Radiations Regulations 1999 (staff safety and equipment) and the Ionising Radiation (Medical Exposure) Regulations 2000 (patient protection). Guidance notes on the use of radiation in general dental practice, summarising this legislation, are available to all dentists.

Ionising radiation includes X-rays, gamma rays and cosmic rays. These are all high-energy, short-wavelength, high-frequency electromagnetic radiations. They exist as tiny packets of energy called photons. While gamma rays are used in hospital practice in nuclear medicine, X-rays are the only usual concern of dentists.

X-rays are produced by an electrical process in an X-ray tube (Fig. 196). Electrons, released from a heated tungsten filament, are accelerated in a vacuum by the application of a high voltage (typically 50–75 kV (kilovolts)) and strike a positively charged target. The sudden halt of the electrons releases energy, mainly as heat but also as X-rays. The X-rays are a mixture of photons of different energies, but low-energy (dose-producing) photons predominate.

The X-rays are filtered using aluminium to remove the low-energy photons (Fig. 197). The photons are then shaped into an appropriately sized beam by collimation using steel diaphragms or cylinders (Fig. 198).

Interaction with matter

Three possible interactions can occur at the atomic level when X-rays interact with matter:

- photoelectric interaction
- Compton interaction
- coherent scatter.

The first two result in absorption of all or part of the X-ray photon energy and ionisation of an atom.

In a living cell, ionisation can have damaging effects. We are particularly concerned if the DNA of a cell is damaged. This may occur by a *direct* interaction of X-ray photons with the DNA or *indirectly* when a photon disrupts a water molecule into reactive radicals that go on to damage DNA.

Somatic and genetic effects of X-rays

The irradiation of cells can result in **somatic** effects (i.e. those occurring in the irradiated somatic cells of an individual) or **genetic** effects (i.e. those occurring in the germ cells and transmitted to the offspring of the irradiated individual) because of gonadal exposure. In properly conducted dental radiography, genetic effects are not usually considered because the gonads should not be irradiated.

Somatic effects can be:

- deterministic: e.g. cataract formation, loss of fertility, erythema of the skin, 'radiation sickness'
- stochastic: tumour induction (also occurs in genetic effects).

All deterministic effects have threshold doses below which they do not occur. Above the threshold dose, the effect is certain to occur. In dental radiography these thresholds should never be reached. The risk from dental radiography is for stochastic effects.

Doses and risks in dental radiography

Doses and risks vary enormously according to the type of equipment used, so it is hard to give firm figures, but recent estimations of risk (and radiation dose) are given in Table 17.

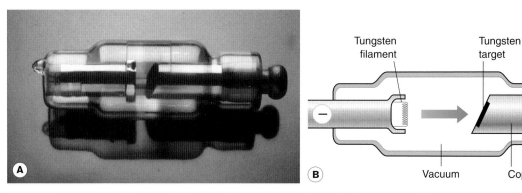

Fig. 196 An X-ray tube insert from a dental X-ray set **(A)** and a diagram **(B)** showing the structure and the direction of electron flow (arrow).

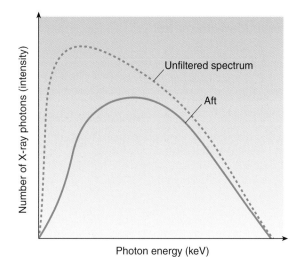

Fig. 197 The effect of filtration on the X-ray beam. Low-energy photons predominate in the unfiltered spectrum. Filtration removes proportionately more of these 'weak X-rays', resulting in a filtered beam with a higher mean energy at the expense of a loss of intensity.

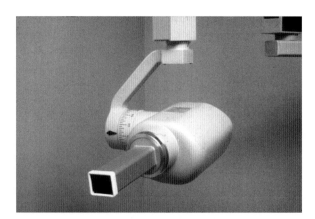

Fig. 198 An X-ray set with rectangular collimation. This beam restriction method results in a dose reduction to patients of about 65% compared with conventional 6-cm-diameter round beams.

Table 17 Estimates of dose and risk in dental radiography

Technique	Effective dose (microsieverts)	Risk of cancer (per million)
Intra-oral (bitewing, periapical)	2–10	0.06–0.7
Panoramic	7–26	0.21–1.9
Lateral cephalogram	3	0.06–0.1
Cone beam CT scan*	50–100	< 50
Computed tomographic scan of mandible for implantology	480–3300	24–242

These risks are calculated for a 30-year-old adult. Risks for children are two to three times greater, while for older patients risk falls until, at 80 years, they are virtually negligible.

*Doses for full field view.

16.2 Radiation protection

Learning objectives

You should:
- know when radiography is justified and which views to use
- know how to limit dosage to patients and staff
- be able to use the equipment in a manner most likely to ensure useable radiographs are produced
- understand the administrative requirements for different members of a dental team.

The aim of radiation protection is to ensure all exposures are kept as low as reasonably achievable (ALARA principle).

Protection of patients

In dental radiography, protection of patients is achieved by three main means:

- justification
- dose limitation
- quality assurance.

Justification

There is a legal requirement that no radiological examination should be used unless there is likely to be a benefit in terms of improved prognosis or management of the patient.

This implies that no X-ray examination is ever 'routine' and that radiographic 'screening' is unacceptable. Instead, radiographs should be prescribed according the clinical needs of the patient.

Selection of bitewing radiographs

The nearest we come to 'routine' radiography in dentistry is with the bitewing radiograph. For dentate patients who are new to the practice (and partially dentate patients where films can be supported in the mouth), most authorities agree that a posterior bitewing examination is justified. Thereafter, the intervals between bitewing examinations should be determined by assessment of caries risk (Table 18).

Obviously bitewing frequency for an individual patient may change if the patient changes caries risk category.

If the dentist feels that a radiographic examination is of help in assessment of bone loss in periodontal disease, then bitewing radiographs will provide the necessary information in the premolar and molar regions, providing geometrically accurate images. Where periodontal probing depths exceed 5 mm, then vertical bitewing radiographs are appropriate.

Selection of periapical radiographs

Periapical radiographs are indicated in the following situations:

1. When dictated by localised symptoms/signs (pain, swelling and tenderness of a tooth).
2. Prior to the extraction of third molars, lone-standing upper molars or where there is reasonable clinical suspicion that problems may arise. The fashion of routine pre-extraction radiographs has arisen in the absence of any scientific evidence of benefit.
3. Prior to preparation of a tooth for a crown or bridge retainer.
4. In endodontics, where basic guidelines suggest radiograph(s) at the following stages:
   a. preoperative
   b. working length estimation
   c. master cone position (precondensation)
   d. postcondensation
   e. At 1 year after treatment completion.
5. Dental trauma.

This list is not exhaustive. Where there is any localised dental or alveolar problem, a periapical radiograph may be appropriate.

Table 18 Intervals between bitewing examinations indicated by caries risk Interval (months) by caries risk category

	Low	Moderate	High
Child	12–18	12	6
Adult	24 or greater	12	6

Selection of panoramic radiographs

In terms of image quality, panoramic radiography is inferior to good intra-oral radiographs. Consequently, for most dental diagnostic uses it is a 'second best' imaging technique. Possible situations where it may be useful include:

- where a bony lesion or unerupted tooth is of a size or position that precludes its complete demonstration on intra-oral radiographs
- in orthodontic assessment when clinically indicated (no 'screening')
- preoperative assessment of third molars, unless other adequate radiographs are available
- when mandibular fracture is suspected.

Routine 'screening' of all new patients is never justifiable; research has shown that the majority of patients who receive a 'screening' panoramic radiograph receive no diagnostic benefit from the examination.

Dose limitation

Doses in dental radiography can be minimised by considering:

- kilovoltage: for intra-oral radiography a minimum of 50 kV is set and 65–70 kV is recommended
- AC/DC generation of X-rays: 'DC' (constant potential) generators lead to fewer low-energy (dose-producing) X-ray photons
- filtration: aluminium filters absorb low-energy X-ray photons
- collimation: on intra-oral X-ray sets, the beam can be restricted to a rectangle of 4 cm by 3 cm, leading to a substantial dose reduction over the conventional 6-cm-diameter round beam; all new equipment should be fitted with rectangular collimation and it should be retro-fitted on older equipment; on panoramic machines, selective field size collimation facilities may be available
- image receptor speed:
- E-speed film needs approximately half the X-ray exposure of D-speed film, with no loss of diagnostic quality
- F-speed films are now available that offer a further 20% reduction in exposure
- digital systems may offer some reduction in exposure time (and hence dose) compared with film
- rare-earth film/screen combinations in cassettes give significant dose reduction compared with calcium tungstate combinations; a combination of ISO speed 400 or better is used. Digital systems for extra-oral radiography offer limited, if any, dose reduction compared with fast rare-earth film/screen combinations
- lead shielding of patients: the only requirement to use a lead apron is when a pregnant woman is being examined using a technique involving a beam that would pass through the fetus. Thyroid shielding can be used if that organ lies in the primary beam of X-rays.

Quality assurance

A poor-quality image means that the patient receives reduced, or no, benefit from the risk of the X-ray examination. Even in the best hands, radiographs may be produced that are 'rejects'. A quality standard of no greater than 10% of radiographs being non-diagnostic has been set for general dental practice. Good quality of radiographs can be addressed by attention to all of the criteria listed in Table 19.

A quality assurance programme of regular checks, cleaning and servicing should be established to maintain high standards and to fulfil the legal requirement.

Protection for staff

While practitioners rightly consider the well-being of patients first, dental staff should not be ignored. Dentists and ancillary staff may be exposed many times each day to X-rays if staff protection is not ensured. The following are the important considerations.

Position

For intra-oral radiography, nobody except the patient should be within the controlled area (Fig. 199) unless specific guidance has been received from a medical physics expert/radiation protection adviser. This controlled area

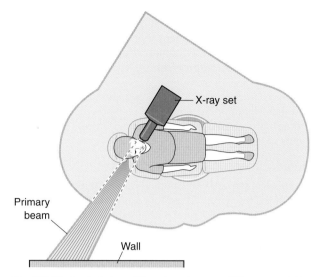

Fig. 199 The 'controlled area'. The primary beam would be unacceptably intense for many metres and we rely on walls to attenuate the X-ray beam to an acceptable level. While this diagram is two-dimensional, remember that the controlled area extends above and below the patient and X-ray set. Ceiling and floor materials may not provide an adequate barrier to limit the controlled area.

has a strict definition; however, safety should be adequate outside an area of radius 2 m centred on the patient and, for intra-oral radiography, never in line of the primary beam.

Workload

While it is probably impossible for a member of dental staff to receive a dose approaching the limits set by law for workers, radiation dose monitoring has been recommended for anyone taking more than 100 intra-oral or 50 panoramic radiographs per week.

Local rules

Every dental practice has to have a set of local rules for radiation safety. By reading these and adhering to them, radiation safety of staff should be assured.

'Good practice' guidelines

Guidelines on the safe use of radiation are produced by the UK Department of Health.

Administration of radiation protection

The process of radiology in medicine/dentistry is divided into specific 'roles'.

Employer (legal person)

The employer (e.g. NHS Trust, Health Authority, principal in general dental practice) has legal responsibility to ensure that regulations are followed. The employer must ensure that referrers have written guidance (referral/selection criteria) on referral of patients for X-ray examination.

Referrer

The referrer is a registered medical/dental practitioner. The duty of the referrer is to supply adequate clinical

Table 19 Methods of assuring good-quality radiographs

Area	Improving methods
Radiographic technique	Use of film-holding/beam-aiming devices for intra-oral radiography Careful positioning for panoramic radiography Careful selection and instruction of patients
X-ray set	Regular maintenance and servicing, as recommended by the manufacturer Triennial survey of radiation safety by appropriately trained person
Film and cassettes	Use film before expiry date; store in cool dry conditions, handle with care Ensure cassettes are light tight and that intensifying screens are cleaned
Darkroom	Must be light tight and have correct safelights Clean work surfaces
Manual processing	Use a thermometer and timer and use time/temperature processing Fix and wash films adequately Change chemicals as advised by manufacturer
Automatic processing	Clean and service regularly Change chemicals as advised by manufacturer
After-care	Mount, name and date radiographs

Viewing box essential: magnification extremely valuable for intra-oral radiographs.

information to allow the practitioner to justify the examination. In general practice, the referrer is the dentist.

Practitioner

The practitioner is an individual who is qualified to justify radiological examinations. In hospitals, this is the radiologist or, depending on local arrangements, the radiographer. In general dental practice, it is the dentist.

Operator

The operator is the person who carries out the radiological examination. In hospitals this is the radiographer. In general dental practice, it is the dentist or a *suitably qualified* therapist, hygienist or dental nurse.

Radiation Protection Supervisor

The Radiation Protection Supervisor is an individual who takes the role of checking that legal requirements and 'good practice' are being followed. In general dental practice, this is usually a dentist.

Radiation Protection Adviser

All facilities, including general dental practices, must appoint a Radiation Protection Adviser. This is a medical physicist who provides expert support in ensuring that regulations are followed and good practice is maintained.

16.3 Further reading

You are recommended to read the following to supplement this chapter:

European Commission 2004 Radiation Protection No 136 *European Guidelines on Radiation Protection in Dental Radiology*. Luxembourg: Office for Official Publications of the European Communities (http://ec.europa.eu/energy/nuclear/radioprotection/publication/doc/136_en.pdf)

National Radiological Protection Board (NRPB) and Royal College of Radiologists 1994 *Guidelines on Radiology Standards for Primary Dental Care*. Documents of the NRPB Vol 5 (3). London: NRPB

National Radiological Protection Board 2001 Guidance notes for dental practitioners on the safe use of X-ray equipment. London: Department of Health (http://www.hpa.org.uk/radiation/publications/misc_publications/dental_guidance_notes.pdf)

Pendlebury ME, Horner K, Eaton KA 2004 *Selection Criteria for Dental Radiography*, 2nd edition. London: Faculty of General Dental Practitioners (UK), Royal College of Surgeons of England

Sixteen

Self-assessment: questions

Multiple choice questions

1. The following are ionising radiation:
   a. X-rays
   b. Radiowaves
   c. Microwaves
   d. Gamma rays
   e. Cosmic rays

2. The following are everyday risks to patients in dental radiography:
   a. Deterministic effects
   b. Somatic stochastic effects
   c. Genetic stochastic effects
   d. Salivary gland cancer
   e. Cataract formation

3. The dose of radiation from a panoramic radiograph is:
   a. About the same as 1 to 4 days of background radiation
   b. Much less than the dose from a chest radiograph
   c. Equivalent to that from a set of posterior bitewing radiographs
   d. Always 7–26 μSv (microsieverts)
   e. Associated with a risk of cancer typically higher than that from a lateral cephalogram

4. A lower radiation dose for a periapical radiograph can be achieved by:
   a. Using a 50 kV X-ray set rather than a 70 kV X-ray set
   b. Using a constant potential (DC) X-ray set rather than a pulsating potential (AC) X-ray set
   c. Using a lead apron
   d. Using D-speed film
   e. Using a digital radiography system

Extended matching items

EMI 1

Options:

A Old film stock
B Too low an X-ray exposure
C The radiographic cassette leaks light
D Poor patient positioning
E Light fogging during automatic processing
F Poor film/screen contact
G Incorrect processing
H Patient movement during exposure
I Static electricity discharge
J Excessive X-ray exposure

Lead in: Poor quality radiographs lead to the need for repeat exposures, thus increasing radiation dose to patients. Match each panoramic radiographic film fault below to the 'diagnosis' (cause of the fault) above. There may be more than one possible cause for some film faults.

1. Localised areas of 'black' (high density) along the edge of the radiograph.
2. Areas of the radiograph show 'blurring' (reduced image sharpness).

3. Lower border of mandible is distorted ('up and down' shape).
4. Low density and contrast throughout the image.
5. Wide front teeth.
6. Uniformly dark, low contrast image.
7. Narrow, 'matchstick' front teeth.
8. A mixture of small black spots and thin zig-zag lines over the image.
9. The film steadily increases in density and loses contrast from one end to the other.
10. All radiographs show low contrast and, notably, metal restorations look grey.

EMI 2

Options:

A Bitewing examination
B Periapical radiograph(s)
C Occlusal radiograph(s)
D Panoramic radiograph
E Lateral cephalometric radiograph
F CT or cone beam CT examination
G Magnetic resonance imaging
H Radioisotope imaging
I Ultrasound examination
J No radiological investigation needed

Lead in: One of the simplest means of radiation protection of patients is the use of referral criteria to select the appropriate radiological investigation, thus minimising X-ray examinations that do not alter management of the patient's problem. Select the most likely radiological investigation(s) from the list above that would be appropriate to the case histories below. More than one investigation may be appropriate for some cases.

1. A patient has gingivitis and probing suggests some early loss of periodontal attachment throughout the mouth.
2. A patient presents with a symptomatic internal disc derangement of a temporomandibular joint that has proved unresponsive to conservative treatment.
3. A patient presents with recurrent, severe, sharp toothache of 10 minutes' duration, precipitated by hot stimuli. The causative tooth is difficult to localise clinically.
4. A 14-year-old patient has a retained maxillary canine and no sign of the permanent successor.
5. A patient presents with a painless, clicking temporomandibular joint.
6. A patient presents with an acute pericoronitis on an erupting wisdom tooth. This is the first occasion it has occurred.
7. A 12-year-old patient who has mild crowding, a Class I malocclusion and a skeletal Class 1 pattern wants and seems suitable for orthodontic treatment using a simple upper removable appliance.

8. A patient requires endosseous implants in the posterior maxilla.
9. A patient presents with a large, painless hard bony swelling in the lower first molar region.
10. A 12-year-old patient, with Index of Orthodontic Treatment Need (Dental Health Component) > 4 and a severe Class 2 skeletal pattern requires and seems suitable for upper and lower fixed appliances.

Essay questions

1. The risk to patients from dental radiography is so low as to be negligible. Discuss.
2. How would you carry out radiographic quality assurance in a dental practice?

Viva questions

1. When should you use a lead apron in dental radiography?
2. Where should the operator stand when exposing a patient for an intra-oral radiograph?
3. How would you respond to a patient who expressed concern about the X-ray exposure from a dental radiograph?
4. How would you improve the risk/benefit when exposing a patient for a panoramic radiograph?
5. Why are X-rays considered to be dangerous?
6. How do you assess when a patient should have a set of bitewing radiographs?

Self-assessment: answers

Multiple choice answers

1. a. **True.** These are produced by bombarding a positively charged target with electrons.
   b. **False.** Low frequency and, therefore, have insufficient energy to ionise atoms.
   c. **False.** Low frequency and, therefore, have insufficient energy to ionise atoms.
   d. **True.** Naturally occurring radiation from radioactive materials.
   e. **True.** Cosmic rays come from outer space but contribute a substantial part of our natural background radiation.

   All of these radiations are electromagnetic (EM) radiation. EM radiation exists as photons, tiny packets of energy with a waveform (they have a frequency and a wavelength). The higher the frequency, the greater the energy in each photon. X-rays, gamma rays and cosmic rays are all high-frequency EM radiation and can ionise atoms.

2. a. **False.** These effects have threshold doses considerably higher than that which might be received during dental radiography. They may, however, occur during radiotherapy.
   b. **True.** These effects (tumour induction) have no threshold dose. However, the risk is believed to be directly related to the dose. With low doses associated with dental radiography, the risk is low.
   c. **False.** It is generally accepted that gonadal doses in dental radiography are so low as to be negligible. This is particularly plausible when considering panoramic radiography (the beam is highly collimated and is angled slightly upwards) and intra-oral radiography using film holders (paralleling techniques) and rectangular collimation.
   d. **True.** There is published evidence of an association between dental radiography and salivary gland (and brain) tumours. However, this work refers back to a time of higher radiation doses and it must be remembered that the risks are small.
   e. **False.** Cataract formation is a deterministic effect that should never occur as a consequence of dental radiography.

3. a. **True.** The annual average dose to the UK citizen from all forms of radiation is 2500 µSv (microsieverts). The doses from dental radiography can be related to this. Using the doses given in the text of this chapter, a panoramic radiograph would be equivalent to approximately this number of days.
   b. **False.** Doses from chest radiography vary but a typical range is 20–40 µSv, in the same general range as panoramic radiographs.
   c. **True.** Using the dose ranges given in this chapter, two bitewing films is around the same level of dose

as a panoramic radiograph. However, the ranges involved mean that this may not always be the case.
   d. **False.** The dose range given assumes 'good practice' and up-to-date equipment. Many older machines with higher doses are used in dental practices, and the common practice of overexposing to compensate for underdevelopment during processing means that doses may be considerably higher.
   e. **True.** Looking at the figures quoted in the text of this chapter, you will see that the risk from a panoramic radiograph is believed to be typically an order of magnitude greater than that of a lateral cephalogram.

4. a. **False.** Lower voltages give a higher proportion of weaker X-rays. Weak X-rays are more likely to undergo absorption (photoelectric interactions) in the patient's tissues.
   b. **True.** A 'DC' X-ray set produces a smaller proportion of weak X-rays.
   c. **False.** Using standard 'good practice' technique (paralleling technique and rectangular collimation) none of the primary beam should be directed towards the trunk of the patient. Scattered radiation is principally internal and would be unobstructed by a lead apron.
   d. **False.** This is the slower of the two intra-oral film speeds usually available.
   e. **True.** Both types of digital intra-oral system (CCD-based and photostimulable phosphors) can produce a periapical radiograph using a substantially lower X-ray exposure.

Extended matching items answers

EMI 1

1. **C.** Old cassettes may get damaged during years of use and start to leak light. Light fogs the film, leading to irregular areas of black at the edge of the radiograph in a position corresponding to the leak. This fault will occur on every radiograph.
2. **F.** Radiographic cassettes contain a light-sensitive film sandwiched between two intensifying screens. The intensifying screens fluoresce when exposed to X-rays and this produces the image on the radiograph. A sharp image is only produced if the components are squeezed tightly together. Poor contact between films and screens (usually due to cassette damage) leads to all or parts of the image losing sharpness, without distortion of shape.
3. **H.** Patient movement is usually seen most easily as a distortion of the line of the lower border of the mandible. In some cases this can look like a sharp step (like a fracture), while in others an up-and-down wave effect can occur, corresponding to the timing and duration of the movement.

4. **B** and **G**. Low density and contrast means either insufficient exposure or under-development during processing. If this fault occurs, you should always assume the latter cause, as turning up the exposure to compensate for under-development is bad radiation protection practice!

5. **D**. This fault is almost always due to the patient being positioned too far back in the panoramic machine (or focal plane too far forward). It is one of the commonest faults in panoramic radiography. Occasionally the same fault could be due to the patient moving, but there would probably also be distortion of the lower border shape also (see answer 3). The use of bite blocks and positioning lights should reduce the risk of this fault.

6. **G** and **J**. High density and low contrast means either excessive exposure or over-development during processing.

7. **D**. This fault is always due to the patient being positioned too far forward in the panoramic machine (or focal plane too far back). The use of bite blocks and positioning lights should reduce the risk of this fault.

8. **I**. Static electricity can build up when pulling a film out of the box. At some point this may discharge across the film and, if this occurs before development, will produce fine black lines and spots. Classically, the artefacts can look like a negative version of lightning in the sky.

9. **E**. This gradual change in image quality from one side of the radiograph to the other invariably means that there has been light fogging. As the film is fed into an automatic processor, the leading edge enters quickly and is not fogged, but the trailing edge is left for some time outside the processor and gets fogged. This often occurs with processors that have are positioned under a bright light; the daylight hood affords some protection, but is not perfect. If the processor is in a darkroom, it suggests that there may be white light leaking into the room, or that the safelights are faulty or too close to the processor.

10. **A**. This description fits best with fogging of the film stock. This is usually a consequence of age (all film has a 'use by' date), although poor storage can accelerate the process.

EMI 2

1. **J**, or possibly **A**. With such uniform, shallow, periodontal probing depths, a radiograph is unlikely to reveal any additional information. Bitewing radiographs may, however, have already been taken for caries diagnosis and can be examined for periodontal bone support as an added bonus.

2. **G**. The disc position and condition can only be seen using magnetic resonance imaging (or arthrography). Obviously, MR does not use ionising radiation, and is thus without known risk.

3. **A**, and probably **B**. The symptoms fit with a clinical diagnosis of acute pulpitis from an unidentified tooth. In such instances, a bitewing radiograph will be useful as this may demonstrate caries, or a particularly deep restoration, that would help identify the causative tooth. A periapical radiograph would be useful if endodontic treatment is being considered, as this will show the pulpal anatomy. If extraction is planned, then it can be argued that no periapical radiograph is needed, unless there are clinical concerns about the difficulty of extraction, e.g. a third molar.

4. **B** or **C** as a first-line investigation. Depending on the likely treatment, D could be added to the list if a complete orthodontic assessment is required and can be used with C to localise the permanent canine by parallax.

5. **J**. Clicking temporomandibular joints are essentially normal variants. The click is due to disc displacement with reduction (see Ch. 15). A plain radiograph would not, of course, show the interarticular disc in any case.

6. **J**. If this is the first occasion of pericoronitis, then wisdom tooth removal will not be a consideration (see NICE Guidelines in Ch. 6). As such, radiographic examination is unlikely to alter management.

7. **D**. The panoramic radiograph is ideal for viewing the developing dentition and most orthodontists would say they need one. Interestingly, research shows that in simple cases, clinical examination supplemented by study models, without radiography, is often sufficient for treatment planning. British Orthodontic Society Guidelines (reproduced in European Guidelines, referenced in Further Reading) give clear guidance as to when a cephalometric radiograph is useful in orthodontic treatment. For a simple orthodontic treatment such as this, it is very unlikely that a cephalogram could add anything useful to treatment planning.

8. **F**. In this anatomical situation, it would be sensible to obtain cross-sectional images, which can be obtained using either conventional CT or cone beam CT, in order to define accurately the available bone quantity and the anatomical relationship of the maxillary sinus. Most implantologists would have already taken D for such patients as part of the decision-making process about whether implants were appropriate.

9. **D** and **C** would be the first choice radiographs. The occlusal view would be a 'true' occlusal, giving an image at a right-angle to the panoramic radiograph. In a dental practice situation with limited radiological facilities, B might be the only radiographic option.

10. **D** and **E**. The panoramic radiograph is ideal for viewing the developing dentition. British Orthodontic Society Guidelines (reproduced in European Guidelines, referenced in Further Reading) give clear guidance as to when a cephalometric radiograph is useful in orthodontic treatment. This patient satisfies the criteria for cephalometric examination.

Essay answers

1. The essay plan would cover:

   Define the risk. Exposure to X-rays carries with it risks. X-rays are ionising radiation that cause ionisation of atoms by photoelectric and Compton interactions. Ionisation can damage important molecules such as DNA in cells, leading to cell death or mutations. With dental radiography, the risk is of somatic stochastic effects (tumour induction). The chance of these effects is directly related to dose; there is no threshold dose below which they are sure not to occur.

   Quantify the risk. Risks are related to doses. Doses in dental radiography are variable, depending on many factors, but typical ranges are 2–10 μSv for intra-oral radiographs and 7–26 μSv for extra-oral. These relate to cancer risks of 0.06–0.7 per million and 0.21–1.9 per million, respectively. Doses are a fraction of annual average exposures to the UK population and risks are less than those of dying from other causes, such as accidents at work. Risks are higher in children, who are, therefore, a group of greater concern.

   Is risk negligible? It is important to remember that radiography is not a 'normal' part of someone's life. It is an additional risk. It is something carried out by clinicians 'to' a patient and a tangible benefit must be demonstrable. However low the risk, every effort must be made to maximise the benefit and minimise the risk through justification, dose limitation and quality assurance.

2. The essay plan would cover:

   Definition. Quality assurance (QA) can be defined as the organised effort of staff to ensure the consistent production of high-quality radiographs at the lowest possible cost with minimum exposure of patients and personnel to radiation. QA is an essential component of radiation protection.

   Identifying problems. Begin with a staff meeting to discuss issues related to radiography and try to instil an appreciation of the importance of good quality in diagnosis and radiation protection. Try to identify any existing, known, problems by discussion. Audit film quality to see whether you reach the quality standard of no more than 10% unsatisfactory radiographs. Carry out a 'film reject analysis' to identify the principal problems. For example, if 'pale' low-contrast radiographs are a problem then this could be caused by poor exposure selection, a faulty X-ray machine or (most likely) underdevelopment. If the main problem is 'blurred' panoramic radiographs, then examine the films to determine whether this is caused by positioning faults, movement or poor intensifying screen/film contact.

   Action. Address first the problems identified by film reject analysis. For example, if a major problem was underdevelopment, make a fresh start with processing by cleaning the processing tanks and using fresh solutions. Monitor processing times and check developer temperature.

   QA programme. Establish a programme of regular checks. In your essay answer give a possible programme. There is no 'correct' make-up of a QA programme as this would be tailored to the particular dental practice, but demonstrate that you understand the principles:

   Daily activities
   - Maintain a log of film quality
   - Check developer temperature and process test film using test object
   - Clean X-ray viewer
   - Clean darkroom work surfaces.

   Weekly activities
   - Check film stock
   - Clean intensifying screens.

   Two-weekly activities
   - Change developer and process reference film.

   Monthly activities
   - Check darkroom light-tightness and safelights (Coin test).

   Annual activities
   - Have X-ray sets serviced.

   Tri-annual activities
   - Survey X-ray sets for radiation safety.

Viva answers

1. When a fetus is in the line of the primary (main) X-ray beam.

2. Outside the controlled area. This area is defined as in the line of the primary beam until it is attenuated by distance (well beyond the confines of any dental surgery) and a space around the patient and X-ray set in all other directions with a 2 m radius (see Fig. 199). Strictly, the dimensions are set by the Radiation Protection Adviser.

3. First, explain that radiographs are only prescribed when they are justified (when they will give a clinical benefit). Second, explain that doses are kept 'as low as reasonably achievable' by using well-maintained equipment and the best materials (this should be the case!). It may be worth discussing dose levels, in particular relating the likely X-ray dose to the annual average radiation exposure to the UK population.

4. Reduce the risk by using up-to-date equipment and a rare-earth screen/film combination. Carefully select the exposure and use accurately monitored processing of film. Maximise the benefit by only exposing the patient when it is clinically justified and by systematically examining the radiograph to identify all abnormalities of relevance to treatment.

5. X-rays are high-energy radiation that cause ionisation of atoms. Ionisation can disrupt important molecules in the cells of living tissue, in particular DNA. This can lead to cell death or mutations. Mutation may lead to tumour formation.

6. No radiographic examination should be performed until a full history and complete clinical examination have been performed. Posterior bitewing examination should be carried out for all new dentate/partially dentate patients unless approximal surfaces can be directly visualised clinically. Frequency of subsequent bitewing examinations should be based upon caries risk status (see Table 18). Caries risk should be reassessed at each course of treatment so that (for example) an individual is not 'condemned' to a permanent high-risk category.

Index

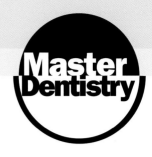

Please note that page references relating to non-textual content such as Boxes, Figures or Tables are in *italic* print. Question and Answer sections are indicated in the form of 54Q/58A.